AF389101

Multi-Functional Collagen-Based Biomaterials for Biomedical Applications

Multi-Functional Collagen-Based Biomaterials for Biomedical Applications

Editors

Nunzia Gallo
Marta Madaghiele
Alessandra Quarta
Amilcare Barca

MDPI • Basel • Beijing • Wuhan • Barcelona • Belgrade • Manchester • Tokyo • Cluj • Tianjin

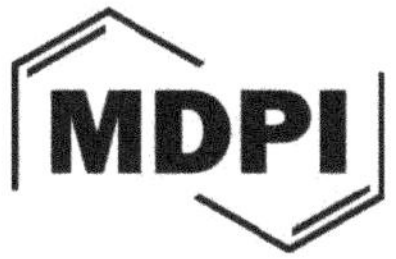

Editors

Nunzia Gallo
Department of Engineering
for Innovation
University of Salento
Lecce
Italy

Marta Madaghiele
Department of Engineering
for Innovation
University of Salento
Lecce
Italy

Alessandra Quarta
Institute of Nanotechnology
CNR NANOTEC
Lecce
Italy

Amilcare Barca
Department of Biological and
Environmental Sciences and
Technologies
University of Salento
Lecce
Italy

Editorial Office
MDPI
St. Alban-Anlage 66
4052 Basel, Switzerland

This is a reprint of articles from the Special Issue published online in the open access journal *Polymers* (ISSN 2073-4360) (available at: www.mdpi.com/journal/polymers/special_issues/multi_functional_collagen_based_biomaterials_for_biomedical_applications).

For citation purposes, cite each article independently as indicated on the article page online and as indicated below:

LastName, A.A.; LastName, B.B.; LastName, C.C. Article Title. *Journal Name* **Year**, *Volume Number*, Page Range.

ISBN 978-3-0365-7073-0 (Hbk)
ISBN 978-3-0365-7072-3 (PDF)

© 2023 by the authors. Articles in this book are Open Access and distributed under the Creative Commons Attribution (CC BY) license, which allows users to download, copy and build upon published articles, as long as the author and publisher are properly credited, which ensures maximum dissemination and a wider impact of our publications.
The book as a whole is distributed by MDPI under the terms and conditions of the Creative Commons license CC BY-NC-ND.

Contents

Preface to "Multi-Functional Collagen-Based Biomaterials for Biomedical Applications"

Polymeric biomaterials represent an essential tool in the biomedical field. Their high biocompatibility and ability to provide adequate regenerative support are fundamental for the development of new therapeutic devices. In particular, biomaterials derived from living organisms exhibit not only structural roles but are also implicated in cellular processes. Among them, type I collagen plays a dominant role in maintaining the biological and structural integrity of various tissues. In recent years, with the goal of developing multi-functional collagen-based devices able to better promote the functional recovery of damaged tissues, numerous studies focused on novel techniques, and methods for the development of innovative and advanced high-performance formulations. The ability to tune collagen-based biomaterials performance is an extremely important knowledge to acquire when specific multi-functionalities are sought.

The present Special Issue collected 12 peer-reviewed interdisciplinary contributions on the broad topic of multi-functional collagen-based biomaterials for biomedical applications, with a focus on their development and customization methods as well as their functions enhancement. An update on the clinical efficacy and safety of collagen-based injectables for aesthetic and regenerative medicine applications was done by Salvatore et al., while the most recent outcomes of collagen matrices for endodontic treatment were provided by Sugiaman et al. To finely control material-cell interaction, collagen-fibronectin binding domains were identified by Liu et al. and the interaction between material-related parameters and the resulting performance was investigated by Ludolph et al.. Since various factors affect the network structure, Maher et al. investigated the effect of different collagen forms on hydrogel-forming properties. The network structure of collagen matrices was also subjected to optimization for corneal regeneration. In this context, Osidak et al. developed and in vivo tested a collagen membrane for replacing damaged corneal stroma and Montalvo-Parra et al. for the treatment of corneal opacities. To further improve collagen bioactivity and make multifunctional collagen-based constructs, Kilb et al. developed an antibiotic-enriched collagen laminate for the treatment of hard-to-heal wounds. Melo et al. developed a new approach to the treatment of severe osteoporotic fractures, by combining biomaterials with biofabrication techniques. Lastly, new collagen sources were investigated to both find more effective formulations for certain applications and overcome issues related to mammal-derived collagens. Gallo et al. extracted collagen from fish skin in pure and native form. Similarly, Anohova et al. demonstrated the possibility of using squid collagen for biomedical applications. Chen et al. developed a fish scale-derived collagen/hydroxyapatite membrane for bone regeneration.

Nunzia Gallo, Marta Madaghiele, Alessandra Quarta, and Amilcare Barca
Editors

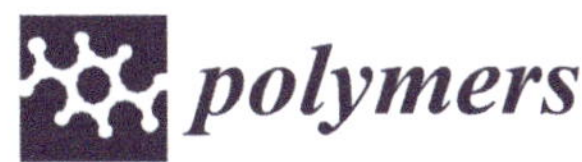 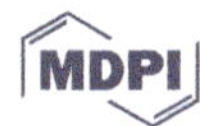

Review

An Update on the Clinical Efficacy and Safety of Collagen Injectables for Aesthetic and Regenerative Medicine Applications

Luca Salvatore [1], Maria Lucia Natali [1,2], Chiara Brunetti [1], Alessandro Sannino [2] and Nunzia Gallo [1,2,*]

[1] Typeone Biomaterials S.r.l., Muro Leccese, 73100 Lecce, Italy
[2] Department of Engineering for Innovation, University of Salento, 73100 Lecce, Italy
* Correspondence: nunzia.gallo@unisalento.it

Abstract: Soft tissues diseases significantly affect patients quality of life and usually require targeted, costly and sometimes constant interventions. With the average lifetime increase, a proportional increase of age-related soft tissues diseases has been witnessed. Due to this, the last two decades have seen a tremendous demand for minimally invasive one-step resolutive procedures. Intensive scientific and industrial research has led to the recognition of injectable formulations as a new advantageous approach in the management of complex diseases that are challenging to treat with conventional strategies. Among them, collagen-based products are revealed to be one of the most promising among bioactive biomaterials-based formulations. Collagen is the most abundant structural protein of vertebrate connective tissues and, because of its structural and non-structural role, is one of the most widely used multifunctional biomaterials in the health-related sectors, including medical care and cosmetics. Indeed, collagen-based formulations are historically considered as the "gold standard" and from 1981 have been paving the way for the development of a new generation of fillers. A huge number of collagen-based injectable products have been approved worldwide for clinical use and have routinely been introduced in many clinical settings for both aesthetic and regenerative surgery. In this context, this review article aims to be an update on the clinical outcomes of approved collagen-based injectables for both aesthetic and regenerative medicine of the last 20 years with an in-depth focus on their safety and effectiveness for the treatment of diseases of the integumental, gastrointestinal, musculoskeletal, and urogenital apparatus.

Keywords: collagen; injectable collagen; medical devices

Citation: Salvatore, L.; Natali, M.L.; Brunetti, C.; Sannino, A.; Gallo, N. An Update on the Clinical Efficacy and Safety of Collagen Injectables for Aesthetic and Regenerative Medicine Applications. *Polymers* **2023**, *15*, 1020. https://doi.org/10.3390/polym15041020

Academic Editors: Jianxun Ding and Donatella Duraccio

Received: 19 December 2022
Revised: 19 January 2023
Accepted: 13 February 2023
Published: 17 February 2023

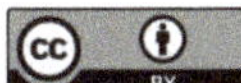

Copyright: © 2023 by the authors. Licensee MDPI, Basel, Switzerland. This article is an open access article distributed under the terms and conditions of the Creative Commons Attribution (CC BY) license (https://creativecommons.org/licenses/by/4.0/).

1. Introduction

Soft tissues loss could be due to iatrogenic, traumatic, pathological, or physiological reasons. Aside from significantly affecting patients' quality of life, their surgical management requires targeted, costly and sometimes constant interventions. With the average life increase, a proportional increase of age-related soft tissues diseases has been witnessed. Due to this, recent decades have seen a tremendous demand for soft tissue reconstruction strategies and one step resolutive procedures. Intense scientific and industrial research has been conducted to develop innovative approaches or optimize current solutions. Among them, in the last two decades injectable formulations have attracted even more interest for both aesthetic and regenerative surgery for their versatility and multifunctionality (Figure 1). Indeed, injectable scaffolds could be used in large and irregularly shaped lesions for a huge variety of damaged tissues, as well as providing temporary pain relief and functional improvement with a single treatment. Thus, injectable formulations could reduce the number of surgical procedures, costs, times and accelerate healing rate and quality.

The popularity of minimally invasive techniques increased rapidly for several reasons. A principal factor is the acceptance of soft tissue fillers among patients that are not ready for permanent treatments [1]. In the case of patients not wishing to undergo surgery, an easier procedure would generally be more accepted. Moreover, compared to undergoing more invasive surgery, fillers offer the patient less discomfort and a shorter recovery time, making them very practical in the resolution of minor-serious disease and allowing patients to return immediately to their daily routine [1,2]. Minimally invasive therapies would give a better quality of life also for that part of population that would otherwise not survive the trauma induced by conventional surgeries. Moreover, they could delay the execution of invasive surgical procedures for the implantation of permanent devices [3]. In the case of a staged surgical intervention, the use of injectable systems may avoid the need for multiple invasive operations, thus reducing the related morbidities and negative aesthetic effects associated with repeated procedures [4]. With regard to aesthetic treatments, minimally invasive therapies are preferred as they are less impacting and give a more natural look. Moreover, the lack of an external incision or an autologous tissue donor site is preferred because the absence of scarring is usually socially and psychologically more accepted.

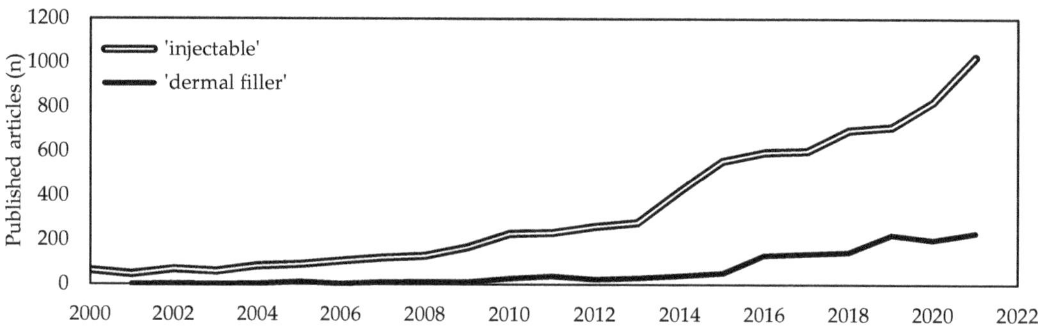

Figure 1. The increasing research interest in injectable formulations and dermal filler. Articles indexed in Scopus (www.scopus.com) with the keywords 'injectable' and 'dermal filler' and published from 2000 to 2022 (last accessed on 27 May 2022).

From the surgeon's point of view, the advantages of minimally invasive procedures include principally the need for fewer resources (e.g., operating room, staff, equipment, and time). Being simpler, transcutaneous injections require less operating room staff and time. The pro-regenerative action of injectables would reduce operating room time also because they would be able to restore physiological conditions with a single injection. However, it should not be forgotten that simpler procedures are not less exhausting and do not require less experience. Like any surgical procedure, minimally invasive therapies require adequate knowledge in order to reach the best outcome and avoid unwanted adverse events.

Thus, not only clinicians' but especially patients' preference for fewer invasive and expensive procedures has undoubtedly promoted their use [4–10]. An injectable formulation for soft tissues reconstruction currently relies on two main approaches, involving autologous tissue displacement (e.g., lipofilling, platelet-rich plasma) or biomaterials-based filling [5]. Both approaches have some advantages and drawbacks. Autologous materials provide the most physiological solution (no adverse events or immune reactions) but suffer from donor site morbidity, volume resorption rate variability, and double surgery requirements. Moreover, their harvesting is a time-consuming procedure that requires double intervention. Alternatively, biomaterials offer an off-the-shelf solution with immediate results and should be distinguished as non-resorbable and resorbable, depending on their half-life. Non-resorbable solutions (e.g., silicone, poly(methyl methacrylate), polyvinylpyrrolidone, polyacrylamide), are permanent (last more than 2 years) but usually suffer from mild-severe adverse reactions (i.e., granuloma, implant encapsulation, persistent pain or rejection) that limit patient satisfaction and could require implant removal surgery [6–12]. Contrarily, resorbable formulations are usually based on natural biomaterials (i.e., collagen, hyaluronic acid, calcium hydroxyl apatite) and last 6–18 months [13–16]. Their durability depends on many factors such as the raw material type, product cross-linking degree, lost tissue extension, disease site and etiology, and patient metabolism, age and co-morbidities. The most used resorbable dermal fillers are collagen or hyaluronic acid based.

Collagen is the most abundant structural protein of vertebrate connective tissues [17–25] and plays a crucial structural role for the maintenance of tissues' architecture, shape and mechanical properties [20]. Moreover, by mediating a fundamental inter- and intracellular signaling it dictates specialized regulatory functions, especially during development and repair processes [26–32]. Type I collagen is one of the most widely used biomaterials in the health-related sectors, including medical care and cosmetics [17–25,33]. Several collagen-based injectable products have been approved for clinical use and used in many clinical settings.

This review will specifically focus on the clinical efficacy of collagen-based injectables for both aesthetic and regenerative medicine from 2000 until today. In particular, collagen extraction sources for injectables development and relative applications are discussed. To the best of our knowledge, we collected and discussed all pertinent research reports, commercial products data, and clinical trials about approved collagen-based injectable formulations, in order to underline the advantages and disadvantages related to their use. Accordingly, the available clinical results of the last 20 years about some of the leading collagen-based approved products were gathered and discussed according to the body site and pathology. In particular, this review focused on collagen-based injectables currently used for the regeneration of the musculoskeletal, urogenital, gastrointestinal, and integumental systems as well as for non standard clinical applications by presenting exemplary attempts to improve tissues' regenerative performance. Finally, collagen-based products adverse events rate and their regulation are discussed.

2. Methodology

A deep search was undertaken on studies about injectable collagen alone or in combination with other materials for cosmetic and medical applications. The electronic search engines used were PubMed (https://pubmed.ncbi.nlm.nih.gov, accessed on 4 January 2023), ScienceDirect (https://www.sciencedirect.com, accessed on 4 January 2023), Google Scholar (https://scholar.google.com, accessed on 4 January 2023) and U.S. National Library of Medicine (https://clinicaltrials.gov/, accessed on 22 December 2022). The keywords used were 'injectable' and 'collagen'. Several synonyms were searched for each component (i.e., injection, hydrolysate, gelatin, dermal filler, solution, colloid, infusion, hydrogel). The search included all studies related to injectable collagen-based formulations, including clinical trials, prospective case series, retrospective reviews, and case reports, independently from their level of evidence. A total of 125 studies were screened from 2000 to 2022 and reviewed.

3. Collagen as Biomaterial

Collagen is the most abundant structural protein of vertebrate connective tissues, and accounts for about the 30% of the total body protein content [17–25]. The collagen family is a group of proteins that share a unique molecular fingerprint that is characterized by the presence of a right-handed triple-helical domain formed by three left-handed polyproline-II helices [26,34,35]. This superfamily accounts for 28 members, named from type I to XXVIII according to the discovery order [34,36]. Type I collagen was the first to be discovered and accounts for the 70% of the total collagen found in the human body [26]. This protein is a hetero trimer of about 400 kDa consisting of two identical $\alpha 1$ (≈ 139 kDa) chains and one $\alpha 2$ (≈ 129 kDa) chain of about 1000 amino acid residues [20,37]. Both chains are characterized by the repetition of the Glycine-X-Y triplet, where the X and Y positions are usually represented by proline and hydroxyproline, respectively [34,37]. Hydroxylation of proline residues is a typical modification of collagen and, because it accounts for about 11–14% of total residues, it is commonly used as a marker to detect and quantify collagen in tissues [35,38]. Another peculiarity of fibril-forming type I collagen molecules is their ability to spontaneously assemble to form fibrils in which molecules are quasi-hexagonally packed and super-twisted in a right-handed structure along the longitudinal axis of the fibril [39–41]. Thus, collagen molecules are aligned parallel to one another with a staggering of about 67 nm (D-banding) and can assemble into fibrils that can be greater than 500 µm in length and 500 nm in diameter [25,34,42,43]. Then, fibrils assemble in fibers whose 3D arrangement is tissue specific.

Type I collagen not only covers a crucial structural role in tissue architecture maintenance but is actively involved in several biological and pathological processes [44]. The involvement of collagen in numerous cellular processes prompted research towards the use of collagen as biomaterial for the development of simplified ECM-like structures [20,35]. To this, several companies isolate medical-grade type I collagen from several sources (Table 1) and manufacture collagen-based implantable devices that are currently used in many clinical settings. Besides its advantages in term of biocompatibility for its physiological structural and non-structural functions, the use of collagen as biomaterial offers several advantages including low immunogenicity, tunable properties, and biodegradability. The low evolutionary gap and the high conservation of type I collagen amino acid composition among vertebrates make that homology up to 95% [19,45–48].

Table 1. Most important world companies producing clinical grade collagen and related extraction sources.

Animal Source	Extraction Tissue	Company
Equine	Tendon	Euroresearch S.r.l. (Milan, Italy) www.euroresearch.it, accessed on 14 February 2023
	Tendon	Opocrin Spa (Formigine, Italy) www.opocrin.it, accessed on 14 February 2023
	Tendon	Typeone Biomaterials S.r.l. (Calimera, Italy) www.typeone.it, accessed on 14 February 2023
Bovine	Corium, tendon, membranes	Bovine collagen products (Branchburg, NJ, USA) www.bovinecollagenproducts.com, accessed on 14 February 2023
	Corium, tendon	Collagen solution (Eden Prairie, MN, USA) www.collagensolutions.com, accessed on 14 February 2023
	n. d.	Royal DSM (Heerlen, The Netherlands) www.dsm.com, accessed on 14 February 2023
	Tendon	Integra LifeScience Corp. (Princeton, NJ, USA) www.integralife.com, accessed on 14 February 2023
	Dermis	Koken Co., Ltd. (Tokyo, Japan), www.kokenmpc.co.jp, accessed on 14 February 2023
	Dermis	Devro Plc (Moodiesburn, UK) www.devro.com, accessed on 14 February 2023
	Tendon	Getinge (Göteborg, Sweden) www.getinge.com, accessed on 14 February 2023
	Dermis	Symatese (Chaponost, France) www.symatese.com, accessed on 14 February 2023
	Hide	Advanced Biomatrix (Carlsbad, CA, USA) www.advancedbiomatrix.com, accessed on 14 February 2023
Swine	Skin	Ubiosis (Gyeonggi-do, Republic of Korea) www.ubiosis.com, accessed on 14 February 2023
	Skin	Botiss Biomaterials GmbH (Zossen, Germany) www.botiss-dental.com, accessed on 14 February 2023
Jellyfish	n. d.	Jellagen (Cardiff, UK) www.jellagen.co.uk, accessed on 14 February 2023
Plant	Leaves	CollPlant (Rehovot, Israel) www.collplant.com, accessed on 14 February 2023

The possibility to define specific scaffolds properties (i.e., by tuning protein concentration, solvent type and concentration, protein molecular weight, superficial morphology, 3D organization, and by pre- and post-production processing) offers a great opportunity to modulate the structure-related biological activity of the scaffolds in order to optimize their capability to induce and sustain tissue regeneration [20,35,43,49–55]. Moreover, the use of collagen is advantageous for regenerative medicine and tissue engineering applications because, being recognized as a self-molecule, it is metabolized by the natural body enzymatic apparatus that gradually breaks down collagen molecules and substitutes it with newly synthetized one. Molecular pathways that mediate collagen degradation are several and are tissue and cell specific [39]. In general, the human body has several collagen degrading enzymes including the matrix metalloproteinases (in particular, matrix metalloproteinase 1), and cathepsins and neutrophil elastase that cleave collagen molecules which undergo a successive proteolytic process that depends on several factors (i.e., triple helix stability, protein amino acid sequence, crosslinking) [56–61]. Generally, collagen fragments resulting from the action of collagenases are further degraded by gelatinases and non-specific proteases. Thus, the presence of an accurate and complex degradation system for the endogenous collagen makes the exogenous collagen highly biodegradable and low immunogenic. Recently, the attention on collagen degradation pathways has grown for the even more evident collagen critical role in tissue homeostasis [39]. Evidence about collagen and its degradation products could also be helpful in promoting the restoration of tissue structure and function [62].

4. Historical Overview on Collagen-Based Injectable Formulations

The history of biomaterials used as soft tissues filler dates from before the 19th century. The first injectable filler, which was autologous fat, was used in 1893 for forearm scar filling [63]. Since then, several materials have been used for the development of injectable formulations. Some of them were abandoned because of the development of medium-severe adverse reactions (e.g., paraffin: embolization, granuloma formation, migration; silicone: granuloma formation; teflon: inflammatory reaction) [15,64]. Among them, autologous fat is still used as filler for its biocompatibility, availability and low cost. However, its long-term variable and unpredictable results limited its employment [10,15].

A strong turning point happened in 1981 with the development and Food and Drug Administration (FDA) approval of the first collagen filler, Zyderm® (Inamed Corporation, Santa Barbara, CA, USA). A new aesthetic procedure category of injectable treatments known as "fillers" was created. This paved the way for research into and development of biomaterials-based injectable formulations. However, the risk of immunogenic and hypersensitivity reactions soon decreased the popularity of animal-derived collagen fillers [64]. Moreover, the fear that the protein extracted from some animal tissues can be a vector for prion infections precluded their use. However, it should be taken into account that the first registered adverse events were not only related to material properties but also to the implantation methods. Proper patient selection and optimal methods of treatment delivery are crucial factors for therapeutic success and patient satisfaction [65]. Unfortunately, due to this, in the 1990s many collagen injection therapies failed because of the lack of data. Thereafter, surgeons were even more reluctant to perform collagen injections because they were commonly considered as ineffective therapies.

Thus, despite the growth of research interest in new fillers development, Zyderm® remained the only FDA approved injectable formulation until 2003 when the first hyaluronic acid based dermal filler, Restylane® (Galderma, Fort Worth, TX, USA, www.galderma.com, accessed on 14 February 2023), was approved. Since 2003, there has been an exponential increase in the number of FDA approved fillers. Indeed, both permanent (e.g., poly(methyl methacrylate), polyacrylamide, polyvinylpyrrolidone) and resorbable (e.g., collagen, hyaluronic acid, calcium hydroxyl apatite, poly(L-lactic acid) materials-based fillers were developed and clinically approved. Although synthetic compounds gained popularity as soft-tissue augmentation for their cost-effectiveness, mass production, limited immunogenicity and long-term effects, they also raised concerns over their long-term safety due to the growing data on long-term side effects or adverse events such as tissue necrosis, infection, granulomas, chronic inflammatory reaction [6–12].

In this context, resorbable fillers caught on even more for their relative safety in terms of local immunological reactions and ability to actively restore soft tissues volume. Indeed, the advantages offered by the use of minimally invasive therapies and the spread of the idea of regenerating damaged tissues pushed towards the development of temporary injectable hydrogels with specific properties. In particular, as argued by Cho et al., injectable bioactive formulations should: (i) be biocompatible without toxicity or immunogenic phenomenon after degradation; (ii) have mechanical properties compliant with the targeted tissue; (iii) be able to keep drugs and cells in the injected area; (iv) have adequate permeability, pore size and interconnectivity for mass transport and cell colonization; (v) be cost-effective; (vi) be easily handled; (vii) be biodegradable, allowing replacement by the newly formed functional tissue [66]. Indeed, an ideal injectable formulation should form a natural open pore 3D scaffold that should allow cell migration, and slowly break down stimulating growth factors and cytokines to promote neocollagenesis, elastic fiber production, neovascularization, and the wound healing response/repair [67]. Thus, ideal injectables should not only provide immediate and stable results, but also recreate natural-like extracellular matrix (ECM) for bio-dermal restoration and a long-lasting effect. However, one of the main disadvantages of resorbable filler is their short half-life. An inadequate reabsorption rate may not be sufficient to support the regenerative processes and therefore may lead to form loss. Thus, resorbable fillers-based approaches may require multiple applications to maintain their effect.

For this reason, in the last two decades, type I collagen-based products and derivates (i.e., hydrolysates, gelatin, peptides) came back into vogue because of the spreading idea of developing multifunctional fillers able to fill soft tissue defects and restore deficient tissue physiological functions [4,12,14,32,66,68,69]. The use of heterologous collagen as a medical product spread also as results of the development of both accurate extraction processes and effective sterilization procedures that improved their safety profile. Indeed, advances in purification processes allowed creation of collagen preparations with minimum immunogenicity and infection risks, with high purity levels [19,25]. Moreover, with the definition of adequate implantation protocols, collagen-based injectable therapies were re-evaluated as a minimally invasive and effective strategies for the treatment of different types of diseases. Therefore, on account of collagen's intrinsic structural and non-structural properties due to which it is historically considered as the "gold standard" material for the development of health-care related products, collagen-based injectable formulations have proved to be a promising strategy in many applicative areas. Despite the well-known effectiveness of collagen in tissue regeneration, the recent discovery of new ECM homeostasis molecular mechanisms raised again the interest in the mechanism of action of collagen. Indeed, lately it has been discovered that type I collagen operates a traction on the type VI collagen fibrils, which forms a network of fibrils in the immediate vicinity of the cell membranes [70]. The mechanical stress that results on the cells stimulates the production of new ECM (mechano-transduction process).

5. Collagen-Based Injectable Formulations

More than 60 kinds of collagen-based fillers are available on the market, according to the end-use and they have routinely been introduced in many clinical settings (Table 2). The most common collagen extraction sources for the manufacture of collagen based injectable formulations are bovine, swine, porcine, equine and human derived, whose advantages and disadvantages are described in depth elsewhere [19,20,25]. Bovine collagen is one of the most commonly used fillers for effectively reducing wrinkles and other facial imperfections. More famous branded bovine-based collagen fillers are Zyderm®, Zyplast®, Contigen® (Allergan Inc., Dublin, Ireland), Artefill® (Suneva Medical, San Diego, CA, USA), and Artecoll® (Canderm Pharma Inc., Saint-Laurent, QB, Canada). Others include CHondroGrid® (Bioteck Spa, Arcugnano, Italy), Integra Flowable Wound Matrix® (Integra LifeScience Corp., Princeton, NJ, USA), Resoplast® (Rofil Medical International, Breda, The Netherlands), Atelocell® (KOKEN Co., Ltd., Bunkyo-ku, Tokyo, Japan). However, bovine collagen is known to be exposed to zoonosis (e.g., the foot and mouth disease and the group of the bovine spongiform encephalopathies, among which the most dangerous for humans is the transmissible spongiform encephalopathy) and to trigger allergies (about 2–4% of population) [71–73]. In addition to the strict regulation to which all implantable products are subjected, two consecutive negative patient skin tests at 6 and 2 weeks are required before use [73,74]. This sensitivity has been considered generally acceptable for implants for human use and actually bovine collagen is principally used for the treatment of the integumental [6,75–96] (NCT01060943) and musculoskeletal apparatus [97–112] and to a minor extent for the gastrointestinal [113–120], urinary [65,121–125] and cardiovascular [126–128] systems. Recently, bovine collagen in fibrillar form has been employed as an organ protection system during thermal ablation of hepatic malignancies [129].

Porcine collagen is the second most used. There are several products derived from porcine collagen, including GUNA® (GUNA, Milan, Italy) products, CartiRegen® (Joint Biomaterials S.r.l., Mestre, Italy), COLTRIX CartiRegen® and TendoRegen® (Ubiosis, Gyeonggi-do, Republic of Korea), CartiFill®, CartiZol®, RegenSeal® and TheraFill® (Sewon Cellontech Co., Ltd., Seoul, Republic of Korea), Dermicol-P35 (Evolence, Ortho Dermatologics, Skillman, NJ, USA), Fibroquel® (Aspid S.A. de C.V., Mexico City, Mexico), Fibrel® (Mentor Corporation, Santa Barbara, CA, USA), Permacol® (Tissue Science Labs., Aldershot, UK) and RPC Pure Collagen® (EternoGen LLC, Columbia, MO, USA). Among them, Dermicol-P35®, was withdrawn from the market in 2009. Compared to other animal derived collagens, porcine collagen-based injections are said to be rather painful and may cause allergic reactions [17]. While bovine collagen is used for many purposes, porcine collagen is almost exclusively used for the treatment of diseases belonging to the musculoskeletal apparatus [130–146] (NCT02539030, NCT02519881, NCT02539095), followed by the integumental apparatus [67,76,86,87,147–152] (NCT03844529, NCT00891774, NCT00929071) and gastrointestinal apparatus [116,117,153–159]. Only recently porcine collagen potential has been explored for the treatment of facial nerve palsy [160] and for the treatment of COVID-19 due hyperinflammation [161,162] (NCT04517162). However, despite their wide use and effectiveness, bovine and porcine collagens suffer from cultural or religious concerns (bovine collagen: Sikh, Buddhism; porcine collagen: Jewish, Islamic faiths), which restricted their applicative potential [18,19].

Equine collagen is the third most used collagen. It is free from the risks of triggering immune reaction and of zoonosis transmission, as reported elsewhere [19]. This kind of collagen is less used than bovine and porcine derived collagen for the manufacture of injectable formulations because of its naturally high hierarchical organization that made it more compliant for other applications (i.e., sponges, thin substrates). Thus, less injectable products from horse collagen are available but recently discovered advantages deriving from its use [19] are driving the development of new equine collagen-based products. Among them, Nithya®, Linerase® (Euroresearch, Milan, Italy), Salvecoll-E® (Nearmedic Italy S.r.l., Como, Italy), Biocollagen® and ActivaBone® (Bioteck Spa, Arcugnano, Italy) are commercially available and are mainly used for the treatment of diseases belonging to the integumental [163,164], urogenital [165] and gastrointestinal [160] apparatus. Its potential has also been recently explored for the treatment of periodontal tissues, with encouraging outcomes [166,167].

Human collagen fillers were developed in the early 2000s and are principally used for the integumental apparatus (e.g., facial soft tissues augmentation, wrinkles, scars, fat atrophy, diffuse depressions, paralyzed lips and tongues, nasolabial folds, and others) [6,168–172] and have been investigated for diseases of the gastrointestinal apparatus (e. g., vocal folds) [118,173–175]. In particular, there are three kinds of human collagen based injectables: autologous reconstituted collagen formulation (Autologen® and Dermologen®, Collagenesis, Inc., Beverly, MA, USA) [173], autologous collagen formulations from in vitro cultured cells (Isolagen therapy® from Fibrocell Science, Exton, Pennsylvania, USA,; Cosmoplast® and Cosmoderm® from Inamed Corporation, Santa Barbara, CA, USA)(NCT00655356)[6,169], and reconstituted collagen formulation from deceased humans

(Fascian® from Fascia Biosystem, Beverly Hills, CA, USA; Dermalogen® and Cymetra® from Life Cell Corp., Branchburg, NJ, USA) [6,118,168,170–173]. Autologous reconstituted collagen formulations are produced from collagen harvested from patients' skin small biopsy, harvested during an earlier procedure, and liquefied for future re-injection. Two square inches of donor material are required to formulate a 1-mL syringe of injectable material, which can be stored for 6 months [176]. This procedure was developed by Collagenesis Inc. (Beverly, MA, USA) and is commercially known as Autologen®. As previously noted, human collagen fillers can also be derived from in vitro cultured autologous cells. In particular, skin cells from behind the human ear could be harvested, cloned, and derived collagen could be then harvested, liquefied, and injected. This procedure was developed by Fibrocell Science Inc. (Exton, PA, USA) and is commercially known as azfibrocel-T (formerly Isolagen Therapy®). Being autologous collagen, these kinds of formulations are allergy free, making them an excellent alternative to animal-derived treatments. Apart from general mild disorders (bruising 5%, erythema 15%, hemorrhage 10%, with numbers comparable to placebo groups), this kind of human derived formulation does not trigger serious adverse events (NCT00655356). Human collagen fillers could also be prepared from deceased human donors, with the main advantages of extensive raw material availability and the reduced preparation time compared to both autologous reconstituted collagen formulation and autologous collagen formulations from patients' own in vitro cultured cells. Injectables from human donors (Dermalogen®) were firstly developed by Life Cell Corporation (Branchburg, NJ, USA). Because Dermalogen® originates from humans, also the deceased human-derived collagen-based injectables do not need an allergy test. Although human-derived collagens proved to be a good alternative, they have some disadvantages such as long preparation times, non-availability of sufficient donor tissue and high management costs (i.e., harvesting, donor tissue availability, isolation, manufacturing, need for highly specialized teams and instruments, refrigerated and limited storage, shipping) [7,176,177]. Moreover, while no efficacy differences emerged between the use of autologous collagen and animal-derived collagen, a 2–3 folds greater injection of cadaveric collagen is needed for similar augmentation results to those achieved with bovine collagen [176]. Thee mentioned drawbacks, together with the insubstantial difference in terms of efficacy compared to animal-derived collagen-based injectables, led to the progressive abandonment of human collagen for large scale applications and its exclusive use for patients with hypersensitivity to animal derived collagens.

In the last decade, new solutions were offered by recombinant collagens. Indeed, two injectable fillers, consisting of collagen, hyaluronic acid and carboxymethylcellulose, are now commercially available. In particular, Fillagen® (Monodermà, Milan, Italy), made with recombinant polypeptide of collagen α1-chain from silkworm [178], and Karisma® (Taumed, Rome, Italy), made with unspecified recombinant collagen were proposed. More recently a photocurable collagen-based regenerative dermal and soft tissues filler was developed by CollPlant Biotechnologies Ltd (Rehovot, Israel, www.collplant.com, accessed on 14 February 2023), comprising a recombinant type I collagen from tobacco plant (not currently commercially available).

Table 2. Summary of clinically available type I collagen-based injectable formulations.

Source	Manufacturer	Product	Additives	Applications	Ref.
Equine	Euroresearch S.r.l. (Milan, Italy) www.euroresearch.it, accessed on 14 February 2023	Nithya	–	Integumental	[163]
		Linerase	–	Integumental	[164–167,179]
	Nearmedic Italy S.r.l. (Como, Italy) www.salvecoll.com, accessed on 14 February 2023	Salvecoll-E	–	Integumental	[60]
	Bioteck Spa (Arcugnano, Italy) www.bioteck.com, accessed on 14 February 2023	Biocollagen gel	Type III collagen, bone spongy powder	Musculoskeletal	–
		Biocollagen crunch	Type III collagen, bone powder, bone spongy chips	Musculoskeletal	–
		ActivaBone CLX gel	Bone powder, exur, Vitamin C	Musculoskeletal	–
		ActivaBone Injectable Paste	Demineralized bone matrix, bone powder, exur, Vitamin C	Musculoskeletal	–
		ActivaBone modulable paste	Demineralized bone matrix, bone powder, bone cortical and spongy granules, exur, Vitamin C	Musculoskeletal	–
		ActivaBone Crunch	Demineralized bone matrix, bone powder, cortical and spongy chips, exur, Vitamin C	Musculoskeletal	–
Bovine	Bioteck Spa (Arcugnano, Italy) www.bioteck.com, accessed on 14 February 2023	CHondroGrid	–	Musculoskeletal	[112]
	Integra LifeScience Corp. (Princeton, NJ, USA) www.integralife.com, accessed on 14 February 2023	Integra Flowable Wound Matrix	Glycosaminoglycans	Integumental	[88]
		Helitene	–	Soft tissues	[129]
	Rofil Medical International (Breda, The Netherlands)	Resoplast	Lidocaine hydrochloride	Integumental	–
	Suneva Medical (San Diego, CA, USA) www.sunevamedical.com, accessed on 14 February 2023	ArteFill	Polymethylmethacrylate, lidocaine	Integumental	[75,77–85]
	Datascope Corp., (Montvale, NJ, USA)	VasoSeal	–	Cardiovascular	[128]
	BioMimetic Therapeutics, LLC (Franklin, TN, USA) www.biomimetics.com, accessed on 14 February 2023	Augment	β-tricalcium phosphate, recombinant human platelet-derived growth factor-BB	Musculoskeletal	[97,99–111]
	KOKEN Co., Ltd. (Bunkyo-ku, Tokyo, Japan) www.kokenmpc.co.jp, accessed on 14 February 2023	Atelocell	Type III collagen	Integumental, gastrointestinal	[86,87,113,114], NCT01060943
	B. Braun (Crissier, Switzerland) www.bbraun.com, accessed on 14 February 2023	Gelofusine	–	Cardiovascular	[126,127]
	Allergan, Inc. (Dublin, Ireland) www.abbvie.it, accessed on 14 February 2023	Zyplast	Glutaraldehyde	Integumental	[6,76,83,89–92,95,96,98,116,117,119,180]
		Zyderm	–	Integumental	[6,83,89,90,93,94,118,120,180]
		Contigen	glutaraldehyde	Gastrointestinal and genitourinary	[115,121–125]

Table 2. *Cont.*

Source	Manufacturer	Product	Additives	Applications	Ref.
	GUNA (Milan, Italy) www.guna.com, accessed on 14 February 2023	Dental Skin BioRegulation	Vitamin C, magnesium gluconate, pyridozine chlorhydrate, riboflavin, thiamine chlorhydrate	Skin	[181]
		Dental ATM BioRegulation	Hypericum	Musculoskeletal	[130]
		MD-HIP	Calcium phosphate	Musculoskeletal	[131]
		MD-ISCHIAL	Rhododendron	Musculoskeletal	[132]
		MD-KNEE	Arnica	Musculoskeletal	[133,143,144]
		MD-LUMBAR	Hamemelis	Musculoskeletal	[132,134,135]
		MD-NECK	Silicio	Musculoskeletal	–
		MD-SHOULDERS	Iris	Musculoskeletal	[145,146]
		MD-SMALL JOINTS	Viola	Musculoskeletal	–
		MD-THORACIC	Cimifuga	Musculoskeletal	–
		MD-MATRIX	Citric acid, nicotinamide	Soft tissues	[135,136,160]
		MD-MUSCLE	Hypericum	Musculoskeletal	[130,132–137,146,160]
		MD-POLY	Drosera	Musculoskeletal	–
		MD-NEURAL	Citrullus	Musculoskeletal	[132,134,160]
		MD-TISSUE	Ascorbic acid, magnesium gluconate, pyridoxine chlorhydrate, riboflavin, thiamine chlorhydrate	Soft tissues	–
	Joint Biomaterials S.r.l. (Mestre, Italy) www.joint-biomateriali.it, accessed on 14 February 2023	CartiRegen	Fibrin glue	Musculoskeletal	–
	Ubiosis (Gyeonggi-do, Republic of Korea) www.ubiosis.com, accessed on 14 February 2023	COLTRIX CartiRegen	–	Musculoskeletal	–
		COLTRIX TendoRegen	–	Musculoskeletal	–
Swine	Sewon Cellontech Co., Ltd. (Seoul, Republic of Korea) www.swcell.com, accessed on 14 February 2023	CartiFill	Glucose, CaCl, amino acids, vitamin B, fibrin glue	Musculoskeletal	[138,139], NCT02539030, NCT02519881
		CartiZol	Glucose, CaCl, amino acids, vitamin B	Musculoskeletal	[140], NCT02539095
		RegenSeal	–	Musculoskeletal	[141]
		TheraFill	–	Integumental	[86,87]
	Sunmax Biotechnology Co., Ltd. (Tainan, Taiwan) www.sunmaxbiotech.com, accessed on 14 February 2023	Facial Gain	Lidocaine	Integumental	NCT03844529
		Collagen Implant I	–	Integumental	–
	Evolence (Skillman, NJ, USA)	Dermicol-P35	Ribose	Integumental	[2,147–149], NCT00929071, NCT00891774
	Mentor Corp. (Santa Barbara, CA, USA)	Fibrel	–	Integumental	[150,151]
	Tissue Science Labs. (Aldershot, UK)	Permacol	–	Gastrointestinal	[153–159]
	EternoGen, LLC (Columbia, MO, USA)	RPC Pure Collagen	Ethylenediamine tetraacetic acid	Integumental	[67]
	Aspid S.A. de C.V. (Mexico City, Mexico) www.aspidpharma.com, accessed on 14 February 2023	Fibroquel	Polyvinylpyrrolidone	Musculoskeletal	[161,162], NCT04517162
	ColBar LifeScience Ltd. (Tel Aviv, Israel) www.ortho-dermatologics.com, accessed on 14 February 2023	Evolence	Ribose	Integumental	[147,152]

Table 2. *Cont.*

Source	Manufacturer	Product	Additives	Applications	Ref.
	Fascia Biosystem (Beverly Hills, CA, USA)	Fascian	Lidocain	Integumental	[6,168,171]
	Fibrocell Science (Exton, PA, USA) www.fibrocell.com, accessed on 14 February 2023	Isolagen therapy	–	Integumental	NCT00655356
Human	Inamed Corporation (Santa Barbara, CA, USA) www.inamed-cro.com, accessed on 14 February 2023	Cosmoplast	Glutaraldehyde, lidocaine hydrochloride	Integumental	[6,169]
		Cosmoderm	lidocaine hydrochloride	Integumental	[6,169]
	Life Cell Corp. (Branchburg, NJ, USA)	Dermalogen	Type and VI collagen, elastin, fibronectin, chondroitin sulfate, and other proteoglycans	Integumental	[170]
		Cymetra	Elascin, glycosaminoglycans, Lidocaine hydrochloride	Integumental	[6,118,172–175]
	Collagenesis, Inc., (Beverly, MA, USA)	Autologen	Elastin, fibronectin, glycosaminoglycans	Integumental	–
		Dermologen	–	Integumental	[173]
Plant	Vesco Pharmaceutical Co. Ltd. (Bangkok, Thailand) www.vescopharma.com, accessed on 14 February 2023	Collagen C 1000	Vitamin C	Integumental	–
Silkworm	Monodermà (Milan, Italy) www.monoderma.com	Fillagen	I-yaluronic acid, carboxymethylcellulose	Integumental	[178]
n. d.	Taumed (Rome, Italy) www.taumed.it, accessed on 14 February 2023	Karisma	I-yaluronic acid, carboxymethylcellulose	Integumental	–
n. d.	LABO International S.r.l. (Padova, Italy) www.labosuisse.com, accessed on 14 February 2023	Fillerina con 3D collagen	Hyaluronic acid	Integumental	–
n. d.	Hebey Mepha Pharm Group Co., Ltd. (Shandong, Hebei, China) www.mephacn.com, accessed on 14 February 2023	Collagen Plus	–	Integumental	–
n. d.	Pierre Mulot Laboratories (Paris, France)	Neutroskin	Vitamin C	Integumental	–
n. d.	Elements Pharmaceuticals (Shijiazhuang, Hebei, China) www.elementspharma.com, accessed on 14 February 2023	Ele-collagen	Vitamin C, Vitamin B6	Integumental	–
n. d.	Globus Medical (Audubon, PA, USA) www.globusmedical.com, accessed on 14 February 2023	Kinex Bioactive gel	Bioglass, hyaluronic acid	Musculoskeletal	–

6. Clinical Efficacy of Collagen-Based Injectable Implants

Collagen-based formulations are mainly used for the treatment of several kind of diseases belonging mainly to the musculoskeletal (i.e., hip or knee osteoarthritis [112,131,133,140,142,144,182], sprained knee pain [143], injured cartilage [138,141], piriformis syndrome [136], ankle and hindfoot arthritis [103] or fusion [100,106–109], lumbar spinal fusion [99], myofascial pain syndrome [130,137], chronic pain [132], acute lumbar spine pain [134], partial-thickness rotator cuff tears [141,146,183], plantar fasciitis [184], calcific supraspinatus tendinitis [145], pain [130,132,134,137]), urogenital (i.e., urinary incontinence [122,124,125,185–189], neurogenic urinary incontinence [190], lichens sclerosus [165], intrinsic sphincter deficiency [191–193], post-prostatectomy incontinence [65,123,194–197], retrograde ejaculation [198]), gastrointestinal (i.e., glottic insufficiency [113,114,116,118,119,173,199–203], rectal fistula [153,154,156,157], fecal incontinence [69,115,155,204]), and integumental (i.e., nasolabial folds [2,67,76,86,87,96, 149,163,172,205–208], nasojugal folds [152], lip [2,77,95,148,169,172], cheek and temple area [172], glabellar groove [77], post-rhinoplasty dorsal irregularities [77,209], depressed acne scars [77,172,210] augmentation, post-burn hands malfunction [88] and vitiligo [164]) systems, as well as for non standard clinical applications (i.e., facial nerve rehabilitation after palsy [160,211], organ protection during thermal ablation [129], COVID-19 associated hyperinflammation [161,162] (NCT04517162), vitiligo [164], ovarian function after premature ovarian failure [212], the closure of artery aneurysms [128,213] and blood volume augmentation [127,214]) (Figure 2).

However, many manufacturers have chosen to not publish their findings but keep their data privately on file. Thus, no public clinical efficacy research results are available for many injectable solutions, meaning that the limited information available restricts the discussion on the efficacy and safety of collagen-based formulations for healthcare applications.

6.1. Integumental Apparatus

Type I collagen is the main component of skin (85–90% type I collagen, 10–15% type III collagen). Fibrillar collagen types I, III, and V self-assemble into larger collagen fibers that form the dermis 3D network [215].

To improve the appearance of aged skin many non-invasive (i.e., topical formulations, oral supplements), minimally invasive (i.e., dermal fillers) and surgical treatments (i.e., blepharoplasty) were developed. Although a multitude of topical treatments are available for the improvement of aged skin appearance, these procedures appeared to have minimal ability to remodel dermal ECM [215]. However, collagen supplements originating from various animal sources such as marine, bovine, and porcine were revealed to be able to partially improve skin integrity. Thus, injectables became more popular for their immediate effect. As previously noted, several biomaterials (i.e., collagen, hyaluronic acid, calcium hydroxyl apatite, carboxy methyl cellulose, poly (methyl methacrylate), poly(L-lactic acid) were employed for the development of skin filler, each of which has some advantages and drawbacks.

Among them, collagen is the most promising for its low adverse effects rate and natural filling effect. The return to favor of collagen injectables for aesthetic medicine could be due to the acquired knowledge about chronological skin aging processes. Wrinkles formation is caused by collagen density decrease due to its turn-over slowing-down [215]. Its decreased synthesis and replacement rate causes matrix loss and thus skin collapse and loss of elasticity, which in turn leads to the appearance of wrinkles, folds, and facial contour changes, as masterfully described by Fisher et al. 2008 [215]. Due to this, several commercial collagen-based products are available and are used principally for facial contouring, such as for nasolabial folds [2,67,76,86,87,96,149,163,172,205–208], nasojugal folds [152], lip [2,77,95,148,169,172], cheek and temple area [172], glabellar groove [77], post-rhinoplasty dorsal irregularities [77,209], depressed acne scars [77,172, 210], augmentation [96,172].

Usually, collagen injectable formulations for antiaging treatments are supplied in the form of dry powder to be resuspended in a suitable buffer (e.g., NaCl 0.9%) or in liquid form in ready-to-use syringes with a final collagen concentration of 30–35 mg/mL. A total of 2–5 mL is injected to reach the desired effect. In particular, a volume of about 0.9–3.0 mL [67,86,95, 149,205–208] is injected in the first session, but because of collagen's rapid degradation, 1–3 touch-up treatments [67,87,96,149,206] of about 0.8–2.1 mL [67,149,206] are usually performed usually after 1–2 week from the first treatment [67,76,86,87,96,149,208] and more rarely after 1 [206] or 6 months [207].

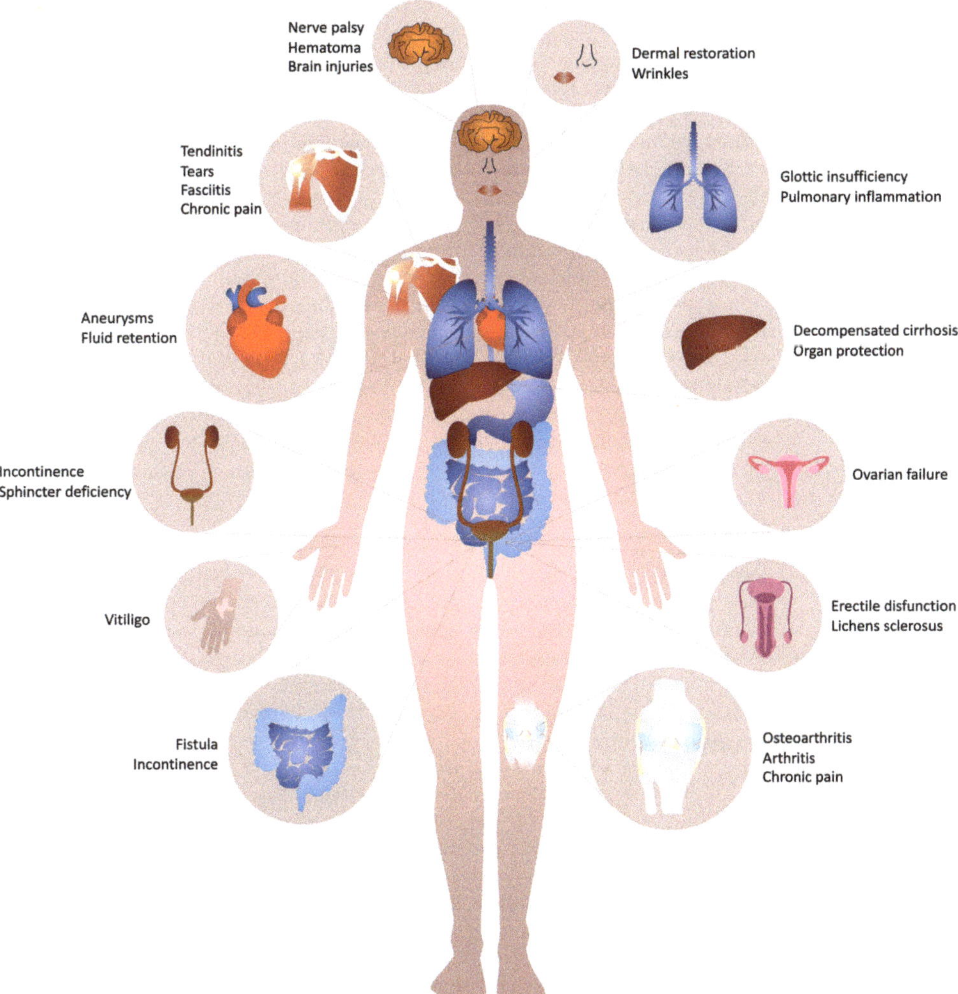

Figure 2. Main collagen-based injectables applications for the treatment of several kind of diseases belonging to the integumental, musculoskeletal, urogenital, gastro-intestinal apparatus, besides for non-standard clinical applications.

An improvement of the Crows' feet severity, Facial Volume Loss Scale (FVLS), and Wrinkle Severity Rating Scale (WSRS) of about 1 point was registered almost always after 6–8 months [86,163]. Accordingly, the improvement of the Global Aesthetic Improvement Scale (GAIS), Merz Aesthetic Scale (MAS) after 12 weeks of at least 1 point was registered in another study [67]. The maximum WSRS improvement of about 0.5–1.0 point was usually reached after 3 months [96,205,206]. However, the WSRS and GAIS score were reduced by about 0.5–1.0 and 1.0–1.5 points respectively after 12–24 months, confirming the biodegradability of collagen fillers and therefore the need to resort to multiple injections to maintain the desired effect [87,96]. Indeed, based on overall Subject Global Evaluation scores, patients reported 96% aesthetic improvement at the week-3 follow-up visit, a value that decreased to 60% at month-3 and to 15% at month-13 post–last treatment visits [205]. However, collagen persistence has been successfully improved by about 2 points of the WSRS scale after 6 months and prolonged with the use of crosslinked collagen (Dermicol-P35) up to 1 year with 1 touch-up after 1 week without immediate or delayed positive hypersensitivity reactions [149,208]. Collagen filler injected volume or its animal extraction may not be the influencing factor of collagen efficacy or side effects. Several studies reported how injected volume did not differ significantly between porcine collagen formulation (i.e., 2.03–2.11 mL for nasolabial fold, 0.90 mL for lip) and bovine collagen formulation (i.e., 1.8–2.1 mL for nasolabial fold, 0.85 mL for lip) nor were statistically significant differences registered in WSRS and GAIS score improvement, patients' satisfaction and adverse events [86,87,95]. Collagen fillers (Dermicol-P35, Artecoll®, Cymetra) demonstrated their effectiveness also in cases of depressed acne scars since they allowed to reach a high degree of correction, with no adverse events and high patient satisfaction level [77,172,210]. Although the acne scars were not completely removed, their appearance was greatly improved [210].

Collagen filler is generally considered safe. As shown in Table 3, fillers were well tolerated and there were no serious adverse reactions [67,87,96,163,216]. Indeed, serious adverse events that were not injection site related usually not occur [67]. However, all injection site reactions were mild to moderate in severity and resolved in 1–2 weeks without sequalae [2,86], except for some rare cases. Usually, 80% of participants had at least 1 injection site reaction after the initial injection [67]. Light/moderate bruises appear on the injection points that totally disappeared within 5–10 days [163]. Only one severe bruising was reported after 1-week follow-up and resolved after 4 weeks [67]. A case of mild induration after 4 weeks resolved in 6–12 weeks [67].

As previously mentioned, with the spreading idea of regenerating lost tissues rather than repairing them, collagen formulations started to be employed not only for aesthetic medicine but also for regenerative medicine. Only recently, collagen fillers started to be used for the treatment of other integumentary apparatus diseases such as the post-burn hands malfunction [88] and vitiligo [164]. Indeed, the potential of a collagen-glycosaminoglycans matrix (INTEGRA™ Flowable Wound Matrix) has been investigated for post-burn hands treatment with the idea that its composition was supposed to have the potential to rebuild the lost or injured deep dermal structure and enable soft tissue augmentation [88]. The work of Hirche et al. was the first pilot study using percutaneous injectable collagen-glycosaminoglycans matrix for post-burn dermal augmentation safety and efficiency, and active range of motion (AROM), disabilities of the arm, shoulder and hand (DASH) score, Vancouver scar scale (VSS) score and scar quality improvement were registered after 6 months [88]. Despite the encouraging results, further studies on the formulation's long-term efficacy on a higher number of patients are necessary in order to evaluate the possible quality of life and grip strength that appeared to not be changed after 6 observation months [88]. More recently, collagen injections were proposed also for unresolved diseases such as vitiligo. Although a variety of treatments for the re-pigmentation of vitiligo lesions are available (e.g., platelet-rich plasma injections, UV-phototherapy), none of them effectively promote complete and long-lasting re-pigmentation. Thus, the potential synergistic effect of intradermal collagen injections (Linerase®) in combination with UV-phototherapy was investigated and 70% re-pigmentation occurred after six sessions with mild-to-moderate pain and no adverse events [164]. Moreover, no relapses were reported after one year [164].

Table 3. Clinical trials details (i.e., participants, injections number, volume and administration time (weeks (w)) and adverse events recurrence on collagen based injectable formulations for skin rejuvenation from 2000 to 2022.

	Nithya					Dermicol-P35						Permacol	Therafill			RPC Pure-Collagen	Sunmax FacialGain		Zyplast			Artecoll	Koken		CosmoDerm			CosmoPlast	Isolagen
Collagen Source	Equine	Swine																Bovine						Human					
Injection specification – Number (n)	1	2	2	1	1–2	1–2	2	2	1	1	1	1	n. d.	1	1	2	1	1	3	1–3	1	1	1	1	1	1	1	1–4	3
Injection specification – Volume (mL)	2–5	2.2	2	n. d.	n. d.	0.6	1	1	1	n. d.	n. d.	1.5–3.0	1	2	2	2.56	n. d.	1.5–3.0	2	1.6	1	n. d.	1.8	2	1	n. d.	n. d.	1	n. d.
Injection specification – Amount (mg)	80	77	70	n. d.	n. d.	21–42	70	70	35	n. d.	n. d.	52–105	30	60	60	89.6	n. d.	53–105	70–210	56–168	35	n. d.	54	70	35	n. d.	n. d.	n. d.	n. d.
Injection specification – Interval (inj./weeks)	1	0.5/w	0.5/w	n. d.	0.5/w	0.25/w	0.04/w	0.25/w	n. d.	n. d.	n. d.	n. d.	0.5/w	n. d.	n. d.	1/w	n. d.	n. d.	0.8/w	0.5/w	n. d.	n. d.	n. d.	n. d.	n. d.	n. d.	n. d.	0.3/w	0.6/w
Observation time (weeks)	24	48		48	24	32	n. d.	8	1	1	240	48	12	24	48	12	52	48	24	24	12	136	24	48	6	24	6	100	29
Participants (n)	72	148	24	20	172	12	1	1	10	30	1	19	73	57	57	30	n. d.	18	439	138	118	153	57	57	3	n. d.	1	117	110
Adverse events – Severe	0	0	149	0	0	0	0	0	0	0	1	0	n. d.	0	0	1	n. d.	0	0	0	0	0	0	0	0	n. d.	0	0	0
Adverse events – Non severe	n. d.	5	0	16	154	0	0	0	0	38	0	18	n. d.	12	1	0	n. d.	1	n. d.	124	109	n. d.	18	5	1	n. d.	1	42	32
Adverse events – Allergic reaction			n. d.									1																2	
Adverse events – Pain												9		1					58	58								4	
Adverse events – Infection					12							9						1											8
Adverse events – Papule/erythema	v		80		17					14				7		24			391		75		8	1	1		1	4/31	14
Adverse events – Nodule/lumpiness		1		16															369		15	52		1				7	
Adverse events – Bruise	v		27													1			241	66	51	20						1	5
Adverse events – Edema/swelling			42							22				2	1	24			378	101	61		6	3			1	5	
Adverse events – Hemorrhage																												3	10
Adverse events – Itching																24			##		24		1				1	9	
Adverse events – Induration/tenderness		3	36											1					391	88	14		2					1	
Adverse events – Discoloration		1			12									1					149		31							2	
References	[163]	[149]	[208]	[148]	NCT00891774	[209]	[207]	[210]	NCT00929071	[2], NCT00911872	[147]	[95]	NCT01060943	[86]	[87]	[67]	NCT03844529	[95]	[96]	[76]	NCT00876265	[77]	[86]	[87]	[217]	NCT01212809	[217]	[205,206], NCT00444210, NCT00444353	NCT00655356

6.2. Musculoskeletal Apparatus

Aging leads not only to skin texture loss but also to a progressive and gradual reduction of all human capabilities. The loss of muscle or osteochondral mass with advancing age is the major public health problem for the elderly population. Thus, musculoskeletal apparatus-related medical treatments and costs increase with population age (numbers over 50 years). Among invasive and non-invasive currently available treatments, collagen injections are revealed to be quite effective for the treatment of several musculoskeletal diseases such as hip [131] or knee osteoarthritis [112,133,140,142,144,182], sprained knee pain [143], injured cartilage [138,141], piriformis syndrome [134], ankle and hindfoot arthritis [103] or fusion [100,106–109], lumbar spinal fusion [99], myofascial pain syndrome [130,137], chronic pain [132], acute lumbar spine pain [134] and in partial-thickness rotator cuff tears [141,144,183], plantar fasciitis [184], and calcific supraspinatus tendinitis [145] and pain [130,132,134,137].

Osteoarthritis is an inflammatory degenerative disease characterized by the progressive damage of articular cartilage and underlying bone that predominantly affects hip and knee [218]. Interleukin (IL)-1β, tumor necrosis factor (TNF)-α, and IL-6 seem to be the main proinflammatory cytokines involved in the pathophysiology of osteoarthritis, even though others, including IL-15, IL-18, IL-21, leukemia inhibitory factor (LIF), and chemokines are implicated [182,219]. The expression of these inflammation mediators in turn activates the cartilage-degrading enzymes, that are matrix metalloproteinases (MMPs) and A disintegrin metalloproteinase with thrombospondin motifs (ADAMTS) [112,219], that progressively degrade the ECM, including collagen. From this observation, several studies were performed to prove the hypothesis that an exogenous administration of collagen may be beneficial to osteoarthritis damaged cartilage and bone.

Indeed, a total of 12 mL of collagen and polyvinylpyrrolidone based formulation (Fibroquel®) affected the values of the Lequesne index (LKI) by −51%, Western Ontario and McMaster University Index (WOMAC) pain subscale by –51%, WOMAC stiffness subscale by −49%, WOMAC disability subscale by −42%, and the use of analgesics by –83% after 6 months [182]. Moreover, pro-inflammatory cytokine expression was lowered in patients under collagen treatment compared with placebo [192]. Injections of collagen, arnica and hypericum (MD-Knee® and MD-Muscle®) brought a significant reduction of Visual Analogue Scale (VAS) pain at rest with a decrease of the average score for pain during movement of more than two-fold after 12 weeks [133]. Similar results were obtained by Martin et al. who found a LKI and VAS significant improvement 6 months after five weekly injections (a total of 20 mL) of MD-Knee® [144]. More recently, analogous clinical outcomes were obtained with pure collagen formulations, with a reduced number of injections. Indeed, three injections of a hydrolyzed collagen suspension (a total of 6 mL of CHondroGrid®) significantly reduced VAS, LKI, and WOMAC scores [112], by up to about 50% [142].

Because of the avascular, aneural, and immunoprivileged nature of hyaline cartilage, the regenerative potential of cartilage after injury is limited. In this circumstance, collagen injections revealed to be a promising modality for single-stage cartilage repair: collagen augmented chondrogenesis by 50% filling of the microfractures with CartiFill®. This showed a superior VAS improvement rate analysis and a superior filling rate in the cartilage tissues as well as integration with the surrounding tissues 24 months postoperatively compared with that achieved only with microfracture [139].

Peri-articular collagen injections (MD-Knee® and MD-Matrix®) twice/week for 3 consecutive weeks revealed to be effective also for the treatment of sprained knee pain, with a rapid recovery and an excellent control of breakthrough pain without the use of anti-inflammatory drugs [143].

Thus, all clinical outcomes confirmed the benefits in collagen use and allowed to define intra-articular collagen injection as inflammation down-modulator and cartilage regenerator 'biodrug' [182]. Collagen can effectively promote repair processes of the cartilage matrix, interrupting the degenerative process and articular damage, which causes inflammation and pain [144]. The administration of type I collagen after arthroscopic lavage is safe and effective and induced systemic inflammation downregulation [182]. Adverse events are rare, most frequently including site pain that lasts at most 24 h [131,182]. No aseptic acute arthritis, infections after injection or any other complication have ever been registered [112,131,182]. Taking into account that osteoarthritis is the most common form of musculoskeletal disorder with a prevalence of 23% of over 40 people and an annual incidence of 203 per 10,000 person/year [220], it is easy to understand how it has high economic costs and a devastating impact on patient quality of life. The above-mentioned recent studies showed how the benefits associated with the use of collagen make it a very promising non-invasive solution that has begun to find its place among conventional therapies (i.e., corticosteroids, polynucleotides, platelet-rich plasma, hyaluronic acid intra-articular injections). Although today collagen injections are still less popular than hyaluronan, they exert a similar clinical effect, besides being equally well tolerated both locally and at a systemic level, confirming the material non-inferiority [144]. The reduced cost of collagen-based formulations compared to hyaluronic acid-based formulations could bring to the attainment of the intra-articular therapy to a broad range of the population, resulting in the reduction of social cost due to working days lost and caregivers' time off work [144].

Osteochondral disorders are followed by less common but equally disabling muscular and tendon pain. Inflammatory or degenerative process, fracture, radicular syndrome, or nonspecific syndrome are causes of chronic musculoskeletal pain, which is the most common health complaint, with significant social and economic consequences [132,134]. The incidence of musculoskeletal pain increases with age and strongly affects the quality of life of a growing number of affected people [137]. Current medical procedures include conservative methods (i.e., rehabilitation, medications), minimally invasive interventions (e.g., acupuncture) or surgical treatment. However, the huge risk of gastrotoxicity, hepatotoxicity, cardiotoxicity and nephrotoxicity, after long-term and/or high doses of common nonsteroidal anti-inflammatory drugs, pushed researchers toward the investigation of safer options [134]. In this circumstance, the subcutaneous/intramuscular administration of collagen containing products (MD-Lumbar MD®, MD-Muscle®, MD-Neural®) represented a new concept in the treatment of pain, that is based on the strengthening the collagen matrix underlying the musculoskeletal system structures and on the analgesic effects of these products. Although few published data are available, it is clear that collagen-based injections represent a safer treatment option with no adverse events, 54–60% pain relief [130,132], good tolerability [134], and comparable or better efficacy with the standard treatments [130,134].

Only recently the efficacy of collagen injections (RegenSeal®, MD-Shoulder®, MD-Muscle®) for the treatment of tendon tear have been clinically investigated [141,183,184]. The first prospective, randomized clinical trial has been conducted by Kim et al. in 2020 and reported rotator cuff functional outcomes improvement and a decreased tear size in 37% of patients with a single collagen injection (0.5–1.0 mL) [141]. A case study confirmed how multiple intratendinous weekly injections of 2 mL of collagen are able to reduce the partial-thickness tear in three months and to completely heal tendon tear in 18 months, which in addition appeared quite regular and isoechoic [183]. Collagen injections were thus found to be effective to decrease tear size (50–77% complete recovery), pain, increase functional shoulder score and delay tear progression in partial-thickness rotator cuff tears [141,145,146,183]. The precise mechanism of tendon healing after injection of collagen is still unknown. However, two in vivo studies on rabbits proved that injections of collagen in the tissue during the ECM remodeling phase led to better tendon healing and earlier progression to the remodeling phase [141,221,222]. Both histological and biomechanical studies of type I collagen implants facilitated continuity of injured tendons, decreased peritendinous adhesion, and improved muscle activity in Achilles tendons of rabbits [221,222]. Despite their low efficacy rate and their limited use, collagen injections would be more advantageous than traditional surgery for their cost-effectiveness, easy performance and less time-consuming nature.

6.3. Urogenital System

Collagen injections have been revealed to be a minimally invasive and quite effective solution for specific urogenital system diseases such as stress urinary incontinence [122,124,125,185–189], neurogenic urinary incontinence [190], lichens sclerosus [165], intrinsic sphincter deficiency [191–193], post-prostatectomy incontinence [65,123,194–197], retrograde ejaculation [198] and ovarian function after premature ovarian failure [212].

Stress urinary incontinence affects 10–30% of women above 50 years of age [185]. To solve this common issue, in addition to surgical practices (i.e., retropubic bladder neck suspension or slings), biomaterials injections (i.e., teflon, fat, silicone, collagen) have been performed to increase urethral strength and avoid urinary leak. Among them, collagen (Contigen®, Linerase®) has remained the most promising. In a study of Martins et al., either cure or improvement was achieved in 86% of women, with a registered leak pressure increase and reduction in urinary protector use and urine leakage volume [185]. In another study, 48% were totally dry and 31% were socially continent after 2 months [187]. However, because of collagen absorption, stress urinary incontinence recurrence occurred in 41% of patients who achieved continence after 7–8 months [187]. Collagen reportedly degraded completely within 10–19 weeks, although magnetic resonance imaging of the urethra showed the persistence of the implant for as long as 22 months after injection [196]. Thus, repeated injections (2–5) may be necessary [187,188,190]. Hence, reinjections were performed, with a 42% regain of continence, giving a long-term success rate of 58–60% [187]. Totally favorable results, including improvement (40%) and cure (30%), were also recorded for up to 4 years [124]. However, it should be mentioned that elderly patients should be counseled that approximately 40% will experience recurrent leakage, which may not resolve with reinjection [187]. Conversely, Gorton et al. reported the absence of correlation between long-term success and the number of previous operations, body mass index, age, number or total volume of collagen injections [125].

Men's post-prostatectomy incontinence incidence ranges from 2% to 87% [123]. The most commonly performed surgical procedures include the insertion of an artificial urinary sphincter or of injectable bulking agents. In this case, collagen (Contigen®) is the most commonly used and several works reported how 3–4 collagen injections led 8–20% of patients to dryness and 38–39% to significant improvement [123,194]. Treatment was found to be pad related. The highest success rate was reached in patients that fewer than 6 pads per day (72%) a value that lowers up to 29% for patients using more than 6 pads per day [123]. Moreover, in cases of radiation therapy or bladder neck incision after a radical prostatectomy, the success rate is even lower [123]. The success rate of collagen injection strongly decreased in the treatment of urinary incontinence in children with neurogenic bladder dysfunction secondary to myelomeningocele. In this case, only 15% improved and 5% were completely dry [190]. Additionally, the initial improvement in the first 2 months after injection deteriorated thereafter in 80% of children [190]. The first severe case was registered in 2006, when three years after a single sub ureteral collagen injection for the treatment of bilateral vesicoureteral reflux in a 1 year of age girl, hydronephrosis with ureteral stenosis with a knotty sclerosis and a histiocytic and granulomatous reaction occurred and required ureteral reimplantation [223]. Despite the widespread and long-term application of collagen for the treatment of stress urinary incontinence, treatment-related morbidity was minimal. Urinary tract infections occurred in 6% to 25% of cases while transient hematuria and hypersensitivity were occasionally reported [124,125]. No implant migration, nor seroconversion to antibodies that cross-reacted with human collagen, nor symptoms were even registered [123]. However, patients who have required a penile clamp and experienced continuous leakage or those who have undergone transurethral incision of a bladder neck contracture are unlikely to respond well to collagen injection therapy [194].

Recently, collagen injections (Linerase®) have been proposed for the treatment of male genital *lichen sclerosus* and retrograde ejaculation. In the case of lichens sclerosus, it revealed to be safe and effective in 10 days and for up to 12 months [165]. Likewise, two injections of 6 mL of collagen (one per year) were revealed to be effective and complication free in cases of retrograde ejaculation [198].

Collagen-based injections were also found to be effective for the treatment of premature ovarian failure [212]. Indeed, umbilical cord mesenchymal stem cells loaded collagen formulation was found to be able to rescue overall ovarian function, evidenced by elevated estradiol concentrations, improved follicular development, and increased number of antral follicles [212]. Moreover, successful clinical pregnancy was achieved after the transplantation of the cell loaded collagen gel [212].

Thus, collagen injections seemed to be a simple, least morbid, cost-effective, and effective treatment for disease affecting the urinary apparatus, with low failure rates [123].

6.4. Gastrointestinal Apparatus

Injectable collagen has been shown to be effective in the management of gastrointestinal apparatus diseases such as glottic insufficiency [113,114,116–119,173,199–203], rectal fistula [153,154,156,157] and fecal incontinence [115,155,204].

Glottic dysfunctions due to glottic gap, atrophy, paresis, bowing, paralysis and scarring result in voice absence or alteration. The gold standard for the treatment of vocal fold disfunctions is represented by medialization laryngoplasty or arytenoid adduction, surgical treatments that could significantly improve glottal adduction and phonation. Recently, to reach a better postoperative voice in the long term, biomaterials injection (i.e., autologous fat, silicone, collagen, hyaluronic acid, carboxymethylcellulose) [116,224,225] has been additionally performed. However, autograft represent the known advantages of a double surgery, but means double surgery time and costs. Instead, xenografts are an attractive alternative for supplementing arytenoid adduction, because of their noninvasiveness, ready availability, and possibility to be performed under local anesthesia. Among them, collagen injectable formulations proved to be effective for vocal fold management. Patients treated with 1–2 mL of selected collagen injectable formulations (Koken®, AlloDerm®, Zyplast®) showed at least some improvement in vocal function after the treatment, according to the Grade, Roughness, Breathiness, Asthenia, Strain (GRBAS) scale, Maximum phonation time, Mean flow rate, Relative glottal area. In particular, perceptual and objective voice quality improvement (less weak and breathy) was registered, with an increase of the mean maximum phonation time from around 8–11 s to 13–15 s, and a reduction of the mean flow rate from 322–564 mL/s to 223–385 mL/s and of the glottal gap [113,114,200], for at least up to 2 years after operation [114]. Thus, from the moment in which the safety and efficacy of collagen injections for the treatment of the vocal cords was affirmed by Ford and Bless in 1993 [202], the injection of heterologous material started to be even more required, given the positive feedback and long-term results [118]. Although collagen injections were quite effective, and serious adverse events were rare [113,114,117,202], documented complications included local abscess, migration of the implant, hypersensitivity reactions, stiffening, fusiform collagen mass, nodules [116,173] principally related to the procedure and injection site [113]. Indeed, if properly injected, the complication rate after collagen injection would decrease [200].

Anal fistula is a tunnel that connects an infected cavity in the anus, to an opening on the skin. Usually, fistulas are surgically removed by fistulotomy, which is the gold standard procedure (37–98% success rate). However, complex fistula fistulotomy may result in variable degrees of anal sphincter apparatus impairment. Several alternative treatments were proposed and among them a trans anal rectal advancement flap represents the most effective treatment for complex anal fistulas allowing the successful closure of the internal opening. However, the recurrence rate is approximately 30% [157]. The interest in biomaterials use increased for their simple and repeatable application, preservation of sphincter integrity, and minimal patient's discomfort [157]. Among biomaterials, fibrin glue and collagen injections were proposed. Fibrin glue was soon abandoned for its high rates of recurrences. Conversely, collagen injections (Permacol®) were revealed to be effective to treat anal fistula. In particular, no complications occurred and complete healing was reached after 3–15 months upon surgery [156–158]. The treatment success rate varies among studies, with a 56% of success rate at 12 months of follow up in a more recent study [156]. However, it should be mentioned that patients' characteristics play a key role in the healing rate since a significant correlation with age was registered by Giordano et al. [156], with an increased chance of healing as age increased. While some authors confirmed the complete safety of the procedure and of the collagen injections [153,154,157,158], others registered middle-serious adverse events, including abscess (3%), bleeding (3%) and pain (7%) [156]. Although reports suggest that collagen injections are quite safe, minimally invasive, healing promoters for the sphincter-preserving procedure, and well tolerated by patients, further studies are needed for confirming their effectiveness in the treatment for complex anal fistulas.

Similarly, collagen injections were revealed to be quite effective for the treatment of fecal incontinence [115,155]. As reported by Stojkovic et al., after 2 months 5% of patients were completely continent, 58% had an improved incontinence score and 37% had no change or a worse score [115]. Healing was discovered to be strictly dependent on the incontinence etiology: a significant improvement of the incontinence score was indeed registered in case of idiopathic fecal incontinence and in older people while no improvements were observed in case of neuropathic or traumatic incontinence [115]. Despite the partial positive 1–2 years positive follow up, the disadvantage of collagen as filler agent is that degradation occurs over a period of 12–30 months [115] that obliges at least one repeat injection.

6.5. Others

New experimentations using collagen-based formulations were performed for non-standard clinical applications such as facial nerve rehabilitation after palsy [160,211], organ protection during thermal ablation [129], COVID-19 related hyperinflammation [161,162] (NCT04517162), artery aneurysms closure [128,213], blood volume augmentation [127,214] and the treatment of chronic ischemic heart diseases [226].

Given the absence of experiences with collagen-based injections in the field of facial palsy rehabilitation, the aim of a recent pilot randomized study was to test the short-term effectiveness of a collagen-based treatment (MD Neural®, MD Matrix® and MD Muscle®) on patients complaining of long-standing facial nerve axonotmesis with the possible expectation of collagen redirecting and guiding reinnervation/reorganization processes [160,211]. Although the recovery outcomes are difficult to interpret because of the presence of several confounding factors (i.e., palsy etiology, time from disease onset, patients' age, association of medical treatment), a significant improvement of both electrophysiological and questionnaire scores in the duration of voluntary activity was found in patients treated with in situ collagen injections [160,211].

Another recent application field for collagen-based injectable formulations is in the surrounding organ protection during tumor thermal ablation [129]. Organ protection is usually performed by using fluids (e.g., dextrose) or gas (e.g., CO_2) displacement but because of their physical properties they distribute freely in the injection site and decrease the durability of separation. The injection of a highly viscous fibrillar collagen (Helitene®) focally interposed between the liver and adjacent structures prior to hepatic microwave ablation made the organ separation durable, low cost, well tolerated, facilitated hemostasis and healing besides making thermal ablation technically successful without complication [129].

A collagen-based injectable formulation was found to be a potential drug in the treatment of symptomatic COVID-19 patients for its immunomodulatory properties, in relation to IL-1β, IL-8, TNF-α, TNF-β1, IL-17, cyclooxygenase 1 (Cox-1), endothelial leucocyte adhesion molecule 1 (ELAM-1), vascular cell adhesion molecule 1 (VCAM-1), intercellular adhesion molecule 1 (ICAM-1) downregulation, tissues fibrosis reduction, and IL-10 and T cells upregulation. Intramuscular injection of collagen (Fibroquel®) was able to significantly decrease the interferon gamma-induced protein 10 (IP-10), IL-8, macrophage colony-stimulating factor (M-CSF), high-sensitivity C-reactive protein (hsCRP), D-dimer and lactate dehydrogenase (LDH) levels, in the first week of treatment [162] (NCT04517162). Moreover, collagen injections were associated with better oxygen saturation values and shortened symptom duration, extubation and reduced inflammation when compared to placebo [161,162] (NCT04517162). Thus, collagen-based injections were considered safe and well-tolerated and did not induce liver damage, infections, impairment of hematopoiesis or blood alterations [161,162] (NCT04517162).

Interestingly, collagen intravenous injections (Gelaspan®, Gelofusione®) were successful for blood volume expansion in cases of dehydration, illness, trauma or severe sepsis/septic shock related surgery and were found to be more effective in achieving hemodynamic stability in critically ill patients compared to standard plasma volume replacement products, with no side effects [127,214].

In cases of complications due to percutaneous transfemoral catheter procedures, vascular surgery is necessary after the failure of the ultrasound-guided compression repair attempt [128]. A less invasive method to percutaneously close a femoral artery pseudoaneurysm was found by injecting collagen and inducing clotting within the aneurysm, with a 98% success rate [128]. The hemostatic power of collagen is due to the fact that the collagen hydrogel forms an 3D network which triggers the hemostatic cascade (i.e., platelet aggregation, adherence, and activation) [213]. Moreover, upon contact with blood, the collagen expands its physical mass resulting in mechanical occlusion of the vessel puncture site and tissue tract [213].

Despite all the functional improvements that collagen is able to support in several diseases, neither improvement nor adverse events were observed in patients with chronic ischemic heart disease treated with mesenchymal stromal cells in a collagen gel vehicle compared with control patients and patients treated with mesenchymal stromal cells alone [226].

Thus, as emerged in this section, collagen-based injectable formulations can be very useful in the treatment of unresolved issues and open the way for new solutions and less invasive approaches. Based on this evidence, even more research has been performed and accordingly, even more clinical studies have been planned. Hence, besides the discussed clinical outcomes, several clinical studies aiming at improving functional recovery of liver in cases of decompensate cirrhosis (NCT02786017), brain in cases of intracranial hematoma (NCT02767817), erectile function in men with type I or II diabetes mellitus (NCT02745808), blood volume during surgery (NCT02808325, NCT01515397) and fluid retention in cases of breast cancer (NCT04637308) are ongoing (Table 4).

Table 4. New applications of collagen based injectable formulations.

Formulation	Study Aim	Status	Outcomes	ClinicalTrials.gov Identifier
Injectable Collagen Scaffold™ HUC-MSCs	Improvement of erectile function in men with diabetes	Unknown	n. d.	NCT02745808
Injectable Collagen Scaffold™ HUC-MSCs	Improvement of liver function in cases of decompensated cirrhosis	Unknown	n. d.	NCT02786017
Injectable Collagen Scaffold™ MCSs	Improvement of functional brain recovery in cases of brain injury	Unknown	n. d.	NCT02767817
Gelofusine	Fluid retention prevention in patients with breast cancer	Completed	n. d.	NCT04637308
Gelofusine	Improvement of blood volume in patients scheduled for abdominal or pelvic surgery	Completed	n. d.	NCT02808325
Gelofusine	Improvement of blood volume for intravascular volume compensation during surgery	Completed	n. d.	NCT01515397

7. Adverse Reactions to Collagen-Based Injectable Implants

All types of fillers may trigger an early tissue response to the injected material. Regardless of the filler material, frequently reported side effects are bruising, redness, swelling, induration, erythema pain, tenderness, itching and, in the most severe cases, violaceous plaque and granulomas [227–229]. These side effects are usually mild and transient and resolve spontaneously after a short time. Only a few cases of severe and permanent complications have been registered.

Although compared with other injectables collagen-based formulations have many advantages, it does not mean that they are absolutely safe. Indeed, severe and non-severe adverse reactions to collagen treatments may occur. To the best of our knowledge, based on harvested and available data on adverse reactions registered after collagen-based commercial product applications (Table 5), severe adverse events accounted for 8.2% (211 cases on 2587 patients), while mild adverse events accounted for about 5.3% (137 cases on 2587 patients) of those receiving the treatment.

With a focus on collagen extraction sources, it emerged that severe adverse events accounted for 12.1% (211 cases on 1742 patients) and mild events for 3.8% (67 on 1742 patients) when bovine collagen was used. In particular, severe adverse events were addressed to the use of one collagen-based product that was Augment®, an injectable formulation composed of bovine collagen, β-tricalcium phosphate and recombinant human platelet-derived growth factor-BB [102] (NCT01305356, NCT00583375). Leaving aside the Augment® severe adverse reactions (211 on 1742 procedures), the other analyzed bovine collagen-based products (i.e., ChondroGrid, Atelocell, Zyderm, Zyplast, Contigen, Gelofusine, Flowable wound matrix and Helitene) were not associated with such issues [88,113,114,116,118,127,129,142,187,188,190,214,230] (NCT02808325, NCT04637308, NCT02715466, NCT01515397, NCT02631356, NCT00868062). Since bovine collagen appeared to be safe, these events could be ascribable to other Augment components, without certainty. As regards mild adverse reactions, they were registered only when using Augment, Chondrogrid or Zyderm [101,106,118,142].

Porcine derived collagen-based products (i.e., Cartifil, Cartizol, Fibroquel, Permacol and MD products) revealed to not trigger severe adverse events (no cases on 751 procedures) and to be responsible for the 9.2% of mild adverse events (69 cases on 751 procedures) [131–136,138,140,141,143,145,146,153–157,160–162,182,204] (NCT02539030, NCT02539095, NCT04019782, NCT03323567, NCT02539082, NCT01528995, NCT04517162, NCT04353908). Mild adverse events could be due both to collagen type or to other components (i.e., glucose, CaCl, amino acids, vitamin B, fibrin glue for Cartifil/Cartizol; polyvinylpyrrolidone for Fibroquel) or to the injection procedure. However, data were not enough to identify the causes. Definitely though, the low mild adverse events rate of the MD product could be clearly ascribable to the presence of other bioactive compounds (such as calcium phosphate, rhododendron, arnica, hamemelis, silicon, iris, viola, cimifuga, citric acid, nicotinamide, hypericum, drosera, citrullus, ascorbic acid, magnesium gluconate, pyridoxine chlorhydrate, riboflavin, thiamine chlorhydrate) that had a strong impact on patients' post intervention events. As regards Permacol, since it is not characterized by the presence of other components, adverse events triggered by its use could be attributed to collagen type, to the injection procedure, to the disease or to the patient specific response. In this case, available data do not allow clearly attribution of responsibility. However, mild adverse event usually resolved spontaneously or required minimal, not invasive intervention [131,140,141,156,160,162,204] (NCT04353908, NCT04517162, NCT01528995, NCT02539030).

The third most used collagen type Is equine derived collagen, whose use is very recent and thus limited compared to bovine and porcine derived injectable products. Indeed, it has been reported to be used (i.e., Linerase, Savecoll-E) only on 94 patients, with no adverse events and only one registered mild reaction (1.1%) [60,164–166]. Thus, although this percentage seems to be very low compared to other products, the limited number of executed procedures with equine collagen prevented the assessment of this collagen type as safer. This consideration could be applied also for human collagen derived products (i.e., Cymetra, Dermologen) for which two severe and zero mild adverse events were registered on the only patients [173,202]. However, these data and these considerations are only indicative because not all studies reported participant number and adverse event occurrence.

As regards aesthetic applications, collagen injectables are generally considered as safe because serious adverse events that were not injection site related usually not occur [67]. Indeed, severe adverse events rate accounted for 0.1% of the total (2 cases on 2063 patients). In particular, severe adverse events occurred only when using porcine derived collagen Dermicol-P35 (with ribose as crosslinker) and RPC Pure Collagen (with ethylenediamine tetraacetic acid) [67,147]. However, two cases occurring on 780 injections were not enough to relate the adverse events to collagen type or other components. Contrarily, non-severe adverse reactions always occur (Table 3) and accounted for 28% (577 cases on 2063 patients). They may be categorized into early and late reaction [16,231]. Usually, injection site reactions were mild to moderate in severity and resolved in 1–2 weeks without sequelae [2,86], except for some rare cases. About 80% of participants had at least 1 injection site reaction after the initial injection [67]. This kind of adverse reaction is localized and may be associated with transient systemic symptoms on rare occasions [232]. Early complications occur immediately up to several days after treatment and completely auto-resolve in a few months, without treatment [217,227,229]. They can be divided into non-hypersensitive and hypersensitive reactions. Non-hypersensitive reactions, which can occur with any filler, include local injection site reactions (i.e., erythema, edema, pain, tenderness, bruising, itching), discoloration (i.e., redness, whiteness, or hyperpigmentation), infections (i.e., herpes virus reactivation or bacterial contamination), skin necrosis (vascular occlusion), and misplacement [231]. Hypersensitive reactions are due to the material and depend on patient immune system reactivity and hypersensitivity. Late complications occur after 2–12 months and consist in foreign body granulomatous reaction, granulomas, and abscess formation [231]. Among non-severe adverse events, pain (13.9%), nodule (11.0%), bruises (11.1%), edema (11.3%), erythema (17.8%), itching (5.8%), swelling (6.0%), tenderness (3.0%), lumpiness (1.4%), induration (12.0%), discoloration (5.3%) were the most common. Very rare were cold sores, infections, blistering, papules, and hemorrhages (>0.5%). Contrary to what might be expected, allergic reactions occurred only in 0.1% of cases.

In terms of collagen extraction source, bovine (48%) and porcine (38%) derived formulations were the most used, followed by human (11%) and equine derived (4%). Accordingly, Dermicol-P35 and Zyplast were the most used products, followed by Therafil, Artecol, Koken, Isolagen therapy, CosmoPlast, Nithya, RPC Pure-Collagen, Permacol, Sunmax FacialGain, and CosmoDerm. Non severe events were registered to happen with all collagen types, except for equine derived collagen-based formulations. Indeed, bovine and swine derived collagen-based formulations triggered 12.5% and 11.8% non-severe events (257 and 244 cases on 2063 injections, respectively), followed by human derived with about 3.7% (76 cases on 2063 injections). Equine collagen injectables were revealed to be adverse events free but it should be taken into account that reported data were referred to only one study performed on 72 people [163]. Thus, Nithya, RPC Pure Collagen and Artecol reported no adverse events [67,77,163]. The non-severe adverse events rate was reported to be of 39.2% for Dermicol-P35 (213 cases on 544 injections) [2,147–149,207,209,210] (NCT00891774, NCT00929071, NCT00911872), 94.7% for Permacol (18 cases on 19 injections) [95], while for the others the rate was about 7–36%. In particular, it was 32.8% for Zyplast (13/187 injections) [96] (NCT00876265), 20.2% for Koken (23/114 injections) [87], 29.1% for the Isolagen therapy (32/110 injections) (NCT00655356), 36.4% for Cosmoplast (43/118 injections) [205,206] (NCT00444210, NCT00444353), 33.3% for Cosmoderm (1/3 injections) [217] (NCT01212809) and 7% for Therafil, (13/187 injections) [87] (NCT01060943). In this case, the relatively low number of executed procedures prevented the assessment of product safety profiles and their comparison.

Although non-severe adverse reactions are neither life nor health threatening and thus are not of medical significance, they are cosmetically unacceptable. Nowadays, several tricks and improvements of the injection techniques have been made in order to avoid reactions caused by materials and procedures as much as possible [233]. Hypersensitive reactions are historically defined as the most common. Although it is rare (3% of the world population), some individuals develop allergic reactions to injected products when the body responds with an exaggerated immune response to a foreign substance. Allergic reactions generally occur within minutes of exposure, but delayed hypersensitivity can occur several months or years after injection [9]. Allergy to bovine derived collagen is genetically regulated by the lack of the HLA-DR4 antigen [234]. To avoid allergic reaction, skin testing now is mandatory. However, despite skin testing, hypersensitivity can occur in 1–6% of single skin test negative patients and in about 0.5% of double skin test negative patients [16,227–229]. Thus, a double skin testing is suggested before soft tissue augmentation [228,235]. Although double skin testing does not eliminate all adverse events, most of them were avoided because the great majority of adverse reactions occurred on the first injection session after a single skin test [232]. Collagen antigenicity is related to its molecular structure and is linked to its antigenic determinants that are located on the triple helix (i.e., dependent on the helix conformation), the polypeptide sequence (i.e., independent of the helices organization) and terminal (i.e., telopeptides) dependent [71,236–238]. However, it must be underlined that while collagen antigenicity has been attributed mostly to the terminal telopeptides, the location of the major antigenic sites depends on the specific donor/recipient species pair [71]. Alternatively, human collagen-based fillers offer a solution for their theoretical zero risk of allergic reaction. Nevertheless, erythema and hypersensitivity to human collagen was registered [217].

Foreign body granulomatous reaction and granulomas occurred in 0.01% of cases after 6–9 months after the treatment [231]. However, it must be taken into account that most of this kind of complication occurred with Artecoll®/Artefill®, probably due to the reaction to the poly(methyl methacrylate) microspheres rather than the collagenous component. However, the late adverse reactions to poly(methyl methacrylate) microspheres together with bovine collagen may have increased the immune system response.

Apart from the selected collagen formulation, as with any surgical or minimally invasive procedure, the result obtained with the injection therapy heavily depends on proper patient selection, expertise in performing the procedure, adequate knowledge of facial or other site's anatomy, and use of specialized equipment [13,123]. Only recently, the development of adequate implantation protocols permitted re-evaluation of collagen-based injectable therapies as a minimally invasive and effective strategies for the treatment of different types of diseases. Indeed, as preparation and administration techniques have become increasingly standardized, the frequency of post-injection complications has also decreased. Moreover, the selection of the appropriate filler, which depends on patient factors, including degree of volume loss, disease, age, cost, preference, and surgical candidacy was revealed to be crucial for the implant success [1], underscoring the need for product-specific training. Regardless of materials safety, appropriate handling and adequate experience are mandatory for minimizing the risk of complications and achieving the desired effect. An accurate guide on how to avoid and treat dermal filler complications has been developed by Lemperle et al. [233].

Swelling and bruising, which usually resolves within 4–10 days [163], could be attenuated by icing the area prior to treatment or by avoiding aspirin-containing compounds and anticoagulants, nonsteroidal anti-inflammatory drugs, and various vitamin supplements (e.g., vitamin E, fish oils) for 7–10 days before the procedure [152,231]. Only one severe bruising was reported after 1-week follow-up and resolved after 4 weeks [67]. A case of mild induration after 4 weeks resolved in 6–12 weeks [67].

The gauge of the needle, that depends on both the viscosity of the filler and the size of the particle, directly greatly contributes to the extent of superficial trauma and infections. Larger needle size can lead to a larger epithelial tear and greater disruption of dermal structures, with subsequent capillary leakage, edema, inflammation and sometimes infections [9].

Infection and abscess formation are rare complication of collagen fillers and can occur early on or can be delayed for several weeks to months after injection [231]. Early infections could be prevented by cleaning the treatment area with an antiseptic agent (e.g., isopropyl alcohol, chlorhexidine) while late infections could be treated by broad-spectrum antibiotics or anti-viral prophylaxis [231]. Herpes was registered in 1 case on approximately 15,000 injections [168]. Abscess formation is also rare (4 out of 10,000 patients) and occurs between 7 days to 22 months after treatment and may persist for weeks and periodically recur for months [16].

The occurrence of complications is also dependent on the injection site. Sensitive areas, such as around the mouth or beneath a muscle, heighten the risks for unwanted side effects. A bluish discoloration is associated with vascular injury due to injection. Vascular interruption also heightens the risk for local necrosis. Skin necrosis from mechanical disruption or occlusion of the vascular supply can rarely occur (9 out of 100,000 patients) [16]. Iatrogenic blindness is a rare but possible risk caused by misplaced intravascular injection. The risk is correlated to the complex vascular anatomy of the face interconnecting the extracranial and intracranial vascular network [13]. This tragic complication occurs when the filler is wrongly injected in the ophthalmic artery. Nowadays, several precautions can be taken to avoid necrosis. When injecting, attention should be paid to avoiding arteries, to aspirate before injecting, to use low volumes of products over more sessions as opposed to using high volumes over one session and to use only products that are manufactured for more superficial placement [231]. Moreover, warm compresses, massage, and tapping on the area were revealed to facilitate vasodilation and blood flow [231].

Improper distribution of injected products can also lead to lumps and nodules post-injection, besides facial shape deformity and asymmetry [9]. Denton et al. reported that it is very important to massage the product immediately after placement to mold and smooth the contour [152]. In case of over-injected or under-injected areas, palpation and massage should be performed to evenly distribute the material [86].

Table 5. Collagen injection specifications (number, volume and time), adverse events recurrence (severe and non-severe) and other details from most recent clinical trials on musculoskeletal, gastro-intestinal, urinary, circulatory apparatus and others from 2000 to 2022.

Application	Product	Disease	Number (n)	Injection Specification Volume (mL)	Inj./Time (w)	Observation Time (Weeks)	Participants (n)	Adverse Events Severe	Adverse Events Mild	Ref.
Musculoskeletal apparatus	Augment	Non fused foot and ankle	1	3–6	1	36	14	0	36	[108]
			1	6–9	1	12	7	0	0	[110]
			1	1–9	1	52	26	0	0	[109] NCT00583375
			1	n. d.	1	52	132	75	27	[101], NCT01305356
		Arthritis	1	1–9	1	52	394	136	n. d.	[102], NCT00583375
	Cartifill	Knee cartilage	1	1	1	96	52	0	5	[139], NCT02539030
		Cartilage lesion	1	3	1	6	1	0	0	[138]
	CartiZol	Osteoarthritis	1	3	1	24	101	0	7	[140]
		Chondromalacia, osteoarthritis	1	n. d.	1	n. d.	n. d.	n. d.	n. d.	NCT02539095
	ChondroGrid	Osteoarthritis	3	2	0.5/w (2 w), 0.25/w (1 w)	24	70	0	3	[142]
			3	6		32	20	0	0	[112]
	Fibroquel	Osteoarthritis	3	1.5	1/w	24	n. d.	n. d.	n. d.	NCT04019782
			5	2	1/w	24	10	0	n. d.	[182]
	Linerase	Gingival recession	3	14	1.5/w	n. d.	18	0	0	[167]
	MD-Hip	Osteoarthritis	1	2	1	96	24	0	1	[131]
	MD-Knee, MD-Muscle	Osteoarthritis	10	n. d.	2/w (2 w), 1/w (6 we)	12	30	0	0	[133]
	MD-Lumbar, MD-Muscle, MD-Neural	Lumbar spine pain	5	20	2/w (2 w), 1/w (1 w)	6	73	0	0	[134]
	MD-Knee, MD-Matrix	Sprained knee	6	n. d.	2/w	3	10	0	0	[143]
	MD-Muscle or MD-Matrix	Piriformis syndrome	1–3	n. d.	n. d.	n. d.	28	0	0	[136]
	MD-Lumbar, MD-Ischial	Chronic pain due to arthrosis, myalgia	1	1	1	10	71	0	0	[132]
	MD-Lumbar, MD-Matrix	Back pain	10	n. d.	2/w (2 w), 1/w (6 w)	8	1	0	0	[135]
	MD-Lumbar, MD-Muscle, MD-Matrix	Lumbar joint block	9	n. d.	2/w (2 w), 1/w (5 w)	7	1	0	0	[135]
	MD-Muscle, MD-Neural	Muscle pain	1	1	1	10	53	0	0	[132]
	MD Shoulder	Calcific supraspinatus tendinitis	4	n. d.	1/w	6	10	0	0	[145]
	MD-Shoulder, MD-Muscle	Shoulders periarthritis	10	n. d.	2/w (2 w), 1/w (6 w)	8	22	0	0	[146]
	MD Muscle	Myofascial pain	2	2	1/w	2	18	0	9	[130], NCT03323567
	RegenSeal	Plantar fasciitis	n. d.	n. d.	n. d.	n	n. d.	n. d.	n. d.	NCT02539082
		Rotator cuff tears	1	1	1	48	62	0	0	[141]
	n. d.	Rotator cuff tears	4	8	1/w	72	1	0	0	[183]
	n. d.	Osteoarthritis	1	2	1	24	n. d.	n. d.	n. d.	NCT04998188
Gastro-intestinal apparatus	Atelocell	Vocal folds paralysis	1	0.5–1.3	1	12	155	0	0	[114]
			1	0.5–1.3	1	12	40	0	0	[113]
	Cymetra	Vocal folds paralysis	1	1	1	4	8	0	0	[203]
			1	n. d.	1	2	1	1	0	[173]
	Dermologen	Laryngoplasy	2	n. d.	0.7/w	4	1	1	0	[173]
	Permacol	Fecal incontinence	1	1.5	1	6	28	0	8	[204], NCT01528995
			n. d.	n. d.	n. d.	48	14	0	0	[155]
			1	n. d.	1	36	11	0	0	[157]
		Anal fistula	1	n. d.	1	48	28	0	7	[156]
			1	n. d.	1	12	1	0	0	[153]
		Rectovaginal fistula	1	n. d.	1	8	1	0	0	[154]
	Salvecoll-E	Anorectal fistula	1	2	1	48	70	0	0	[60]
	Zyderm	Laryngeal paralysis	1	0.2–0.5	1	24	7	0	1	[118]
	Zyplast	Laryngoplasy	1	n. d.	1	24	100	0	0	[116]

Table 5. *Cont.*

Application	Product	Disease	Number (n)	Injection Specification		Inj./Time (w)	Observation Time (Weeks)	Participants (n)	Adverse Events		Ref.
				Volume (mL)					Severe	Mild	
urinary system	Contigen	Sphincter incontinence	1–5	2–4		0.05/w	84	63	0	0	[188]
		Urethra hypermobility	1–4	14		1	172	58	0	0	[187]
		Neurogenic bladder dysfunction	1–4	n. d.		n. d.	192	20	0	0	[190]
	Linerase	Lichen sclerosus	6	27		2/week (2 w), 1/8 w	8	1	0	1	[165]
	n. d.	Retrograde ejaculation	2	6		1/year	96	1	0	0	[198]
	n. d.	Bilateral vesicoureteral reflux	1	2.5		1	144	1	1	0	[223]
	n. d.	Stress urinary incontinence	1–2	n. d.		0.25/w	36	40	0	1	[185]
	n. d.	Premature ovarian failure	1	n. d.		1	12	8	0	0	[212], NCT02644447
	n. d.	Erectile disfunction	n. d.	n. d.		n. c.	n. d.	n. d.	n. d	n. d.	NCT02745808
Circulatory system	Gelofusine	Blood volume	1	n. d.		1	n. d.	n. d.	n. d.	n. d.	NCT02808325
		Fluid retention	1	500		1	n. d.	n. d.	n. d.	n. d.	NCT04637308
		Severe sepsis	1	500		1	13	608	n. d.	n. d.	[127], NCT02715466
		Abdominal surgery	n. d.	n. d.		n. d	n. d.	n. d.	n. d.	n. d.	NCT01515397
		Blood volume	1	10 mg/k		1	n. d.	5	0	0	[230], NCT02631356
		Blood volume	1	1 L.		1	4 h	12	0	0	[214], NCT00868062
others	Fibroquel	COVID-19 due hyperinflammatory syndrome	10	15		14/w (3 days), 12/w (4 days)	12	45	0	33	[162], NCT04517162
			7	10.5		7/w	1	35	0	0	[161], NCT04517162
	Flowable Wound Matrix	Hand scar due to severe burns	1	3–6		1	24	8	0	0	[88]
	Helitene	Organ protection during ablation	1	10–30		1	12	3	0	0	[128]
	Linerase	Vitiligo	6	27		0.5/w	12	5	0	0	[164]
	MD Neural, MD Matrix, MD Muscle mix	Facial nerve palsy	16	13		2/w	8	21	0	8	[160], NCT04353908
	n. d.	Decompensated cirrhosis	n. d.	n. d.		n. d.	n	n. d.	n. d.	n. d.	NCT02786017
	n. d.	Brain injury	1	n. d.		1	n. d.	n. d.	n. d.	n. d.	NCT02767817
	n. d.	Ischemic cardiomyopathy	1	n. d.		1	48	50	1, heart failure	0	[226], NCT02635464

8. Regulation

Resorbable injectable soft tissue fillers can be classified as medical devices, medicinal products, or cosmetic products. Injectable formulations are defined as medical devices if their therapeutic effect comes from their intrinsic structure, because their physical, chemical, or mechanical effects are the primary mechanism of action for their therapeutic function. The addition of any cells or cell-stimulating therapeutics into the injectable medical device results in their classification as medicinal products and in the following of other regulations. Indeed, medicinal product regulations require a more thorough investigation of the biocompatibility and therapeutic effect before approval for clinical application. Although medicinal products would be more effective, the translational barriers and the time before patients can benefit from them strongly increase.

In the United States, resorbable injectable soft tissue fillers have long been classified as medical devices while in Europe, dermal fillers have been marketed as medical devices, medicinal products, or cosmetics until now. However, with the entry into force of the new Medical Device Regulation (MDR) 2017/745 on 26 May 2021, all fillers (both for cosmetic and for medical purposes) are classified as class III risk medical devices. This means that all injectable products must be CE certified by a notified body if marketed after 26 May 2020. Thus, manufacturers required documentation including a device master record (technical documentation) and product clinical evaluation in accordance with MEDDEV 2.7/1 as well as an appropriate quality management system according to the Medical Devices Directive (MDD) ISO 13485. As regards injectable soft tissue fillers for cosmetic purposes, because of the absence of an intended medical purpose, they do not require a clinical efficacy investigation, but they are subject to a clinical evaluation regarding safety. Additionally, for materials of animal origin, such as collagen, manufacturers have to comply also with Regulation EU 722/2012.

9. Concluding Remarks

Forerunner fillers were plagued by frequent unwanted side effects and serious complications (i.e., migration of injected filler, granulomatous inflammation, tissue necrosis, and hypersensitivity reactions). With the advancement of research, a new generation of fillers has been developed that have overcome some of the many existing earlier problems. The steps forward regarding safety and the refinement of injection techniques brought an exponential increase in and use of soft tissue filler products and procedures. This growth was fueled by the increased availability of new dermal filler products and by their improved safety profiles.

Injectable systems hold great promise in tissue engineering applications as they can potentially provide for an adequate temporal environment for the injured site regeneration, as well as delivering water soluble drugs, growth factors and cells for better outcomes. Thus, the injectable formulations must have both structural (i.e., filling role) and biological (i.e., pro-regenerative action) impermanent functions. In particular, the hydrogel should not only structurally support tissue regeneration but also stimulate its regeneration and be gradually digested and replaced by the newly synthetized tissue, resulting in a new functional tissue. The success of any injectable system is strongly determined by the framework the hydrogel provides. The 3D network should provide mechanical support compliant with the injured tissue, adequate pore size and interconnectivity to allow mass transport and regenerative processes, and eventually, must provide for the controlled release of bioactive molecules. In clinical setting, injectable materials hold the promise of being an effective minimally invasive treatment for mild-severe defects. The delivery of cells, bioactive factors, and support materials via an injectable system within the context of an endoscopic, arthroscopic, laparoscopic, or radiologically guided procedure is feasible and potentially successful. With the growing knowledge and technology in biomedical and materials sciences, the innovation of injectable biomaterials to fulfill unmet clinical needs is expected to thrive in the near future [14]. Indeed, a high number of bioactive injectable biomaterials have been developed and approved for clinical use.

Among them, multifunctional collagen products are effective in some clinical applications. However, there are some points to be clarified and obstacles to overcome in order to develop disease specific products. As the outcomes of research move toward clinical translation, the elucidation of the mechanisms of interactions between an injectable biomaterial and its surroundings is necessary to reach optimal material performance. However, the interaction between the host tissue and the material is unknown due to the lack of accurate and adequate in vivo evaluation. The scarcity of tools for the in vivo evaluation of injectable biomaterials has posed numerous difficulties in fully understanding injection consequences [14] but, nowadays, new advanced investigation techniques such as cone beam and micro computed X-ray tomography, immunohistochemistry, small-angle X-ray scattering, X-ray diffraction, and the more recent fluorescent labelling of abundant reactive entities, optical photothermal infrared microscopy and infrared atomic force microscopy, fluorescence lifetime imaging microscopy and Raman spectroscopy will allow us to overcome this issue and deeply understand the material's action mechanism over time [3]. These techniques will also allow us to tune the properties of injectable materials according to patient specific disease requirements and comorbidities in order to develop personalized therapies. Moreover, the deep in vivo investigation of the material-tissue interaction will allow us to overcome another important issue of injectable formulations, that is, the effectiveness of mass transport. Clinically available collagen injectables efficacy is hindered by the absence of nutrients necessary to support cell regenerative processes that could be responsible for delayed and deficient integration with the host tissue, especially in the case of large defect regions [68]. To overcome these limits, Alnojeidi et al. developed a new in situ cross-linkable injectable formulation of cross-linked bovine type I collagen, chondroitin sulfate and polyvinyl alcohol, that contains the optimum concertation of necessary amino acids, vitamins, and minerals required for cell growth and proliferation [68].

In addition, the high costs associated with the development and manufacture of medical-grade injectable biomaterials (i.e., basic and applied research on medical device design, raw material extraction, material properties assessment, sterile device production, package and storage condition assessment) or with the incorporation of therapeutic agents are another hindrance to be overcome [14]. Sensitivity analyses showed that surgery would be less costly and more successful than collagen injection if the postoperative length of hospital stay was reduced to 1 day or if the number of injections required to treat patients were more than two for treatment successes and more than four for treatment failures [186]. Endoscopic injection of collagen is effective in many cases, but its cost effectiveness depends on the number of re-injections required. In the treatment for vesicoureteral reflux single collagen injections were very effective and may effectively reduce health care management costs of about $7544 per renal unit (collagen injection cost: $1599, reimplantation cost: $9144) [239]. In the treatment of the stress urinary incontinence, collagen injection is more cost effective than surgery if one application resolves the problem [123]. Instead, surgery (i.e., artificial genitourinary sphincter placement) is more cost effective than collagen injection when more than three collagen injections are required (collagen injection cost: $4300–6021; artificial genitourinary sphincter placement $11,933–15,400) [123,240]. In the case of aesthetic surgery, fillers would be less costly than surgical rhytidectomy ($15,181) in cases of small facial area. In cases of large volume, the medical cost for surgery would be the lowest cost option among the other treatments over the course of several years [1].

Indeed, when developing a new injectable, materials factors such as product cost, scalability and maneuverability should be considered together with safety and quality profiles before proceeding with its pre-clinical and clinical evaluation. Many promising collagen-based materials have been designed and intensely investigated from the physical, chemical, mechanical, morphological and biological (both in vitro and in vivo) point of view but did not attain clinical translation. The consideration of the clinical potential of the material is nowadays mandatory to receive the regulation body approval besides expecting its clinical success [3]. This approach will reduce the tremendous discrepancy between the huge quantity of academic research and the number of products that have been clinically translated [3].

Therefore, much research still needs to be carried out before minimally invasive strategies equal or surpass in terms of effectiveness the currently performed surgical procedures. However, the complete replacement of time-consuming and costly surgeries with injections does not seem to be so far away. In fact, even more collagen-based products are demonstrating their effectiveness in one or more sessions and in various injured body structures. Furthermore, actual preclinical and clinical research is not only confirming their assessed efficacy, but it is improving both formulations and injection techniques, as well as testing them for new, challenging, unresolved diseases.

In achieving this ultimate goal, the collaboration and transparency between researchers, clinicians, patients and companies has proved to be the only constructive way to successfully develop innovative and functional products capable of truly improving human health and making such treatments viable on a large-scale, accessible to the majority of the population and offering patients a long-term quality of life.

Funding: This research received no external funding.

Institutional Review Board Statement: Not applicable.

Data Availability Statement: Not applicable.

Conflicts of Interest: The authors declare no conflict of interest.

References

1. Go, B.C.; Frost, A.S.; Friedman, O. Using Injectable Fillers for Midface Rejuvenation. *Plast. Aesthetic Res.* **2021**, *8*, 39. [CrossRef]
2. Solish, N.J. Assessment of Recovery Time for the Collagen Products Dermicol-P35 27G and 30G. *J. Am. Acad. Dermatol.* **2010**, *62*, 824–830. [CrossRef] [PubMed]
3. Øvrebø, Ø.; Perale, G.; Wojciechowski, J.P.; Echalier, C.; Jeffers, J.R.T.; Stevens, M.M.; Haugen, H.J.; Rossi, F. Design and Clinical Application of Injectable Hydrogels for Musculoskeletal Therapy. *Bioeng. Transl. Med.* **2022**, *7*, e10295. [CrossRef] [PubMed]
4. Kretlow, J.D.; Young, S.; Klouda, L.; Wong, M.; Mikos, A.G. Injectable Biomaterials for Regenerating Complex Craniofacial Tissues. *Adv. Mater.* **2009**, *21*, 3368–3393. [CrossRef] [PubMed]
5. Béduer, A.; Genta, M.; Kunz, N.; Verheyen, C.; Martins, M.; Brefie-Guth, J.; Braschler, T. Design of an Elastic Porous Injectable Biomaterial for Tissue Regeneration and Volume Retention. *Acta Biomater.* **2022**, *142*, 73–84. [CrossRef]
6. Eppley, B.L.; Dadvand, B. Injectable Soft-Tissue Fillers: Clinical Overview. *Plast. Reconstr. Surg.* **2006**, *118*, 98–106. [CrossRef]
7. Buck, D.W.; Alam, M.; Kim, J.Y.S. Injectable Fillers for Facial Rejuvenation: A Review. *J. Plast. Reconstr. Aesthetic Surg.* **2009**, *62*, 11–18. [CrossRef]
8. Requena, L.; Requena, C.; Christensen, L.; Zimmermann, U.S.; Kutzner, H.; Cerroni, L. Adverse Reactions to Injectable Soft Tissue Fillers. *J. Am. Acad. Dermatol.* **2011**, *64*, 1–34. [CrossRef]
9. Luebberding, S.; Alexiades-Armenakas, M. Safety of Dermal Fillers. *J. Drugs Dermatol.* **2012**, *11*, 1053–1058.
10. Cheng, L.; Sun, X.; Tang, M.; Jin, R.; Cui, W.; Zhang, Y.-G. An Update Review on Recent Skin Fillers. *Plast. Aesthetic Res.* **2016**, *3*, 92–99. [CrossRef]
11. Ginat, D.T.; Schatz, C.J. Imaging Features of Midface Injectable Fillers and Associated Complications. *Am. J. Neuroradiol.* **2013**, *34*, 1488–1495. [CrossRef]
12. Lemperle, G. Injectable Dermal Fillers—Resorbable or Permanent? In *Aesthetic Surgery of the Facial Mosaic*; Springer: Berlin/Heidelberg, Germany, 2007; pp. 650–664.
13. Oranges, C.M.; Brucato, D.; Schaefer, D.J.; Kalbermatten, D.F.; Harder, Y. Complications of Nonpermanent Facial Fillers: A Systematic Review. *Plast. Reconstr. Surg. Glob. Open* **2021**, *9*, e3851. [CrossRef] [PubMed]
14. Zhou, H.; Liang, C.; Wei, Z.; Bai, Y.; Bhaduri, S.B.; Webster, T.J.; Bian, L.; Yang, L. Injectable Biomaterials for Translational Medicine. *Mater. Today* **2019**, *28*, 81–97. [CrossRef]
15. Attenello, N.H.; Maas, C.S. Injectable Fillers: Review of Material and Properties. *Facial Plast. Surg.* **2015**, *31*, 29–34. [CrossRef]
16. Cockerham, K.; Hsu, V. Collagen-Based Dermal Fillers: Past, Present, Future. *Facial Plast. Surg.* **2009**, *25*, 106–113. [CrossRef]
17. Silvipriya, K.S.; Krishna Kumar, K.; Bhat, A.R.; Dinesh Kumar, B.; John, A.; Lakshmanan, P. Collagen: Animal Sources and Biomedical Application. *J. Appl. Pharm. Sci.* **2015**, *5*, 123–127. [CrossRef]
18. Avila Rodriguez, M.I.; Rodriguez Barroso, G.L.; Sanchez, M.L. Collagen: A Review on Its Sources and Potential Cosmetic Applications. *J. Cosmet. Dermatol.* **2018**, *17*, 20–26. [CrossRef] [PubMed]
19. Gallo, N.; Natali, M.L.; Sannino, A.; Salvatore, L. An Overview of the Use of Equine Collagen as Emerging Material for Biomedical Applications. *J. Funct. Biomater.* **2020**, *11*, 79. [CrossRef] [PubMed]

20. Salvatore, L.; Gallo, N.; Natali, M.L.; Terzi, A.; Sannino, A.; Madaghiele, M. Mimicking the Hierarchical Organization of Natural Collagen: Toward the Development of Ideal Scaffolding Material for Tissue Regeneration. *Front. Bioeng. Biotechnol.* **2021**, *9*, 644595. [CrossRef]

21. Sandri, M.; Tampieri, A.; Salvatore, L.; Sannino, A.; Ghiron, J.H.L.; Condorelli, G. Collagen Based Scaffold for Biomedical Applications. *J. Biotechnol.* **2010**, *150*, 29. [CrossRef]

22. Lee, C.H.; Singla, A.; Lee, Y. Biomedical Applications of Collagen. *Int. J. Pharm.* **2001**, *221*, 1–22. [CrossRef] [PubMed]

23. Dong, C.; Lv, Y. Application of Collagen Scaffold in Tissue Engineering: Recent Advances and New Perspectives. *Polymers* **2016**, *8*, 42. [CrossRef] [PubMed]

24. Chattopadhyay, S.; Raines, R.T. Review Collagen-Based Biomaterials for Wound Healing. *Biopolymers* **2014**, *101*, 821–833. [CrossRef] [PubMed]

25. Sorushanova, A.; Delgado, L.M.; Wu, Z.; Shologu, N.; Kshirsagar, A.; Raghunath, R.; Mullen, A.M.; Bayon, Y.; Pandit, A.; Raghunath, M.; et al. The Collagen Suprafamily: From Biosynthesis to Advanced Biomaterial Development. *Adv. Mater.* **2019**, *31*, e1801651. [CrossRef] [PubMed]

26. Gelse, K.; Pöschl, E.; Aigner, T. Collagens—Structure, Function, and Biosynthesis. *Adv. Drug Deliv. Rev.* **2003**, *55*, 1531–1546. [CrossRef] [PubMed]

27. Ricard-Blum, S. The Collagen Family. *Cold Spring Harb. Perspect. Biol.* **2011**, *3*, a004978. [CrossRef] [PubMed]

28. Parvizi, J.; Kim, G.K. Collagen. In *High Yield Orthopaedics*; Elsevier: Amsterdam, The Netherlands, 2010; pp. 107–109.

29. Goldberga, I.; Li, R.; Duer, M.J. Collagen Structure–Function Relationships from Solid-State NMR Spectroscopy. *Acc. Chem. Res.* **2018**, *51*, 1621–1629. [CrossRef] [PubMed]

30. Owczarzy, A.; Kurasinski, R.; Kulig, K.; Rogoz, W.; Szkudlarek, A.; Maciazek-Juczyk, M. Collagen—Stucture, Properties and Applications. *Eng. Biomater.* **2020**, *156*, 17–23.

31. Arseni, L.; Lombardi, A.; Orioli, D. From Structure to Phenotype: Impact of Collagen Alterations on Human Health. *Int. J. Mol. Sci.* **2018**, *19*, 1407. [CrossRef]

32. Wang, H. A Review of the Effects of Collagen Treatment in Clinical Studies. *Polymers* **2021**, *13*, 3868. [CrossRef]

33. Meyer, M. Processing of Collagen Based Biomaterials and the Resulting Materials Properties. *Biomed. Eng. Online* **2019**, *18*, 1–74. [CrossRef]

34. Shoulder, M.D.; Raines, R.T. Collagen Structure and Stability. *Annu. Rev. Biochem.* **2009**, *78*, 929–958. [CrossRef]

35. Amirrah, I.N.; Lokanathan, Y.; Zulkiflee, I.; Wee, M.F.M.R.; Motta, A.; Fauzi, M.B. A Comprehensive Review on Collagen Type I Development of Biomaterials for Tissue Engineering: From Biosynthesis to Bioscaffold. *Biomedicines* **2022**, *10*, 2307. [CrossRef] [PubMed]

36. Birk, D.E.; Brückner, P. Collagens, Suprastructures, and Collagen Fibril Assembly. In *The Extracellular Matrix: An Overview*; Springer: Berlin/Heidelberg, Germany, 2011; pp. 77–115.

37. Salvatore, L.; Gallo, N.; Aiello, D.; Lunetti, P.; Barca, A.; Blasi, L.; Madaghiele, M.; Bettini, S.; Giancane, G.; Hasan, M.; et al. An Insight on Type I Collagen from Horse Tendon for the Manufacture of Implantable Devices. *Int. J. Biol. Macromol.* **2020**, *154*, 291–306. [CrossRef] [PubMed]

38. Ignat'eva, N.Y.; Danilov, N.A.; Averkiev, S.V.; Obrezkova, M.V.; Lunin, V.V.; Sobol, E.N. Determination of Hydroxyproline in Tissues and the Evaluation of the Collagen Content of the Tissues. *J. Anal. Chem.* **2007**, *62*, 51–57. [CrossRef]

39. Bou-Gharios, G.; Abraham, D.; de Crombrugghe, B. Type I Collagen Structure, Synthesis, and Regulation. In *Principles of Bone Biology*; Elsevier: Amsterdam, The Netherlands, 2020; pp. 295–337.

40. Kadler, K.E.; Holmes, D.F.; Trotter, J.A.; Chapman, J.A. Collagen Fibril Formation. *Biochem. J.* **1996**, *316*, 1–11. [CrossRef] [PubMed]

41. Collins, C.J.; Andriotis, O.G.; Nedelkovski, V.; Frank, M.; Katsamenis, O.L.; Thurner, P.J. Bone Micro- and Nanomechanics. In *Encyclopedia of Biomedical Engineering*; Elsevier: Amsterdam, The Netherlands, 2019; pp. 22–44.

42. Terzi, A.; Gallo, N.; Bettini, S.; Sibillano, T.; Altamura, D.; Madaghiele, M.; de Caro, L.; Valli, L.; Salvatore, L.; Sannino, A.; et al. Sub- and Supramolecular X-Ray Characterization of Engineered Tissues from Equine Tendon, Bovine Dermis and Fish Skin Type-I Collagen. *Macromol. Biosci.* **2020**, *20*, 2000017. [CrossRef] [PubMed]

43. Terzi, A.; Gallo, N.; Bettini, S.; Sibillano, T.; Altamura, D.; Campa, L.; Natali, M.L.; Salvatore, L.; Madaghiele, M.; de Caro, L.; et al. Investigations of Processing–Induced Structural Changes in Horse Type-I Collagen at Sub and Supramolecular Levels. *Front. Bioeng. Biotechnol.* **2019**, *7*, 203. [CrossRef] [PubMed]

44. von der Mark, K. Structure, Biosynthesis and Gene Regulation of Collagens in Cartilage and Bone. In *Dynamics of Bone and Cartilage Metabolism*; Elsevier: Amsterdam, The Netherlands, 2006; pp. 3–40.

45. Exposito, J.-Y.; Cluzel, C.; Garrone, R.; Lethias, C. Evolution of Collagens. *Anat. Rec.* **2002**, *268*, 302–316. [CrossRef]

46. Chu, M.-L.; de Wet, W.; Bernard, M.; Ding, J.-F.; Morabito, M.; Myers, J.; Williams, C.; Ramirez, F. Human Proα1(I) Collagen Gene Structure Reveals Evolutionary Conservation of a Pattern of Introns and Exons. *Nature* **1984**, *310*, 337–340. [CrossRef]

47. Fidler, A.L.; Boudko, S.P.; Rokas, A.; Hudson, B.G. The Triple Helix of Collagens—An Ancient Protein Structure That Enabled Animal Multicellularity and Tissue Evolution. *J. Cell Sci.* **2018**, *131*, jcs203950. [CrossRef] [PubMed]

48. Exposito, J.-Y.; Valcourt, U.; Cluzel, C.; Lethias, C. The Fibrillar Collagen Family. *Int. J. Mol. Sci.* **2010**, *11*, 407–426. [CrossRef]

49. Madaghiele, M.; Salvatore, L.; Sannino, A. *Tailoring the Pore Structure of Foam Scaffolds for Nerve Regeneration*; Woodhead Publishing Limited: Sawston, UK, 2014; ISBN 9780857096968.

50. Salvatore, L.; Madaghiele, M.; Parisi, C.; Gatti, F.; Sannino, A. Crosslinking of Micropatterned Collagen-Based Nerve Guides to Modulate the Expected Half-Life. *J. Biomed. Mater. Res. A* **2014**, *102*, 4406–4414. [CrossRef] [PubMed]
51. Madaghiele, M.; Calò, E.; Salvatore, L.; Bonfrate, V.; Pedone, D.; Frigione, M.; Sannino, A. Assessment of Collagen Crosslinking and Denaturation for the Design of Regenerative Scaffolds. *J. Biomed. Mater. Res. A* **2016**, *104*, 186–194. [CrossRef] [PubMed]
52. Salvatore, L.; Calò, E.; Bonfrate, V.; Pedone, D.; Gallo, N.; Natali, M.L.; Sannino, A.; Madaghiele, M. Exploring the Effects of the Crosslink Density on the Physicochemical Properties of Collagen-Based Scaffolds. *Polym. Test.* **2021**, *93*, 106966. [CrossRef]
53. Parisi, C.; Salvatore, L.; Veschini, L.; Serra, M.P.; Hobbs, C.; Madaghiele, M.; Sannino, A.; di Silvio, L. Biomimetic Gradient Scaffold of Collagen–Hydroxyapatite for Osteochondral Regeneration. *J. Tissue Eng.* **2020**, *11*, 2041731419896068. [CrossRef]
54. Terzi, A.; Storelli, E.; Bettini, S.; Sibillano, T.; Altamura, D.; Salvatore, L.; Madaghiele, M.; Romano, A.; Siliqi, D.; Ladisa, M.; et al. Effects of Processing on Structural, Mechanical and Biological Properties of Collagen-Based Substrates for Regenerative Medicine. *Sci. Rep.* **2018**, *8*, 1429. [CrossRef]
55. Gallo, N.; Natali, M.L.; Curci, C.; Picerno, A.; Gallone, A.; Vulpi, M.; Vitarelli, A.; Ditonno, P.; Cascione, M.; Sallustio, F.; et al. Analysis of the Physico-Chemical, Mechanical and Biological Properties of Crosslinked Type-I Collagen from Horse Tendon: Towards the Development of Ideal Scaffolding Material for Urethral Regeneration. *Materials* **2021**, *14*, 7648. [CrossRef]
56. Yañez-Mó, M.; Barreiro, O.; Gonzalo, P.; Batista, A.; Megías, D.; Genís, L.; Sachs, N.; Sala-Valdés, M.; Alonso, M.A.; Montoya, M.C.; et al. MT1-MMP Collagenolytic Activity Is Regulated through Association with Tetraspanin CD151 in Primary Endothelial Cells. *Blood* **2008**, *112*, 3217–3226. [CrossRef]
57. Kwansa, A.L.; de Vita, R.; Freeman, J.W. Mechanical Recruitment of N- and C-Crosslinks in Collagen Type I. *Matrix Biol.* **2014**, *34*, 161–169. [CrossRef]
58. Adhikari, A.S.; Chai, J.; Dunn, A.R. Mechanical Load Induces a 100-Fold Increase in the Rate of Collagen Proteolysis by MMP-1. *J. Am. Chem. Soc.* **2011**, *133*, 1686–1689. [CrossRef] [PubMed]
59. Adhikari, A.S.; Glassey, E.; Dunn, A.R. Conformational Dynamics Accompanying the Proteolytic Degradation of Trimeric Collagen I by Collagenases. *J. Am. Chem. Soc.* **2012**, *134*, 13259–13265. [CrossRef] [PubMed]
60. Maternini, M.; Guttadauro, A.; Mascagni, D.; Milito, G.; Stuto, A.; Renzi, A.; Ripamonti, L.; Bottini, C.; Nudo, R.; del Re, L.; et al. Non Cross-Linked Equine Collagen (Salvecoll-E Gel) for Treatment of Complex Ano-Rectal Fistula. *Asian J. Surg.* **2019**, *43*, 401–404. [CrossRef] [PubMed]
61. Sandor, M.; Xu, H.; Connor, J.; Lombardi, J.; Harper, J.R.; Silverman, R.P.; McQuillan, D.J. Host Response to Implanted Porcine-Derived Biologic Materials in a Primate Model of Abdominal Wall Repair. *Tissue Eng. Part A* **2008**, *14*, 2021–2031. [CrossRef] [PubMed]
62. Bohn, G.; Liden, B.; Schultz, G.; Yang, Q.; Gibson, D.J. Ovine-Based Collagen Matrix Dressing: Next-Generation Collagen Dressing for Wound Care. *Adv. Wound Care* **2016**, *5*, 1–10. [CrossRef] [PubMed]
63. Neuber, F. Fettransplantation bericht uber die verhandlungen der deutscht gesellsch chir. *Zentralbl. Chir.* **1893**, *22*, 66.
64. Kontis, T.; Rivkin, A. The History of Injectable Facial Fillers. *Facial Plast. Surg.* **2009**, *25*, 067–072. [CrossRef]
65. Cespedes, R.D. Collagen Injection or Artificial Sphincter for Postprostatectomy Incontinence: Collagen. *Urology* **2000**, *55*, 5–7. [CrossRef]
66. Cho, K.-H.; Uthaman, S.; Park, I.-K.; Cho, C.-S. Injectable Biomaterials in Plastic and Reconstructive Surgery: A Review of the Current Status. *Tissue Eng. Regen. Med.* **2018**, *15*, 559–574. [CrossRef]
67. Inglefield, C.; Samuelson, E.U.; Landau, M.; DeVore, D. Bio-Dermal Restoration With Rapidly Polymerizing Collagen: A Multicenter Clinical Study. *Aesthetic Surg. J.* **2018**, *38*, 1131–1138. [CrossRef]
68. Alnojeidi, H.; Kilani, R.T.; Ghahary, A. Evaluating the Biocompatibility of an Injectable Wound Matrix in a Murine Model. *Gels* **2022**, *8*, 49. [CrossRef] [PubMed]
69. Camilleri-Brennan, J. Anal Injectables and Implantables for Faecal Incontinence. In *Fecal Incontinence—Causes, Management and Outcome*; InTech: Vienna, Austria, 2014.
70. Thomas, K.; Engler, A.J.; Meyer, G.A. Extracellular Matrix Regulation in the Muscle Satellite Cell Niche. *Connect. Tissue Res.* **2015**, *56*, 1–8. [CrossRef] [PubMed]
71. Lynn, A.K.; Yannas, I.V.; Bonfield, W. Antigenicity and Immunogenicity of Collagen. *J. Biomed. Mater. Res. B Appl. Biomater.* **2004**, *71*, 343–354. [CrossRef] [PubMed]
72. Ellingsworth, L.R.; de Lustro, F.; Brennan, J.E.; Sawamura, S.; Mc Pherson, J. The Human Immune Response to Reconstituted Bovine Collagen. *J. Immunol.* **1986**, *136*, 877–882. [CrossRef]
73. Charriere, G.; Bejot, M.; Schnitzler, L.; Ville, G.; Hartmann, D.J. Reactions to a Bovine Collagen Implant: Clinical and Immunologic Study in 705 Patients. *J. Am. Acad. Dermatol.* **1989**, *21*, 1203–1208. [CrossRef]
74. Aamodt, J.M.; Grainger, D.W. Extracellular Matrix-Based Biomaterial Scaffolds and the Host Response. *Biomaterials* **2016**, *86*, 68–82. [CrossRef]
75. Lemperle, G.; Morhenn, V.; Charrier, U. Human Histology and Persistence of Various Injectable Filler Substances for Soft Tissue Augmentation. *Aesthetic Plast. Surg.* **2003**, *27*, 354–366. [CrossRef]
76. Narins, R.S.; Brandt, F.; Leyden, J.; Lorenc, Z.P.; Rubin, M.; Smith, S. A Randomized, Double-Blind, Multicenter Comparison of the Efficacy and Tolerability of Restylane versus Zyplast for the Correction of Nasolabial Folds. *Dermatol. Surg.* **2003**, *29*, 588–595. [CrossRef]

77. Solomon, P.; Sklar, M.; Zener, R. Facial Soft Tissue Augmentation with Artecoll®: A Review of Eight Years of Clinical Experience in 153 Patients. *Can. J. Plast. Surg.* **2012**, *20*, 28–32. [CrossRef]
78. Lemperle, G.; Romani, J.J.; Busso, M. Soft Tissue Augmentation With Artecoll: 10-Year History, Indications, Techniques, and Complications. *Dermatol. Surg.* **2003**, *29*, 573–587. [CrossRef]
79. Cohen, S.R.; Holmes, R.E. Artecoll: A Long-Lasting Injectable Wrinkle Filler Material: Report of a Controlled, Randomized, Multicenter Clinical Trial of 251 Subjects. *Plast. Reconstr. Surg.* **2004**, *114*, 964–976. [CrossRef] [PubMed]
80. Haneke, E. Polymethyl Methacrylate Microspheres in Collagen. *Semin. Cutan. Med. Surg.* **2004**, *23*, 227–232. [CrossRef]
81. Kim, K.J.; Lee, H.W.; Lee, M.W.; Choi, J.H.; Moon, K.C.; Koh, J.K. Artecoll Granuloma: A Rare Adverse Reaction Induced by Microimplant in the Treatment of Neck Wrinkles. *Dermatol. Surg.* **2004**, *30*, 545–547. [CrossRef] [PubMed]
82. Rullan, P.P. Soft Tissue Augmentation Using Artecoll: A Personal Experience. *Facial Plast. Surg.* **2004**, *20*, 111–116. [CrossRef] [PubMed]
83. Thaler, M.P.; Ubogy, Z.I. Artecoll: The Arizona Experience and Lessons Learned. *Dermatol. Surg.* **2005**, *31*, 1566–1576. [CrossRef] [PubMed]
84. Solomon, P.; Ng, C.L.; Kerzner, J.; Rival, R. Facial Soft Tissue Augmentation with Bellafill: A Review of 4 Years of Clinical Experience in 212 Patients. *Plast. Surg.* **2021**, *29*, 98–102. [CrossRef] [PubMed]
85. Cohen, S.R.; Berner, C.F.; Busso, M.; Gleason, M.C.; Hamilton, D.; Holmes, R.E.; Romano, J.J.; Rullan, P.P.; Thaler, M.P.; Ubogy, Z.; et al. ArteFill: A Long-Lasting Injectable Wrinkle Filler Material—Summary of the U.S. Food and Drug Administration Trials and a Progress Report on 4- to 5-Year Outcomes. *Plast. Reconstr. Surg.* **2006**, *118*, 64–76. [CrossRef]
86. Moon, S.H.; Lee, Y.J.; Rhie, J.W.; Suh, D.S.; Oh, D.Y.; Lee, J.H.; Kim, Y.J.; Kim, S.M.; Jun, Y.J. Comparative Study of the Effectiveness and Safety of Porcine and Bovine Atelocollagen in Asian Nasolabial Fold Correction. *J. Plast. Surg. Hand Surg.* **2015**, *49*, 147–152. [CrossRef]
87. Lee, J.H.; Choi, Y.S.; Kim, S.M.; Kim, Y.J.; Rhie, J.W.; Jun, Y.J. Efficacy and Safety of Porcine Collagen Filler for Nasolabial Fold Correction in Asians: A Prospective Multicenter, 12 Months Follow-up Study. *J. Korean Med. Sci.* **2014**, *29*, S217–S221. [CrossRef] [PubMed]
88. Hirche, C.; Senghaas, A.; Fischer, S.; Hollenbeck, S.T.; Kremer, T.; Kneser, U. Novel Use of a Flowable Collagen-Glycosaminoglycan Matrix (Integra™ Flowable Wound Matrix) Combined with Percutaneous Cannula Scar Tissue Release in Treatment of Post-Burn Malfunction of the Hand—A Preliminary 6 Month Follow-Up. *Burns* **2016**, *42*, e1–e7. [CrossRef]
89. Kligman, A.M.; Armstrong, R.C. Histologic Respose to Intradermal Zyderm and Zyplast (Glutaraldehyde Cross-Linked) Collagen in Humans. *J. Dermatol. Surg. Oncol.* **1986**, *12*, 351–357. [CrossRef]
90. Stegman, S.J.; Chu, S.; Bensch, K.; Armstrong, R. A Light and Electron Microscopic Evaluation of Zyderm Collagen and Zyplast Implants in Aging Human Facial Skin: A Pilot Study. *Arch. Dermatol.* **1987**, *123*, 1644–1649. [CrossRef]
91. Elson, M.L. Clinical Assessment of Zyplast Implant: A Year of Experience for Soft Tissue Contour Correction. *J. Am. Acad. Dermatol.* **1988**, *18*, 707–713. [CrossRef]
92. Matti, B.A.; Nicolle, F.v. Clinical Use of Zyplast in Correction of Age- and Disease-Related Contour Deficiencies of the Face. *Aesthetic Plast. Surg.* **1990**, *14*, 227–234. [CrossRef]
93. Cooperman, L.S.; Mackinnon, V.; Bechler, G.; Pharriss, B.B. Injectable Collagen: A Six-Year Clinical Investigation. *Aesthetic Plast. Surg.* **1985**, *9*, 145–151. [CrossRef]
94. Castrow, F.F.; Krull, E.A. Injectable Collagen Implant—Update. *J. Am. Acad. Dermatol.* **1983**, *9*, 889–893. [CrossRef]
95. Downie, J.; Mao, Z.; Rachel Lo, T.W.; Barry, S.; Bock, M.; Siebert, J.P.; Bowman, A.; Ayoub, A. A Double-Blind, Clinical Evaluation of Facial Augmentation Treatments: A Comparison of PRI 1, PRI 2, Zyplast® and Perlane®. *J. Plast. Reconstr. Aesthetic Surg.* **2009**, *62*, 1636–1643. [CrossRef]
96. Baumann, L.S.; Shamban, A.T.; Lupo, M.P.; Monheit, G.D.; Thomas, J.A.; Murphy, D.K.; Walker, P.S. Comparison of Smooth-Gel Hyaluronic Acid Dermal Fillers with Cross-Linked Bovine Collagen: A Multicenter, Double-Masked, Randomized, within-Subject Study. *Dermatol. Surg.* **2007**, *33*, 128–135. [CrossRef]
97. Nevins, M.; Giannobile, W.V.; McGuire, M.K.; Kao, R.T.; Mellonig, J.T.; Hinrichs, J.E.; McAllister, B.S.; Murphy, K.S.; McClain, P.K.; Nevins, M.L.; et al. Platelet-Derived Growth Factor Stimulates Bone Fill and Rate of Attachment Level Gain: Results of a Large Multicenter Randomized Controlled Trial. *J. Periodontol.* **2005**, *76*, 2205–2215. [CrossRef]
98. Nevins, A.; Crespi, P. A Clinical Study Using the Collagen Gel Zyplast in Endodontic Treatment. *J. Endod.* **1998**, *24*, 610–613. [CrossRef]
99. Gadomski, B.C.; Labus, K.M.; Puttlitz, C.M.; McGilvray, K.C.; Regan, D.P.; Nelson, B.; Seim, H.B.; Easley, J.T. Evaluation of Lumbar Spinal Fusion Utilizing Recombinant Human Platelet Derived Growth Factor-B Chain Homodimer (RhPDGF-BB) Combined with a Bovine Collagen/β-Tricalcium Phosphate (β-TCP) Matrix in an Ovine Model. *JOR Spine* **2021**, *4*, e1166. [CrossRef]
100. Scott, R.T.; McAlister, J.E.; Rigby, R.B. Allograft Bone: What Is the Role of Platelet-Derived Growth Factor in Hindfoot and Ankle Fusions. *Clin. Podiatr. Med. Surg.* **2018**, *35*, 37–52. [CrossRef]
101. Daniels, T.R.; Anderson, J.; Swords, M.P.; Maislin, G.; Donahue, R.; Pinsker, E.; Quiton, J.D. Recombinant Human Platelet–Derived Growth Factor BB in Combination with a Beta-Tricalcium Phosphate (RhPDGF-BB/β-TCP)-Collagen Matrix as an Alternative to Autograft. *Foot Ankle Int.* **2019**, *40*, 1068–1078. [CrossRef]

102. DiGiovanni, C.W.; Lin, S.S.; Baumhauer, J.F.; Daniels, T.; Younger, A.; Glazebrook, M.; Anderson, J.; Anderson, R.; Evangelista, P.; Lynch, S.E.; et al. Recombinant Human Platelet-Derived Growth Factor-BB and Beta-Tricalcium Phosphate (RhPDGF-BB/β-TCP): An Alternative to Autogenous Bone Graft. *J. Bone Jt. Surg.* **2013**, *95*, 1184–1192. [CrossRef]
103. Daniels, T.; DiGiovanni, C.; Lau, J.T.C.; Wing, K.; Alastair, Y. Prospective Clinical Pilot Trial in a Single Cohort Group of RhPDGF in Foot Arthrodeses. *Foot Ankle Int.* **2010**, *31*, 473–479. [CrossRef]
104. Abidi, N.A.; Younger, A.; Digiovanni, C.W. Role of Platelet-Derived Growth Factor in Hindfoot Fusion. *Tech. Foot Ankle Surg.* **2012**, *11*, 34–38.
105. Hollinger, J.O.; Hart, C.E.; Hirsch, S.N.; Lynch, S.; Friedlaender, G.E. Recombinant Human Platelet-Derived Growth Factor: Biology and Clinical Applications. *J. Bone Jt. Surg.* **2008**, *90*, 48–54. [CrossRef]
106. DiGiovanni, C.W.; Petricek, J.M. The Evolution of RhPDGF-BB in Musculoskeletal Repair and Its Role in Foot and Ankle Fusion Surgery. *Foot Ankle Clin.* **2010**, *15*, 621–640. [CrossRef]
107. Digiovanni, C.W.; Lin, S.; Pinzur, M. Recombinant Human PDGF-BB in Foot and Ankle Fusion. *Expert Rev. Med. Devices* **2012**, *9*, 111–122. [CrossRef]
108. DiGiovanni, C.W.; Baumhauer, J.; Lin, S.S.; Berberian, W.S.; Flemister, A.S.; Enna, M.J.; Evangelista, P.; Newman, J. Prospective, Randomized, Multi-Center Feasibility Trial of RhPDGF-BB versus Autologous Bone Graft in a Foot and Ankle Fusion Model. *Foot Ankle Int.* **2011**, *32*, 344–354. [CrossRef]
109. DiGiovanni, C.W.; Lin, S.S.; Daniels, T.R.; Glazebrook, M.; Evangelista, P.; Donahue, R.; Beasley, W.; Baumhauer, J.F. The Importance of Sufficient Graft Material in Achieving Foot or Ankle Fusion. *J. Bone Jt. Surg. Am. Vol.* **2016**, *98*, 1260–1267. [CrossRef]
110. Solchaga, L.A.; Daniels, T.; Roach, S.; Beasley, W.; Snel, L.B. Effect of Implantation of Augment® Bone Graft on Serum Concentrations of Platelet-Derived Growth Factors: A Pharmacokinetic Study. *Clin. Drug Investig.* **2013**, *33*, 143–149. [CrossRef]
111. Perrien, D.S.; Young, C.S.; Alvarez-Urena, P.P.; Dean, D.D.; Lynch, S.E.; Hollinger, J.O. Percutaneous Injection of Augment Injectable Bone Graft (RhPDGF-BB and β-Tricalcium Phosphate [β-TCP]/Bovine Type i Collagen Matrix) Increases Vertebral Bone Mineral Density in Geriatric Female Baboons. *Spine J.* **2013**, *13*, 580–586. [CrossRef]
112. de Luca, P.; Colombini, A.; Carimati, G.; Beggio, M.; de Girolamo, L.; Volpi, P. Intra-Articular Injection of Hydrolyzed Collagen to Treat Symptoms of Knee Osteoarthritis. A Functional in Vitro Investigation and a Pilot Retrospective Clinical Study. *J. Clin. Med.* **2019**, *8*, 975. [CrossRef]
113. Kimura, M.; Nito, T.; Imagawa, H.; Tayama, N.; Chan, R.W. Collagen Injection as a Supplement to Arytenoid Adduction for Vocal Fold Paralysis. *Ann. Otol. Rhinol. Laryngol.* **2008**, *117*, 430–436. [CrossRef]
114. Kimura, M.; Nito, T.; Sakakibara, K.I.; Tayama, N.; Niimi, S. Clinical Experience with Collagen Injection of the Vocal Fold: A Study of 155 Patients. *Auris Nasus Larynx* **2008**, *35*, 67–75. [CrossRef]
115. Stojkovic, S.G.; Lim, M.; Burke, D.; Finan, P.J.; Sagar, P.M. Intra-Anal Collagen Injection for the Treatment of Faecal Incontinence. *Br. J. Surg.* **2006**, *93*, 1514–1518. [CrossRef]
116. Jamal, N.; Mundi, J.; Chhetri, D.K. Higher Risk of Superficial Injection during Injection Laryngoplasty in Women. *Am. J. Otolaryngol.* **2014**, *35*, 159–163. [CrossRef]
117. Ford, C.N.; Bless, D.M.; Loftus, J.M. Role of Injectable Collagen in the Treatment of Glottic Insufficiency: A Study of 119 Patients. *Ann. Otol. Rhinol. Laryngol.* **1992**, *101*, 237–247. [CrossRef]
118. Hoffman, H.; McCabe, D.; McCulloch, T.; Jin, S.M.; Karnell, M. Laryngeal Collagen Injection as an Adjunct to Medialization Laryngoplasty. *Laryngoscope* **2002**, *112*, 1407–1413. [CrossRef]
119. Luu, Q.; Tsai, V.; Mangunta, V.; Berke, G.S.; Chhetri, D.K. Safety of Percutaneous Injection of Bovine Dermal Crosslinked Collagen for Glottic Insufficiency. *Otolaryngol. Head Neck Surg.* **2007**, *136*, 445–449. [CrossRef] [PubMed]
120. Kamer, F.M.; Churukian, M.M. Clinical Use of Injectable Collagen. *Arch. Otolaryngol.* **1984**, *110*, 93–98. [CrossRef] [PubMed]
121. Homma, Y.; Kawabe, K.; Kageyama, S.; Koiso, K.; Akaza, H.; Kakizoe, T.; Koshiba, K.; Yokoyama, E.; Aso, Y. Injection of Glutaraldehyde Cross-Linked Collagen for Urinary Incontinence: Two-Year Efficacy by Self-Assessment. *Int. J. Urol.* **1996**, *3*, 124–127. [CrossRef] [PubMed]
122. Elsergany, R.; Elgamasy, A.N.; Ghoniem, G.M. Transurethral Collagen Injection for Female Stress Incontinence. *Int. Urogynecol. J.* **1998**, *9*, 13–18. [CrossRef] [PubMed]
123. Cespedes, R.D.; Leng, W.W.; McGuire, E.J. Collagen Injection Therapy for Postprostatectomy Incontinence. *Urology* **1999**, *54*, 597–602. [CrossRef]
124. Corcos, J.; Fournier, C. Periurethral Collagen Injection for the Treatment of Female Stress Urinary Incontinence: 4-Year Follow-up Results. *Urology* **1999**, *54*, 815–818. [CrossRef]
125. Gorton, E.; Stanton, S.; Monga, A.; Wiskind, A.K.; Lentz, G.M.; Bland, D.R. Periurethral Collagen Injection: A Long-Term Follow-up Study. *BJU Int.* **1999**, *84*, 966–971. [CrossRef]
126. Vandenbulcke, L.; Lapage, K.G.; Vanderstraeten, K.V.; de Somer, F.M.; de Hert, S.G.; Moerman, A.T. Microvascular Reactivity Monitored with Near-Infrared Spectroscopy Is Impaired after Induction of Anaesthesia in Cardiac Surgery Patients. *Eur. J. Anaesthesiol.* **2017**, *34*, 688–694. [CrossRef]

127. Marx, G.; Zacharowski, K.; Ichai, C.; Asehnoune, K.; Černý, V.; Dembinski, R.; Ferrer Roca, R.; Fries, D.; Molnar, Z.; Rosenberger, P.; et al. Efficacy and Safety of Early Target-Controlled Plasma Volume Replacement with a Balanced Gelatine Solution versus a Balanced Electrolyte Solution in Patients with Severe Sepsis/Septic Shock: Study Protocol, Design, and Rationale of a Prospective, Randomized, Controlled, Double-Blind, Multicentric, International Clinical Trial: GENIUS—Gelatine Use in ICU and Sepsis. *Trials* **2021**, *22*, 1–12. [CrossRef]
128. Hamraoui, K.; Ernst, S.M.P.G.; van Dessel, P.F.H.M.; Kelder, J.C.; ten Berg, J.M.; Suttorp, J.; Jaarsma, W.; Plokker, H.W. Efficacy and Safety of Percutaneous Treatment of Iatrogenic Femoral Artery Pseudoaneurysm by Biodegradable Collagen Injection. *J. Am. Coll. Cardiol.* **2002**, *39*, 1297–1304. [CrossRef]
129. Majdalany, B.S.; Willatt, J.; Beecham Chick, J.F.; Srinivasa, R.N.; Saad, W.A. Fibrillar Collagen Injection for Organ Protection during Thermal Ablation of Hepatic Malignancies. *Diagn. Interv. Radiol.* **2017**, *23*, 381–384. [CrossRef]
130. Nitecka-Buchta, A.; Walczynska-Dragon, K.; Batko-Kapustecka, J.; Wieckiewicz, M. Comparison between Collagen and Lidocaine Intramuscular Injections in Terms of Their Efficiency in Decreasing Myofascial Pain within Masseter Muscles: A Randomized, Single-Blind Controlled Trial. *Pain Res. Manag.* **2018**, *2018*, 8261090. [CrossRef] [PubMed]
131. Giovannangeli, F.; Bizzi, E.; Massafra, U.; Vacca, F.; Tormenta, S.; Migliore, A. Intra-Articular Administration of MD-HIP in 24 Patients Affected by Symptomatic Hip Osteoarthritis—A 24-Month Cohort Study. *Physiol. Regul. Med.* **2016**, 31–32.
132. Guitart Vela, J.; Folch Ibanez, J. Collagen MDs for Chronic Pain. Efficacy and Tolerability in Chronic Treatment in 124 Patients. *Physiol. Regul. Med.* **2016**, 9–12.
133. Reshkova, V.; Rashkov, R.; Nestorova, R. Efficacy and Safety Evaluation of GUNA Collagen MDs Injections in Knee Osteoarthritis—A Case Series of 30 Patients. *Physiol. Regul. Med.* **2016**, 27–29.
134. Pavelka, K.; Jarosova, H.; Milani, L.; Prochazka, Z.; Kostiuk, P.; Kotlarova, L.; Meroni, A.M.; Slíva, J. Efficacy and Tolerability of Injectable Collagen-Containing Products in Comparison to Trimecaine in Patients with Acute Lumbar Spine Pain (Study FUTURE-MD-Back Pain). *Physiol. Res.* **2019**, *68*, s65–s74. [CrossRef]
135. Massulo, C. Injectable GUNA Collagen Medical Devices in Functional Recovery from Sport. *Physiol. Regul. Med.* **2016**, 3–7.
136. Staňa, J. 3 Years in Luhačovice Spa with Collagen Medical Devices Injections in the Treatment of Piriformis Syndrome. *Physiol. Regul. Med.* **2016**, 19–20.
137. Alfieri, N. MD-Muscle in the Management of Myofascial Pain Syndrome. *Physiol. Regul. Med.* **2016**, 23–24. [CrossRef]
138. Heng, C.H.Y.; Snow, M.; Dave, L.Y.H. Single-Stage Arthroscopic Cartilage Repair With Injectable Scaffold and BMAC. *Arthrosc. Tech.* **2021**, *10*, e751–e756. [CrossRef]
139. Kim, M.S.; Chun, C.H.; Wang, J.H.; Kim, J.G.; Kang, S.B.; Yoo, J.D.; Chon, J.G.; Kim, M.K.; Moon, C.W.; Chang, C.B.; et al. Microfractures Versus a Porcine-Derived Collagen-Augmented Chondrogenesis Technique for Treating Knee Cartilage Defects: A Multicenter Randomized Controlled Trial. *Arthrosc. J. Arthrosc. Relat. Surg.* **2020**, *36*, 1612–1624. [CrossRef] [PubMed]
140. Lee, H.S.; Oh, K.J.; Moon, Y.W.; In, Y.; Lee, H.J.; Kwon, S.Y. Intra-Articular Injection of Type I Atelocollagen to Alleviate Knee Pain: A Double-Blind, Randomized Controlled Trial. *Cartilage* **2021**, *13*, 342S–350S. [CrossRef] [PubMed]
141. Kim, J.H.; Kim, D.J.; Lee, H.J.; Kim, B.K.; Kim, Y.S. Atelocollagen Injection Improves Tendon Integrity in Partial-Thickness Rotator Cuff Tears: A Prospective Comparative Study. *Orthop. J. Sports Med.* **2020**, *8*, 2325967120904012. [CrossRef] [PubMed]
142. Volpi, P.; Zini, R.; Erschbaumer, F.; Beggio, M.; Busilacchi, A.; Carimati, G. Effectiveness of a Novel Hydrolyzed Collagen Formulation in Treating Patients with Symptomatic Knee Osteoarthritis: A Multicentric Retrospective Clinical Study. *Int. Orthop.* **2021**, *45*, 375–380. [CrossRef] [PubMed]
143. Mariconti, P. Usefulness of GUNA Collagen Medical Devices in the Treatment of Knee Pain. *Physiol. Regul. Med.* **2016**, 39–40.
144. Martin Martin, L.S.; Massafra, U.; Bizzi, E.; Migliore, A. A Double Blind Randomized Active-Controlled Clinical Trial on the Intra-Articular Use of Md-Knee versus Sodium Hyaluronate in Patients with Knee Osteoarthritis ("Joint"). *BMC Musculoskelet. Disord.* **2016**, *17*, 1–8. [CrossRef] [PubMed]
145. Uroz, N.Z. Collagen Medical Device Infiltrations in Shoulder Pathologies. Calcific Supraspinatus Tendinitis. *Physiol. Regul. Med.* **2016**, 15–17.
146. Nestorova, R.; Rashkov, R.; Petranova, T. Clinical and Sonographic Assessment of the Effectiveness of GUNA Collagen MDs Injections in Patients with Partial Thickness Tear of the Rotator Cuff. *Physiol. Regul. Med.* **2016**, 35–37.
147. Wolkow, N.; Jakobiec, F.A.; Dryja, T.P.; Lefebvre, D.R. Mild Complications or Unusual Persistence of Porcine Collagen and Hyaluronic Acid Gel Following Periocular Filler Injections. *Ophthalmic Plast. Reconstr. Surg.* **2018**, *34*, e143–e146. [CrossRef]
148. Braun, M.; Braun, S. Nodule Formation Following Lip Augmentation Using Porcine Collagen-Derived Filler. *J. Drugs Dermatol.* **2008**, *7*, 579–581.
149. Narins, R.S.; Brandt, F.S.; Lorenc, Z.P.; Maas, C.S.; Monheit, G.D.; Smith, S.R. Twelve-Month Persistency of a Novel Ribose-Cross-Linked Collagen Dermal Filler. *Dermatol. Surg.* **2008**, *34*, 31–39. [CrossRef]
150. Pollack, S.v. Silicone, Fibrel, and Collagen Implantation for Facial Lines and Wrinkles. *J. Dermatol. Surg. Oncol.* **1990**, *16*, 957–961. [CrossRef] [PubMed]
151. Mittelman, H. Fibrel: A Dermal Implant Comparison With Collagen Implants. *Arch. Otolaryngol. Head Neck Surg.* **1988**, *114*, 1379. [CrossRef]
152. Denton, A.B.; Shoman, N. Porcine Collagen: Evolence. In *Office-Based Cosmetic Procedures and Techniques*; Cambridge University Press: Cambridge, UK, 2010; pp. 68–70. [CrossRef]

153. Samalavicius, N.E.; Kavaliauskas, P.; Dulskas, A. Permacol™ Collagen Paste Injection for the Treatment of Complex Anal Fistula—A Video Vignette. *Color. Dis.* **2020**, *22*, 116–117. [CrossRef] [PubMed]

154. Pescatori, M. Permacol™ Collagen Paste for Treating a Rectovaginal Fistula Following Anterior Rectal Prolapsectomy. *Tech. Coloproctol.* **2017**, *21*, 909–910. [CrossRef] [PubMed]

155. Harran, N.; Herold, J.; Bentley, A.; Bebington, B.D. Efficacy of Porcine Dermal Collagen (PermacolTM) Injection for Passive Faecal Incontinence in a Dedicated Colorectal Unit at the Wits Donald Gordon Medical Centre. *S. Afr. J. Surg.* **2017**, *55*, 10–13. [CrossRef]

156. Giordano, P.; Sileri, P.; Buntzen, S.; Stuto, A.; Nunoo-Mensah, J.; Lenisa, L.; Singh, B.; Thorlacius-Ussing, O.; Griffiths, B.; Ziyaie, D. A Prospective Multicentre Observational Study of Permacol™ Collagen Paste for Anorectal Fistula: Preliminary Results. *Color. Dis.* **2016**, *18*, 286–294. [CrossRef]

157. Sileri, P.; Franceschilli, L.; del Vecchio Blanco, G.; Stolfi, V.M.; Angelucci, G.P.; Gaspari, A.L. Porcine Dermal Collagen Matrix Injection May Enhance Flap Repair Surgery for Complex Anal Fistula. *Int. J. Color. Dis.* **2011**, *26*, 345–349. [CrossRef]

158. Milito, G.; Cadeddu, F. Conservative Treatment for Anal Fistula: Collagen Matrix Injection. *J. Am. Coll. Surg.* **2009**, *209*, 542–543. [CrossRef]

159. Harper, C. Permacol: Clinical Experience with a New Biomaterial. *Hosp. Med.* **2001**, *62*, 90–95. [CrossRef]

160. Micarelli, A.; Viziano, A.; Granito, I.; Antonuccio, G.; Felicioni, A.; Loberti, M.; Carlino, P.; Micarelli, R.X.; Alessandrini, M. Combination of In-Situ Collagen Injection and Rehabilitative Treatment in Long-Lasting Facial Nerve Palsy: A Pilot Randomized Controlled Trial. *Eur. J. Phys. Rehabil. Med.* **2021**, *57*, 366–375. [CrossRef]

161. del Carpio-Orantes, L.; García-Méndez, S.; Sánchez-Díaz, J.S.; Aguilar-Silva, A.; Contreras-Sánchez, E.R.; Hernández, S.N.H. Use of Fibroquel® (Polymerized Type I Collagen) in Patients with Hypoxemic Inflammatory Pneumonia Secondary to COVID-19 in Veracruz, Mexico. *J. Anesth. Crit. Care* **2021**, *13*, 69–73. [CrossRef]

162. Méndez-Flores, S.; Priego-Ranero, Á.; Azamar-Llamas, D.; Olvera-Prado, H.; Rivas-Redonda, K.I.; Ochoa-Hein, E.; Perez-Ortiz, A.; Rendón-Macías, M.E.; Rojas-Castañeda, E.; Urbina-Terán, S.; et al. Effect of Polymerised Type I Collagen on Hyperinflammation of Adult Outpatients with Symptomatic COVID-19. *Clin. Transl. Med.* **2022**, *12*, 1–8. [CrossRef]

163. Sparavigna, A.; Tateo, A.; Inselvini, E.; Tocchio, M.; Orlandini, M.C.; Botali, G. Anti-Age Activity and Tolerance Evaluation of Collagen Micro-Injection Treatment Associated to Topical Application of a Cosmetic Formulation (Investigator-Initiated Multicentre Trial). *J. Clin. Exp. Dermatol. Res.* **2017**, *8*, 1000391. [CrossRef]

164. Gkouvi, A.; Nicolaidou, E.; Corbo, A.; Selvaggi, G.; Tsimpidakis, A.; Mastraftsi, S.; Gregoriou, S. Heterologous Type i Collagen as an Add-on Therapy to Narrowband Ultraviolet b for the Treatment of Vitiligo: A Pilot Study. *J. Clin. Aesthetic Dermatol.* **2021**, *14*, 31–34.

165. Gkouvi, A.; Corbo, A.; Gregoriou, S. Treatment of Male Genital Lichen Sclerosus with Heterologous Type I Collagen. *Clin. Exp. Dermatol.* **2020**, *45*, 388–390. [CrossRef] [PubMed]

166. Klewin-Steinböck, S.; Nowak-Terpi3owska, A.; Adamski, Z.; Grocholewicz, K.; Wyganowska-Swiatkowska, M. Effect of Injectable Equine Collagen Type I on Metabolic Activity and Apoptosis of Gingival Fibroblasts. *Adv. Dermatol. Allergol.* **2021**, *XXXVIII*, 440–445. [CrossRef]

167. Wyganowska-Swiatkowska, M.; Duda-Sobczak, A.; Corbo, A.; Matthews-Brzozowska, T. Atelocollagen Application in Human Periodontal Tissue Treatment—A Pilot Study. *Life* **2020**, *10*, 114. [CrossRef] [PubMed]

168. Burres, S. Soft-Tissue Augmentation with Fascian. *Clin. Plast. Surg.* **2001**, *28*, 101–110. [CrossRef]

169. Bauman, L. CosmoDerm/CosmoPlast (Human Bioengineered Collagen) for the Aging Face. *Facial Plast. Surg.* **2004**, *20*, 125–128. [CrossRef]

170. Fagien, S.; Elson, M.L. Facial Soft-Tissue Augmentation with Allogeneic Human Tissue Collagen Matrix (Dermalogen and Dermaplant). *Clin. Plast. Surg.* **2001**, *28*, 63–81. [CrossRef] [PubMed]

171. Burres, S. Fascian. *Facial Plast. Surg.* **2004**, *20*, 149–152. [CrossRef] [PubMed]

172. Maloney, B.P.; Murphy, B.A.; Cole, H.P. Cymetra. *Facial Plast. Surg.* **2004**, *20*, 129–134. [CrossRef] [PubMed]

173. Anderson, T.D.; Sataloff, R.T. Complications of Collagen Injection of the Vocal Fold: Report of Several Unusual Cases and Review of the Literature. *J. Voice* **2004**, *18*, 392–397. [CrossRef] [PubMed]

174. Bock, J.M.; Lee, J.H.; Robinson, R.A.; Hoffman, H.T. Migration of Cymetra After Vocal Fold Injection for Laryngeal Paralysis. *Laryngoscope* **2007**, *117*, 2251–2254. [CrossRef] [PubMed]

175. Karpenko, A.N.; Meleca, R.J.; Dworkin, J.P.; Stachler, R.J. Cymetra Injection for Unilateral Vocal Fold Paralysis. *Ann. Otol. Rhinol. Laryngol.* **2003**, *112*, 927–934. [CrossRef]

176. Douglas, R.S.; Donsoff, I.; Cook, T.; Shorr, N. Collagen Fillers in Facial Aesthetic Surgery. *Facial Plast. Surg.* **2004**, *20*, 117–123. [CrossRef]

177. Homicz, M.R.; Watson, D. Review of Injectable Materials for Soft Tissue Augmentation. *Facial Plast. Surg.* **2004**, *20*, 21–29. [CrossRef]

178. Rinaldi, F.; Pinto, D.; Trink, A.; Giuliani, G.; Sparavigna, A. In Vitro and in Vivo Evaluation on the Safety and Efficacy of a Brand-New Intracutaneous Filler with A1-R-Collagen. *Clin. Cosmet. Investig. Dermatol.* **2021**, *14*, 501–512. [CrossRef]

179. Lombardi, F.; Palumbo, P.; Augello, F.R.; Giusti, I.; Dolo, V.; Guerrini, L.; Cifone, M.G.; Giuliani, M.; Cinque, B. Type I Collagen Suspension Induces Neocollagenesis and Myodifferentiation in Fibroblasts in Vitro. *Biomed. Res. Int.* **2020**, *2020*, 6093974. [CrossRef]

180. Keefe, J.; Wauk, L.; Chu, S.; DeLustro, F. Clinical Use of Injectable Bovine Collan: A Decade of OExperience. *Clin. Mater.* **1992**, *9*, 155–162. [CrossRef]
181. Randelli, F.; Menon, A.; Via, A.G.; Mazzoleni, M.; Sciancalepore, F.; Brioschi, M.; Gagliano, N. Effect of a Collagen-Based Compound on Morpho-Functional Properties of Cultured Human Tenocytes. *Cells* **2018**, *7*, 246. [CrossRef]
182. Furuzawa-Carballeda, J.; Lima, G.; Llorente, L.; Nuñez-Álvarez, C.; Ruiz-Ordaz, B.H.; Echevarría-Zuno, S.; Hernández-Cuevas, V. Polymerized-Type I Collagen Downregulates Inflammation and Improves Clinical Outcomes in Patients with Symptomatic Knee Osteoarthritis Following Arthroscopic Lavage: A Randomized, Double-Blind, and Placebo-Controlled Clinical Trial. *Sci. World J.* **2012**, *2012*, 342854. [CrossRef]
183. Corrado, B.; Bonini, I.; Alessio Chirico, V.; Rosano, N.; Gisonni, P. Use of Injectable Collagen in Partial-Thickness Tears of the Supraspinatus Tendon: A Case Report. *Oxf. Med. Case Rep.* **2020**, *2020*, 408–410. [CrossRef] [PubMed]
184. Kim, M.; Choi, Y.S.; You, M.-W.; Kim, J.S.; Young, K.W. Sonoelastography in the Evaluation of Plantar Fasciitis Treatment 3-Month Follow-Up After Collagen Injection. *Ultrasound Q.* **2016**, *32*, 327–332. [CrossRef] [PubMed]
185. Martins, S.B.; Oliveira, E.; Castro, R.A.; Sartori, M.G.; Baracat, E.C.; Lima, G.R.; Girao, M.J. Clinical and Urodynamic Evaluation in Women with Stress Urinary Incontinence Treated by Periurethral Collagen Injection. *Int. Braz. J. Urol.* **2007**, *33*, 695–703. [CrossRef] [PubMed]
186. Oremus, M.; Tarride, J.-E. An Economic Evaluation of Surgery versus Collagen Injection for the Treatment of Female Stress Urinary Incontinence. *Can. J. Urol.* **2010**, *17*, 5087–5093.
187. Winters, J.C.; Chiverton, A.; Scarpero, H.M.; Prats, L.J. Collagen injection therapy in elderly women: Long-term results and patient satisfaction. *Urology* **2000**, *55*, 856–860. [CrossRef]
188. Groutz, A.; Blaivas, J.G.; Kesler, S.S.; Weiss, J.P.; Chaikin, D.C. Female urology outcome results of transurethral collagen injection for female stress incontinence: Assessment by urinary incontinence score. *J. Urol.* **2000**, *164*, 2006–2009. [CrossRef]
189. Bomalaski, M.D.; Bloom, D.A.; McGuire, E.J.; Panzl, A. Glutaraldehyde cross-linked collagen in the treatment of urinary incontinence in children. *J. Urol.* **1996**, *155*, 699–702. [CrossRef]
190. Kassouf, W.; Capolicchio, G.; Berardinucci, G.; Corcos, J. Collagen injection for treatment of urinary incontinence in children. *J. Urol.* **2001**, *165*, 1666–1668. [CrossRef] [PubMed]
191. Faerber, G.J.; Richardson, T.D. *Long-Term Results of Transurethral Collagen Injection in Men with Intrinsic Sphincter Deficiency*; Mary Ann Liebert, Inc.: New Rochelle, NY, USA, 1997; Volume 11.
192. Faerber, G.J.; Belville, W.D.; Ohl, D.A.; Plata, A. Comparison of Transurethral versus Periurethral Collagen Injection in Women with Intrinsic Sphincter Deficiency. *Tech. Urol.* **1998**, *4*, 124–127. [PubMed]
193. Richardson, T.D.; Kennelly, M.J.; Faerber, G.J. Endoscopic injection of glutaraldehyde cross-linked collagen for the treatment of intrinsic sphincter deficiency in women. *Urology* **1995**, *43*, 378–381. [CrossRef]
194. Smith, D.N.; Appell, R.A.; Rackley, R.R.; Winters, J.C. Collagen Injection Therapy for Post-Prostatectomy Incontinence. *J. Urol.* **1998**, *160*, 364–367. [CrossRef]
195. Klutke, C.G.; Tiemann, D.D.; Nadler, R.B.; Andriole, G.L. *Antegrade Collagen Injection for Stress Incontinence after Radical Prostatectomy: Technique and Early Results*; Mary Ann Liebert, Inc.: New Rochelle, NY, USA, 1996; Volume 10.
196. Appell, R.A. Collagen Injection Therapy for Urinary Incontinence. *Urol. Clin. N. Am.* **1994**, *21*, 177–182. [CrossRef]
197. Appell, R.A.; Vasavada, S.P.; Rackley, R.R.; Winters, J.C. Percutaneous antegrade collagen injection therapy for urinary incontinence following radical prostatectomy. *Urology* **1996**, *48*, 769–772. [CrossRef]
198. Nagai, A.; Nasu, Y.; Watanabe, M.; Tsugawa, M.; Iguchi, H.; Kumon, H. Analysis of Retrograde Ejaculation Using Color Doppler Ultrasonography before and after Transurethral Collagen Injection. *Int. J. Impot. Res.* **2004**, *16*, 456–458. [CrossRef] [PubMed]
199. Spiegel, J.R.; Sataloff, R.T.; Gould, W.J. The Treatment of Vocal Fold Paralysis with Injectable Collagen: Clinical Concerns. *J. Voice* **1987**, *1*, 119–121. [CrossRef]
200. Remacle, M.; Lawson, G. Results with Collagen Injection into the Vocal Folds for Medialization. *Curr. Opin. Otolaryngol. Head Neck Surg* **2007**, *15*, 148–152. [CrossRef]
201. Remacle, M.; Hamoir, M.; Marbaix, E. Gax-Collagen Injection to Correct Aspiration Problems after Subtotal Laryngectomy. *Laryngoscope* **1990**, *100*, 662–669.
202. Ford, C.N.; Bless, D.M. Selected Problems Treated by Vocal Fold Injection of Collagen. *Am. J. Otolaryngol.* **1993**, *14*, 257–261. [CrossRef] [PubMed]
203. Lundy, D.S.; Casiano, R.R.; McClinton, M.E.; Xue, J.W. Early Results of Transcutaneous Injection Laryngoplasty with Micronized Acellular Dermis Versus Type-I Thyroplasty for Glottic Incompetence Dysphonia Due to Unilateral Vocal Fold Paralysis. *J. Voice* **2003**, *17*, 589–595. [CrossRef] [PubMed]
204. Rydningen, M.; Dehli, T.; Wilsgaard, T.; Rydning, A.; Kumle, M.; Lindsetmo, R.O.; Norderval, S. Sacral Neuromodulation Compared with Injection of Bulking Agents for Faecal Incontinence Following Obstetric Anal Sphincter Injury—A Randomized Controlled Trial. *Color. Dis.* **2017**, *19*, O134–O144. [CrossRef]
205. Brown, S.A.; Rohrich, R.J.; Baumann, L.; Brandt, F.S.; Fagien, S.; Glazer, S.; Kenkel, J.M.; Lowe, N.J.; Monheit, G.D.; Narins, R.S.; et al. Subject Global Evaluation and Subject Satisfaction Using Injectable Poly-l-Lactic Acid versus Human Collagen for the Correction of Nasolabial Fold Wrinkles. *Plast. Reconstr. Surg.* **2011**, *127*, 1684–1692. [CrossRef] [PubMed]

206. Narins, R.S.; Baumann, L.; Brandt, F.S.; Fagien, S.; Glazer, S.; Lowe, N.J.; Monheit, G.D.; Rendon, M.I.; Rohrich, R.J.; Werschler, W.P. A Randomized Study of the Efficacy and Safety of Injectable Poly-L-Lactic Acid versus Human-Based Collagen Implant in the Treatment of Nasolabial Fold Wrinkles. *J. Am. Acad. Dermatol.* **2010**, *62*, 448–462. [CrossRef]
207. Draelos, Z. Case Study of Dermicol-P35 Used in Patient with Past Hypersensitivity to Crosslinked Bovine Collagen Dermal Filler. *Dermatol. Surg.* **2010**, *36*, 825–827. [CrossRef]
208. Narins, R.S.; Brandt, F.S.; Lorenc, Z.P.; Maas, C.S.; Monheit, G.D.; Smith, S.R.; Mcintyre, S. A Randomized, Multicenter Study of the Safety and Efficacy of Dermicol-P35 and Non-Animal-Stabilized Hyaluronic Acid Gel for the Correction of Nasolabial Folds. *Dermatol. Surg.* **2007**, *33*, S213–S221. [CrossRef]
209. Cassuto, D. The Use of Dermicol-P35 Dermal Filler for Nonsurgical Rhinoplasty. *Aesthetic Surg. J.* **2009**, *29*, S22–S24. [CrossRef]
210. Smith, K.C. Repair of Acne Scars With Dermicol-P35. *Aesthetic Surg. J.* **2009**, *29*, S16–S18. [CrossRef] [PubMed]
211. Horvath, K. The Effect of GUNA-MDs in the Therapy Resistant Facial Paresis. In Proceedings of the International Congress of PRM, Low doses therapies, Prague, Czech Republic, 9 November 2013. Trials and Case Reports.
212. Ding, L.; Yan, G.; Wang, B.; Xu, L.; Gu, Y.; Ru, T.; Cui, X.; Lei, L.; Liu, J.; Sheng, X.; et al. Transplantation of UC-MSCs on Collagen Scaffold Activates Follicles in Dormant Ovaries of POF Patients with Long History of Infertility. *Sci. China Life Sci.* **2018**, *61*, 1554–1565. [CrossRef]
213. Bechara, C.F.; Annambhotla, S.; Lin, P.H. Access Site Management with Vascular Closure Devices for Percutaneous Transarterial Procedures. *J. Vasc. Surg.* **2010**, *52*, 1682–1696. [CrossRef] [PubMed]
214. Awad, S.; Dharmavaram, S.; Wearn, C.S.; Dube, M.G.; Lobo, D.N. Effects of an Intraoperative Infusion of 4 Succinylated Gelatine (Gelofusine®) and 6 Hydroxyethyl Starch (Voluven®) on Blood Volume. *Br. J. Anaesth.* **2012**, *109*, 168–176. [CrossRef] [PubMed]
215. Fisher, G.J.; Varani, J.; Voorhees, J.J. Looking Older Fibroblast Collapse and Therapeutic Implications. *Arch. Dermatol.* **2008**, *144*, 666–672. [CrossRef] [PubMed]
216. Watson, W.; Kaye, R.L.; Klein, A.; Stegman, S. Injectable Collagen: A Clinical Overview. *Cutis* **1983**, *31*, 543–546. [PubMed]
217. Nijhawan, R.I.; Cohen, J.I.; Kaufman, J. Persistent Erythema After Human Collagen Filler Injections. *Cosmet. Dermatol.* **2008**, *21*, 90–94.
218. Pereira, D.; Peleteiro, B.; Araújo, J.; Branco, J.; Santos, R.A.; Ramos, E. The Effect of Osteoarthritis Definition on Prevalence and Incidence Estimates: A Systematic Review. *Osteoarthr. Cartil.* **2011**, *19*, 1270–1285. [CrossRef]
219. Kapoor, M.; Martel-Pelletier, J.; Lajeunesse, D.; Pelletier, J.-P.; Fahmi, H. Role of Proinflammatory Cytokines in the Pathophysiology of Osteoarthritis. *Nat. Rev. Rheumatol.* **2011**, *7*, 33–42. [CrossRef]
220. Cui, A.; Li, H.; Wang, D.; Zhong, J.; Chen, Y.; Lu, H. Global, Regional Prevalence, Incidence and Risk Factors of Knee Osteoarthritis in Population-Based Studies. *EClinicalMedicine* **2020**, *29–30*, 100587. [CrossRef]
221. Meimandi-Parizi, A.; Oryan, A.; Moshiri, A. Role of Tissue Engineered Collagen Based Tridimensional Implant on the Healing Response of the Experimentally Induced Large Achilles Tendon Defect Model in Rabbits: A Long Term Study with High Clinical Relevance. *J. Biomed. Sci.* **2013**, *20*, 28. [CrossRef]
222. Suh, D.-S.; Lee, J.-K.; Yoo, J.-C.; Woo, S.-H.; Kim, G.-R.; Kim, J.-W.; Choi, N.-Y.; Kim, Y.; Song, H.-S. Atelocollagen Enhances the Healing of Rotator Cuff Tendon in Rabbit Model. *Am. J. Sport. Med.* **2017**, *45*, 2019–2027. [CrossRef]
223. Kirlum, H.J.; Stehr, M.; Dietz, H.G. Late Obstruction after Subureteral Collagen Injection. *Eur. J. Pediatr. Surg.* **2006**, *16*, 133–134. [CrossRef]
224. Hartl, D.M.; Riquet, M.; Hans, S.; Laccourreye, O.; Vaissière, J.; Brasnu, D.F. Objective Voice Analysis after Autologous Fat Injection for Unilateral Vocal Fold Paralysis. *Ann. Otol. Rhinol. Laryngol.* **2001**, *110*, 229–235. [CrossRef] [PubMed]
225. Hirano, M.; Mori, K.; Tanaka, S.; Fujita, M. Vocal Function in Patients with Unilateral Vocal Fold Paralysis Before and After Silicone Injection. *Acta. Otolaryngol.* **1995**, *115*, 553–559. [CrossRef] [PubMed]
226. He, X.; Wang, Q.; Zhao, Y.; Zhang, H.; Wang, B.; Pan, J.; Li, J.; Yu, H.; Wang, L.; Dai, J.; et al. Effect of Intramyocardial Grafting Collagen Scaffold With Mesenchymal Stromal Cells in Patients With Chronic Ischemic Heart Disease. *JAMA Netw. Open* **2020**, *3*, e2016236. [CrossRef] [PubMed]
227. Swanson, N.A.; Stoner, J.G.; Siegle, R.J.; Solomon, A.R. Treatment Site Reactions to Zyderm Collagen Implantation. *J. Dermatol. Surg. Oncol.* **1983**, *9*, 377–380. [CrossRef] [PubMed]
228. Elson, M.L. The Role of Skin Testing in the Use of Collagen Injectable Materials. *J. Dermatol. Surg. Oncol.* **1989**, *15*, 301–303. [CrossRef]
229. Aragona, F.; D'Urso, L.; Marcolongo, R. Immunologic Aspects of Bovine Injectable Collagen in Humans. *Eur. Urol.* **1998**, *33*, 129–133. [CrossRef]
230. Zhou, Z.; Chen, X.; Zhou, X.; Yang, X.; Lu, D.; Kang, W.; Feng, X. Effects of Intraoperative Gelatin on Blood Viscosity and Oxygenation Balance. *J. PeriAnesthesia Nurs.* **2019**, *34*, 1274–1281. [CrossRef]
231. Lucey, P.; Goldberg, D. Complications of Collagen Fillers. *Facial Plast. Surg.* **2014**, *30*, 615–622. [CrossRef]
232. Cooperman, L.; Michaeli, D.; Alto, P.; Francisco, S. The Immunogenicity of Injectable Collagen. II. A Retrospective Review of Seventy-Two Tested and Treated Patients. *J. Am. Acad. Dermatol.* **1984**, *10*, 647–651. [CrossRef]
233. Lemperle, G.; Rullan, P.P.; Gauthier-Hazan, N. Avoiding and Treating Dermal Filler Complications. *Plast. Reconstr. Surg.* **2006**, *118*, 92S–107S. [CrossRef] [PubMed]
234. Vanderveen, E.E.; McCoy, J.P.; Schade, W.; Kapur, J.J.; Hamilton, T.; Ragsdale, C.; Grekin, R.C.; Swanson, N.A. The Association of HLA and Immune Responses to Bovine Collagen Implants. *Arch. Dermatol.* **1986**, *122*, 650–654. [CrossRef]

235. Klein, A.W. In Favor of Double Testing. *Dermatol. Surg.* **1989**, *15*, 263. [CrossRef] [PubMed]
236. Morgan, K. What Do Anti-Collagen Antibodies Mean? *Ann. Rheum. Dis.* **1990**, *49*, 62–65. [CrossRef]
237. Holmes, R.; Kirk, S.; Tronci, G.; Yang, X.; Wood, D. Influence of Telopeptides on the Structural and Physical Properties of Polymeric and Monomeric Acid-Soluble Type I Collagen. *Mater. Sci. Eng. C* **2017**, *77*, 823–827. [CrossRef] [PubMed]
238. Steffen, C.; Timpl, R.; Wolff, I. Immunogenicity and Specificity of Collagen. V. Demonstration of Three Different Antigenic Determinants on Calf Collagen. *Immunology* **1968**, *15*, 135–144.
239. Leonard, M.P.; Decter, A.; Mix, L.W.; Johnson, H.W.; Coleman, G.U. Endoscopic Treatment of Vesicoureteral Reflux with Collagen: Preliminary Report and Cost Analysis. *J. Urol.* **1996**, *155*, 1716–1720. [CrossRef] [PubMed]
240. Brown, J.A.; Elliott, D.S.; Barrett, D.M. Postprostatectomy Urinary Incontinence: A Comparison of the Cost of Conservative Versus Surgical Management. *Urology* **1998**, *51*, 715–720. [CrossRef]

Disclaimer/Publisher's Note: The statements, opinions and data contained in all publications are solely those of the individual author(s) and contributor(s) and not of MDPI and/or the editor(s). MDPI and/or the editor(s) disclaim responsibility for any injury to people or property resulting from any ideas, methods, instructions or products referred to in the content.

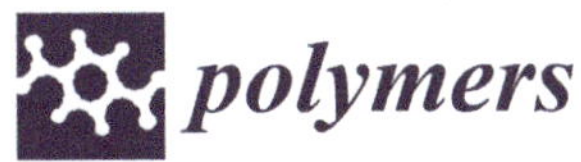 *polymers*

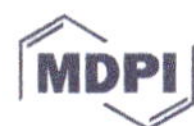

Review

Tissue Engineering with Stem Cell from Human Exfoliated Deciduous Teeth (SHED) and Collagen Matrix, Regulated by Growth Factor in Regenerating the Dental Pulp

Vinna K. Sugiaman [1], Rudy Djuanda [2], Natallia Pranata [1], Silvia Naliani [3], Wayan L. Demolsky [1] and Jeffrey [4],*

1   Department of Oral Biology, Faculty of Dentistry, Maranatha Christian University, Bandung 40164, Indonesia
2   Department of Conservative Dentistry and Endodontic, Faculty of Dentistry, Maranatha Christian University, Bandung 40164, Indonesia
3   Department of Prosthodontics, Faculty of Dentistry, Maranatha Christian University, Bandung 40164, Indonesia
4   Department of Pediatric Dentistry, Faculty of Dentistry, Jenderal Achmad Yani University, Cimahi 40531, Indonesia
*   Correspondence: jeffrey_dent2000@yahoo.com

Abstract: Maintaining dental pulp vitality and preventing tooth loss are two challenges in endodontic treatment. A tooth lacking a viable pulp loses its defense mechanism and regenerative ability, making it more vulnerable to severe damage and eventually necessitating extraction. The tissue engineering approach has drawn attention as an alternative therapy as it can regenerate dentin-pulp complex structures and functions. Stem cells or progenitor cells, extracellular matrix, and signaling molecules are triad components of this approach. Stem cells from human exfoliated deciduous teeth (SHED) are a promising, noninvasive source of stem cells for tissue regeneration. Not only can SHEDs regenerate dentin-pulp tissues (comprised of fibroblasts, odontoblasts, endothelial cells, and nerve cells), but SHEDs also possess immunomodulatory and immunosuppressive properties. The collagen matrix is a material of choice to provide structural and microenvironmental support for SHED-to-dentin pulp tissue differentiation. Growth factors regulate cell proliferation, migration, and differentiation into specific phenotypes via signal-transduction pathways. This review provides current concepts and applications of the tissue engineering approach, especially SHEDs, in endodontic treatment.

Keywords: dentin-pulp complex regeneration; signalling molecules; stem cell from human exfoliated deciduous teeth (SHED); tissue engineering

Citation: Sugiaman, V.K.; Djuanda, R.; Pranata, N.; Naliani, S.; Demolsky, W.L.; Jeffrey. Tissue Engineering with Stem Cell from Human Exfoliated Deciduous Teeth (SHED) and Collagen Matrix, Regulated by Growth Factor in Regenerating the Dental Pulp. *Polymers* **2022**, *14*, 3712. https://doi.org/10.3390/polym14183712

Academic Editors: Dimitrios Bikiaris and Nunzia Gallo

Received: 7 August 2022
Accepted: 2 September 2022
Published: 6 September 2022

Publisher's Note: MDPI stays neutral with regard to jurisdictional claims in published maps and institutional affiliations.

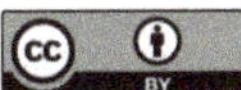

Copyright: © 2022 by the authors. Licensee MDPI, Basel, Switzerland. This article is an open access article distributed under the terms and conditions of the Creative Commons Attribution (CC BY) license (https://creativecommons.org/licenses/by/4.0/).

1. Introduction

Tissue injury can occur when tissue is exposed to various stimuli, including microbial infections, mechanical damage (fractures, cracks, thermal factors), and chemical damage. This condition can cause cell apoptosis or necrosis, as well as microvasculature and stroma damage, leading to the activation of inflammation and wound healing mechanisms. During wound healing, mesenchymal stem cells are recruited to the site of injury to differentiate into stromal cells and replace damaged cells. However, if severe inflammation occurs in the dental pulp, the damaged cells cannot be effectively replaced or healed, a condition called irreversible pulpitis. In this condition, endodontic treatment must be carried out to remove the damaged pulp and prevent the spread of the damage [1–4].

Endodontic treatment involves partial or complete pulp removal (pulp extirpation) and filling the empty root canal with artificial material. Even so, the endodontic treatment causes the tooth to become more fragile, susceptible to caries and periapical infection and more likely to fracture as the tooth losses its vitality due to the absence of blood supply and innervation [5–11].

Therefore, it is crucial to maintain the vitality of the pulp. A tooth without a viable pulp loses its defense mechanism and regenerative ability, making it more prone to severe damage and ultimately leading to extraction. Dentin-pulp complex reconstruction is an ideal approach to restoring pulp vitality by using mesenchymal stem cell or progenitor cells and signalling molecules added to the extracellular matrix to recover fibroblasts, odontoblasts, endothelial cells and nerve fiber functions [8,10–14]. Stem cells can be obtained from various tissues, including teeth, buccal mucosa, skin, fat, and bone [15,16]. The pulp of deciduous teeth, rich in stem cells known as stem cells from human exfoliated deciduous teeth (SHED), is a promising, easy-to-get, and noninvasive source of stem cells for tissue regeneration [17–21]. Not only do they have the regenerative ability to generate dentin-pulp tissues but SHEDs also possess immunomodulatory and immunosuppressive properties [20,22].

Scaffolds are 3-dimensional microstructural materials that provide a biological environment and structural support to facilitate cell growth, desirable interactions, and the formation of functional tissues [8,23,24]. One popular scaffold material is collagen. Collagen is a natural extracellular matrix built from protein and abundant in hard and soft tissues [23]. Collagen is biocompatible, permeable, and biodegradable, so it can function in helping migration, adhesion, proliferation, and cell differentiation [8,12].

Growth factors are polypeptides that play a very important role in the signaling process that occurs during tissue formation and regeneration of the dentin-pulp complex [25,26]. In the dentin-pulp complex regeneration, several growth factors work together through different signalling mechanisms, including Transforming Growth Factor-β (TGFβ), Vascular Endothelial Growth Factor (VEGF),Bone Morphogenic Protein (BMP), Fibroblast Growth Factor (FGF),Platelet-Derived Growth Factor (PDGF), and Nerve Growth Factor(NGF) [25,27,28]. Growth factors will bind to cell surface receptors that subsequently induce cellular processes such as cell proliferation, angiogenesis, neovascularization, and all important steps in the regeneration process [28,29].

Growth Factorplays a role in various stages of the healing process and tissue regeneration, including cell migration, angiogenesis, and neurogenesis [26]. It can also induce odontogenic differentiation through ALK5/Smad2/3, TAK1, p38, and MEK/ERK signalling pathways, supporting cell proliferation and collagen formation [30,31].Tissue engineering applications in endodontic treatment are expected to replace damaged or lost tissue with new natural pulp tissue and reduce the use of artificial materials, making teeth fully functional again [14].

2. Tissue Engineering (TE) in Endodontic Treatment

As mentioned before, one challenge in endodontic treatment is maintaining dental pulp vitality and preventing tooth loss. Regenerative endodontics can overcome this hurdle [32]. According to the American Association of Endodontists, regenerative endodontics is a procedure designed based on biological principles to physiologically replace damaged tooth structures, including root and dentin structures, as well as cells in the pulp-dentin complex [10,32–34].

There are two concepts in regenerative endodontics, namely [35]:(1) guided tissue regeneration (GTR), also known as the revascularization or revitalization approach, and (2) tissue engineering (TE), an interdisciplinary approach to repairing damaged tissue using by combining three components: (1) cells (especially stem cells) capable of forming pulp tissue, root dentin, and tooth-supporting tissues, (2) scaffolds to facilitate cell proliferation and differentiation, and (3) bioactive molecules (generally growth factors) as shown in Figure 1 [28,35–38].

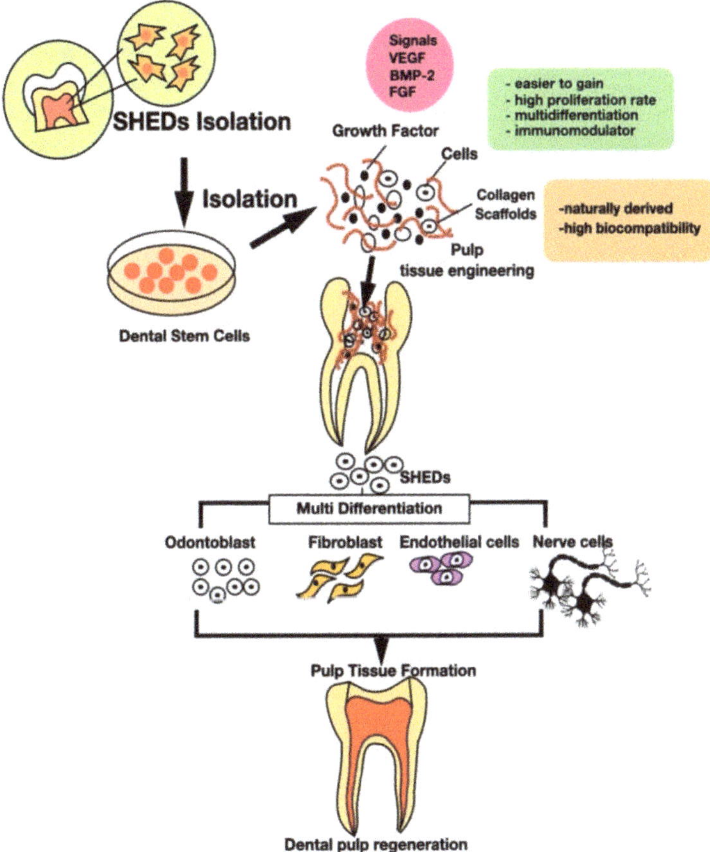

Figure 1. Tissue engineering technology in dental pulp regeneration.

3. Stem Cells

Stem cells are unique cells that possess self-renewal and differentiation properties into another cell type. Based on their differentiation potency, stem cells are divided into the following groups [39–42].

3.1. Totipotent Stem Cells

Totipotent stem cells are stem cells that can generate all types of cells and tissues that exist in organisms and can usually be obtained from embryonic stem cells (from embryos 1–3 days old). Totipotent cells have the highest differentiation potential and allow cells to form embryonic and extra-embryonic structures. An example of a totipotent cell is the zygote, formed after a sperm fertilizes an egg. These cells can later develop into one of the three germ layers or form the placenta. After about four days, the cell mass in the blastocyst becomes pluripotent. This structure is a source of pluripotent cells [35,43].

3.2. Pluripotent Stem Cells

Pluripotent stem cells are stem cells that can generate most cell types (over 200) and tissues found in organisms and have the ability to differentiate into cells of ectodermal, mesodermal, and endodermal origin. They can be obtained from a 5–14 day old blastocyst [35,44,45].

3.3. Multipotent Stem Cells

Multipotent stem cells are stem cells that can generate a limited number of cell and tissue types depending on their origin. These cells can be obtained from cord blood, fetal tissue and postnatal stem cells, including dental pulp stem cells [35,45,46].

3.4. Unipotent Stem Cell

Unipotent stem cells are stem cells that have the narrowest differentiation ability; the can only differentiate into one cell type but are able to divide repeatedly [43,45].

3.5. Induced Pluripotent Cells

Induced Pluripotent Cells are pluripotent stem cells formed by the induction of multipotent cells or adult somatic cells with pluripotent factors such as Oct4, Nanog, Sox2, Klf4, and C-myc [45,47].

There are two approaches to delivering stem cells into the root canal. The first approach is cell transplantation, where autologous or allologous stem cells are applied directly to the root canal. The major obstacle to this process is the immune rejection of allologous stem cells. The second obstacle is cell homing, where stem cells are sent to the injured area; this process is influenced by many factors, such as age, cell number, culture conditions, and method of application. This condition involves the use of chemotactic factors such as stromal cell-derived factor (SDF)-1 are injected into the site of injury to induce stem cell migration from the periapical area to the root canal [27,48].

Based on their stage of development and origin, stem cells can be broadly classified into [32,35,41,47]: (1) embryonic stem cells, which are stem cells derived from embryos, mainly from blastocysts. These cells are capable of dividing and renewing themselves over a long period; (2) adult stem cells, which are stem cells derived from postnatal tissue, can be isolated from various body tissues, such as bone marrow, adipose tissue, encephalon, epithelium, dental pulp, etc.

Tissue injury is always associated with the activation of the immune system or inflammatory cells, including macrophages, neutrophils, CD4+ T cells, CD8+ T cells, and B cells, triggered by cell apoptosis, necrotic cells, microvascular damage, and stroma [40,49–51]. Mesenchymal stem cells can regulate specific and non-specific immune systems by suppressing T cells and dendritic cell maturation, decreasing B cell proliferation and activation, inhibiting NK cell proliferation and cytotoxicity, and increasing T regulatory (Treg) cell formation [49,50].

There are two mechanisms of stem cell immunomodulation: soluble factor secretion and cell-to-cell direct contact. Prostaglandin E2 (PGE2), indoleamine 2,3-dioxygenase (IDO), nitric oxide (NO), interleukin-10 (IL-10), hepatocyte growth factor (HGF), and transforming growth factor 1 (TGFβ1) are secreted factors that have immunomodulatory properties. The cell-to-cell direct contact mechanism involves CD274 (programmed dead ligand 1), vascular cell adhesion molecule-1, and galectin-1 expression. These molecules reduce effector T cell proliferation and increase the proportion of regulatory T cells (Treg) [49,50,52].

Various stem cells can be found in teeth and their associate tissues, such as stem cells from human exfoliated deciduous teeth (SHED), dental pulp stem cells (DPSC), stem cells from the apical papilla (SCAP), periodontal ligament stem cells (PDLC), dental follicle precursor cells (DFPC), dental papilla cells (DPC), dental mesenchymal stem cells (DMSCs), and dental epithelial stem cells (DESCs). For pulp regeneration purposes, SHED, DPSC, and SCAP have strong potential [35,41,53–55].

4. Stem Cells from Human Exfoliated Deciduous Teeth (SHED)

Stem cells from human exfoliated deciduous teeth (SHED) were first obtained by Miura et al. in 2003. SHED expresses cell surface markers STRO-1, CD10, CD29, CD 31, CD44, CD73, CD90, CD105, CD146, CD13, CD166, Nestin, DCX, -tubulin, NeuN, GFAP, S-100, A2B5, CNPaseNanog, Oct3/4 and SSEAs (-3, -4) and does not express CD14, CD15, CD19, CD34, CD45, and CD43 [41,56–59].

SHEDs have two major advantages compared to other stem cells derived from dental tissue: they are easier to gain through noninvasive procedures and have a high proliferation rate [34,41,56,60,61]. SHEDs exhibit higher proliferation rates compared to dental pulp stem cells (DPSCs) and bone marrow-derived mesenchymal stem cells (BMMSCs) [41,45,58,62–64].

SHEDs possess higher potential in forming dentin-pulp complex cells, namely osteoblasts, chondroblasts, adipocytes, endothelial cells, nerve cells, and odontoblasts [57,58,65–67]. The ability of SHEDs to differentiate into odontoblasts is characterized by the expression of dentin matrix protein-1 (DMP-1) and dentin sialophosphoprotein (DSPP) [45,58]. DSPP induces stem cells to odontoblast differentiation through SMAD 1/5/8 phosphorylation and nuclear translocation via the P38 and ERK1/2 pathways. DMP-1 involves maintaining dentin mineralization [68,69].

As for the potential for neural regeneration, SHEDs show more intensive expression of neural differentiation markers than DPSCs, such as b-III-tubulin, and nestin, in neural induction cell culture [37]. SHEDs are also able to increase the angiogenesis process by forming vascular connective tissue structures and expressing and synthesizing VEGF [70].This ability is crucial to maintaining pulp viability as it can supply oxygen and nutrients needed for cell metabolism for tissue regeneration [71].

SHED also functioned as an immunomodulator by suppressing T helper 17 (Th17) cell function and upregulating CD206+ M2 macrophages [57,62]. SHEDs are able to induce the secretion of proinflammatory cytokines, such as interleukin 1b (IL-1b), interleukin 6 (IL-6), interleukin 10 (IL-10), and tumor necrosis factor- a. SHEDs are also capable of inhibiting lymphocyte CD178 expression, suppressing the proliferation of lymphocytes, and decreasing the secretion of IL-4 and IFN-g while sequentially increasing the number of T-reg cells [37,72,73].

5. Collagen Scaffold

Scaffolds are required for regeneration or tissue engineering to facilitate cell growth and functions in the transplanted area [74–76]. Interaction of the cell with the extracellular matrix influences many signalling pathways that change cell behaviours, i.e., adhesion, proliferation, and differentiation [76,77]. Scaffolds can be made of both natural and synthetic materials. Nanoscale proteins are the primary natural scaffolding materials. Nanoscale proteins include collagen, fibronectin, and vitronectin. Synthetic polymers are popular materials because they are biocompatible, biodegradable, mechanically stable, and can be designed in a variety of compositions and shapes [77,78]. These properties enable polymers to biologically affiliate and mimic the natural cell-extracellular matrix [76,79]. Natural scaffolds, such as collagen, have better biocompatibility, whereas synthetic polymers can be controlled for their physicochemical properties, such as their solubility, microstructure, and mechanical strength [76,79].

Nanofibrous scaffolds are more popular than microfiber scaffolds due to their high surface area, interconnected porosity, and positively stimulating extracellular cell-matrix interactions [76]. Nanofibrous scaffolds are made by three methods, namely electrospinning, self-assembly, and separation phase [77]. Electrospinning is the tissue engineering application method most frequently used to synthesize collagen or synthetic scaffolds and/or transport systems for drugs [76].

Collagen is a hydrogel material with high biocompatibility, viscoelasticy similar to soft connective tissue, the ability to transport nutrients and waste, uniform cell encapsulation, in situ gelation ability, and compatibility to be modified by biofunctional molecules or growth factors [80]. Collagen contains arginine-glycine-aspartic acid (RGD) adhesion ligands, which enable cell-biomaterial interactions, leading to cell adhesion [75]. Collagen matrices are compatible with dental pulp stem cell proliferation, adhesion, and differentiation, as shown by the formation of capillary-like microvessels [76,81,82]. Two commercial injectable scaffolds, self-assembling peptide hydrogel and rHCollagen type I, were evaluated. It was found that both of those scaffolds promote SHED cell survival, and when injected into the root canal, these materials promoted odontoblast putative marker expression [83].

Different collagen materials have been compared, such as collagen type I and III, alginate, and chitosan, generating a good result in the proliferative and mineralizing activity of type I collagen. After implanting these cells, the formation of vascularized pulp-like tissue, odontoblast-like cells, and new dentin is produced. SHEDs adhere to PLA cells in dentinal discs [80].

Collagen is a biocompatible material that can be degraded by enzymes; however, natural polymers are difficult to produce and may transmit pathogens from animals (as they are usually produced from animal products) or stimulate an immune response. No scaffold materials have ideal structures and properties that totally resemble natural extracellular matrix as natural ECM comprises complex architecture made up of structural proteins (collagen and elastin), specialized proteins, and glycosaminoglycans. This architecture provides not only structural support for tissue but also a selective dynamic environment that is remodeled via biochemical signals to direct cellular responses [84]. A scaffold should combine the best properties of biomaterials and be as close to the physiological environment of the ECM as possible [80].

6. Growth Factor as Regulator

Regulating molecules are required for SHED to generate endothelial cells, odontoblasts, and neurons that will form the dentin-pulp complex architecture [71,85,86]. They work in signal transduction pathways to regulate cell proliferation, migration, and differentiation into specific phenotypes. BMPs, PDGF, FGF, TGF, EGF, and IGFs are the most common WNT proteins [87–89].

VEGF stimulates SHEDs to undergo endothelial cell differentiation. In an experiment described by Annibali (2014), SHED was incubated in an endothelial cell growth medium (EGM-2MV). This medium contains ascorbic acid, hydrocortisone, rhEGF, FBS, R3-IGF-1, rhbFGF, rhVEGF, and VEGF [71,85]. MEK1/VEGF/ErK, Wnt/VEGF/-catenin, and Notch-EphrinB2/VEGF-DLL4 signaling pathway regulation in response to VEGF stimulation and the expression of VE-Cadherin (endothelial markers), VEGFR2, and CD31 increased dramatically [71,85]. Furthermore, the endothelial-like cells generated by SHEDs could anastomose with the host vascular network, which was demonstrated by an experiment using LacZ tags and galactosidase staining [85].

Odontoblast differentiation was observed after BMP-2 stimulation. This regulatory molecule involves the production of tubular dentin, odontogenesis and morphogenesis. Dentin sialophosphoprotein (DSPP) marker will be abundantly expressed for this distinction [85,90–92]. The production of DSPP is also influenced by two catalytic subunit signaling complexes that target rapamycin complexes 1 and 2 (TORC1 and TORC2). TORC1, which is also required for protein synthesis and translation, regulates and directs cell cycle, growth, and proliferation. Suppression of TORC1 prevented mineralized matrix deposition, which also severely limited the synthesis of DSPP. TORC2 influences both cell survival and cytoskeleton rearrangement. Inhibition of TORC2 promoted mineralization [85,93].

SHED culture in DMEM supplemented with vitamin D3, ascorbic 2-phosphate, dexamethasone, and glycerol phosphate resulted in the expression of odontoblast-specific genes, DMP1 and DSPP. Culture also showed mineralized matrix as visualized using Alizarin red [85,94].

Different techniques for isolating SHEDs revealed various traits for odontoblast differentiation. Despite having functioning odontoblast phenotypes, SHEDs isolated by direct outgrowth showed a decreased rate of mineralization and abnormal cell elongation and polarization due to the vertical orientation of the cell body alongside the dentin-like matrix. SHEDs isolated using enzymatic dissociation quickly formed mineralized tissue and kept their spindle-shaped morphology [85,90]

In immunocompromised mice, the ability of SHEDs to develop into odontoblasts was examined. The dorsum of subcutaneous tissue was implanted with ceramic tricalcium phosphate/hydroxyapatite (TCP/HA) powder and SHED combinations [85].

This resulted in the formation of dentin-like structures. However, the transplant could not form a complete dentin-pulp-like complex. Only 25% of the clones from one of the colony-derived SHED strains transplanted were found to produce ectopic dentin [85].

In another study, slices of extracted third molar teeth were used. To create a porous biodegradable scaffold, poly-L-lactic acid was used to fill the pulp chamber, which was in close contact with the predentin layer. After 1428 days, cells adjacent to the predentin exhibited an active dentin-secreting odontoblast. DSP was also expressed. The cell nuclear location is thought to be polarized eccentrically. The cells displayed cell-cell gap junctions, a well-developed rough endoplasmic reticulum, the Golgi complex, and a large number of vesicles [85].

SHEDs have also been confirmed to be able to develop into neurons. Several neuronal markers, including glutamic acid decarboxylase (GAD), III-tubulin, nestin, $2',3'$-cyclic nucleotide-$3'$phosphodiesterase (CNPase), tyrosine-hydroxylase (TH), polysialylated-neural cell adhesion molecule (PSA-NCAM), and glial fibrillary acidic protein (GFAP) were expressed by SHED-derived neurons.10–12 Several cytokines, including FGF8, SHH, bFGF, and GDNF, influence SHED neuronal regeneration [86,95,96].

FGF8 is responsible for the dorsalization of the anterior neural tube [96]. The notochord secretes SHH during development to induce a general ventral cell destiny in order to generate floor plate and motor neurons. bFGF acts as a proliferation and differentiation regulator. After five days of culture on poly-L-lysine coated dishes without serum, the cells rapidly lost their mesenchymal appearance and took on a more neuronal appearance, including neurite-like outgrowth. Continued injection of SHH/FGF8 generated neurons with developed and extended axon- or dendrite-like structures [85,96].

Upregulation of lncRNA C21orf121 and the downregulation of miR140-5p aid in the differentiation of SHEDs into neuronal cells. lncRNA C21orf121 prevents BMP2 from binding to miR140-5p, which subsequently increases BMP2 production and promotes SHED neurogenesis [86,97]. Table 1 shown several researches that have been conducted using tissue engineering technology in pulp regeneration.

Table 1. Stem cells for dental pulp regeneration [83,98–110].

Article (Author, Year)	Type of Stem Cell	Type of Scaffold	Types of Studies	Evaluation Technique	Outcome
Cordeiro, 2008 [98]	SHED	Poly-L-lactic acid (PLLA)	In-vivo (mice)	Transmission electron microscopy and immunohistochemistry	Odontoblast and endothelial-like cells can be differentiated from SHED
Demarco, 2010 [99]	DPSC	Poly-L-lactic acid (PLLA)	In-vivo (mice)	Immunohistochemistry	Differentiation was determined by evaluation of three putative odontoblastic markers (DSPP, DMP1, and MEPE)
Kodonas, 2012 [100]	DPSCs	- Type I atelocollagen honeycomb sponge (organic) - PLGA (synthetic)	In vivo (mini-pigs)	Histological and immunohistochemistry	The formation of new organic matrix deposits and odontoblast-like cell differentiation occurred.
Rosa, 2013 [83]	SHED	- Self-assembling peptide hydrogel - rhCollagen type I	In vivo (mice)	Histological and immunohistochemistry	Differentiation and proliferative activity to form microvessels and cellular density, expressed odontoblastic differentiation markers(DSPP, DMP-1, MEPE).
Wang Y, 2013 [101]	DPSC	Gelfoam	In vivo (dog)	Radiographic and histologic analyses	Generating pulp-like tissues containing dentin-like tissue and blood vessels.
Iohara K, 2014 [102]	DPSC	Atelocollagen	In vivo (dog)	Immunohistochemically evaluated	Regenerated pulp-like loose connective tissue with vasculature. Odontoblastlike cells attached to the dentinal wall, angiogenesis and re-innervation

Table 1. *Cont.*

Article (Author, Year)	Type of Stem Cell	Type of Scaffold	Types of Studies	Evaluation Technique	Outcome
Qu, 2014 [103]	DPSC	- NF-gelatin/MgP - NF-gelatin	In vitro In vivo (mice)	Immunohistochemical X-ray SEM ALP activity	NF-gelatin/MgP act better as scaffold than Nf-gelatin
Murakami, 2015 [104]	DPSCs/BMMSCs/ADSCs	Atelocollagen	In-vivo (dog)	Immunohistochemistry	Neovascularization occurs, and nerve fibers form in the regenerated pulp tissue. The MDPSC transplantation showed a higher area of vascularization and innervation compared to the MBMSC and MADSC.
Y. S. Kwon, 2015 [105]	DPSC	Collagen hydrogel scaffold cross-linked with cinnamaldehyde (CA)	In vitro	Real-time polymerase chain reaction (PCR) gene expression analysis	Cross-linking of collagen scaffolds with CA is a new strategy for regenerative endodontic therapy regarding hDPC attachment, proliferation and differentiation.
Piva, 2017 [106]	DPSC	Medical-grade poly(L-lactide) (PLLA)	In vivo (mice)	Histology and Immunohistochemistry	Capable of differentiating into endothelial cells,
Widbiller, 2018 [107]	Extraction of dentin matrix protein (eDMP)	- Custom-made fibrin from fibrinogen and thrombin - Fibrin sealant - Self-assembling peptide (SAP) - Plasma rich in growth factor (PRGF)	In vivo (mice)	Histological and immunohistochemistry	eDMP + fibrin and fibrin sealant increased tissue formation than PRGF and SAP
Chang, 2020 [108]	DPSC	Autoclaved treated dentin matrix (a-TDM)	In vivo (mice and goats)	ALP activity spectrophotometer immunohistochemistry	a-TDM + DPSC effective in proliferating and differentiate
Chen H, 2020 [109]	DSC	Matrigel	In vivo (mice)	H&E staining	Microvessel formation, which resembled the natural pulp tissue.
Jang JH, 2020 [110]	DPSC	- Gelatin (GM)- based hemostatic hydrogels (GM) - Fibrin-based hemostatic hydrogels (FM)	In vivo (mini- pig)	Radiographic and histologic	- GM: absence of periapical inflammation and newly formed tertiary dentin with apex maturation - FM: exhibited higher incidences of inflammatory changes (periapical radiolucency and internal root resorption). - Showed microvasculature and odontoblastic layers

7. Dentin Pulp Regeneration

Dentin pulp regeneration aims to revitalize necrotic, infected, or lost pulp teeth by restoring the morphology and function of the pulp. Ideal pulp regeneration should possess natural structures such as nerve fibers and blood vessels, allowing nutritional, defense, sensation, and immunological functions to be restored [10,111]. Growth factors, scaffolds, plasma, or other associated cells such as dentin/odontoblasts, fibroblasts, or endothelial cells may provide regenerative signals in this regeneration process, resulting in cell migration, proliferation, differentiation, angiogenesis and extracellular matrix deposition [28,112].

Endothelial cells differentiate into mesodermal precursor cells (angioblasts) during vasculogenesis, whereas new blood vessels are formed from previously existing blood vessels during angiogenesis. VEGF is the main regulator of angiogenesis and can also increase vascular permeability [28,113]. FGF, another growth factor with an angiogenic role, can attract DPSCs to migrate and proliferate [28]. PDGF can significantly boost cell proliferation, angiogenesis, and odontoblast differentiation [114,115]. BMP7 promotes the formation of dentin (dentinogenesis) [116].

Nerve growth factor (NGF) plays an important role in the nervous system's growth, differentiation, and defense mechanisms by preventing apoptosis and reducing neuronal degradation. NGF expression is typically increased in damaged and developing teeth; this growth factor promotes the proliferation of sensory and sympathetic nerve cells [28]. NGF is also involved in the processes of angiogenesis by inducing VEGF upregulation. NGF binds to tyrosine kinase receptor (TrkA) on the cell surface, resulting in TrkA phosphorylation and activation of multiple signaling pathways, including PI3K/Akt, Ras/Raf/MEK/ERK

1/2, and PLC/PKC. Activation of each of these pathways results in a variety of biological functions, including the prevention of apoptosis [117–119].

In this review, we focus on regenerative endodontic treatment using SHED, collagen scaffold, and growth factors to regenerate dental pulp tissue through tissue engineering technology. The concept of tissue engineering is expected to answer the challenges in dentistry in maintaining the vitality of the dental pulp. Various studies and research are being continuously carried out in order to obtain the best strategy in tissue engineering and regenerative endodontics. This is achieved by understanding the behavior of cells, the suitability of the material with the scaffolds, as well as the growth supporting factors for each specific tissue or organ to be created; these factors are the keys to the success of tissue engineering.

8. Conclusions

In responding to the challenges in dentistry to maintain pulp tissue and prevent tooth loss with irreversible or necrotic pulpitis, regenerative endodontics utilizing tissue engineering technology can be developed. In this technology, the utilization of SHEDs, which have excellent potential with high proliferation speed and ability to differentiate into various cell-forming dental pulp cells, collagen scaffolds as a medium for cell growth and function, and growth factor as a regulator can be utilized to repair and regenerate pulp tissue by regenerating pulp tissue naturally to be fully functional again.

Author Contributions: Conceptualization, V.K.S. and J.; methodology, S.N.; software, R.D.; validation, V.K.S., J. and W.L.D.; formal analysis, N.P.; investigation, V.K.S. and W.L.D.; resources, N.P.; data curation, S.N.; writing—original draft preparation, V.K.S., R.D., N.P., S.N., W.L.D. and J.; writing—review and editing, J. and W.L.D.; visualization, R.D.; supervision, V.K.S.; project administration, J. All authors have read and agreed to the published version of the manuscript.

Funding: This research received no external funding.

Institutional Review Board Statement: Not applicable.

Informed Consent Statement: Not applicable.

Acknowledgments: The authors would like to thank the Faculty of Dentistry, Maranatha Christian University and Faculty of Dentistry, JenderalAchmadYani University.

Conflicts of Interest: The authors declare no conflict of interest.

References

1. Lu, Y.; Liu, Z.; Huang, J.; Liu, C. Therapeutic effect of one-time root canal treatment for irreversible pulpitis. *J. Int. Med. Res.* **2019**, *48*, 0300060519879287. [CrossRef]
2. Guan, X.; Zhou, Y.; Yang, Q.; Zhu, T.; Chen, X.; Deng, S.; Zhang, D. Vital pulp therapy in permanent teeth with irreversible pulpitis caused by caries: A prospective cohort study. *J. Pers. Med.* **2021**, *11*, 1125. [CrossRef] [PubMed]
3. Rechenberg, D.K.; Galicia, J.C.; Peters, O.A. Biological markers for pulpal inflammation: A systematic review. *PLoS ONE* **2016**, *11*, e0167289. [CrossRef] [PubMed]
4. Andreasen, F.M.; Kahler, B. Pulpal response after acute dental injury in the permanent dentition: Clinical implications—A review. *J. Endod.* **2015**, *41*, 299–308. [CrossRef]
5. Goldberg, M. Root Canal Treatment (RCT): From Traditional Endodontic Therapies to Innovating Pulp Regeneration. *J. Dent. Oral Disord. Ther.* **2016**, *4*, 1–6. [CrossRef]
6. Eliyas, S.; Jalili, J.; Martin, N. Restoration of the root canal treated tooth. *Br. Dent. J.* **2015**, *218*, 53–62. [CrossRef] [PubMed]
7. Mazumdar, P.; Choudhury, S.R. Moisture Analysis of Endodontically Treated and Sound Teeth Using Moisture Analyser and Indirect Gravimetric Analysis. *J. Evol. Med. Dent. Sci.* **2020**, *9*, 3721–3725. [CrossRef]
8. Ahmed, G.M.; Abouauf, E.A.; Abubakr, N.; Dörfer, C.E.; El-Sayed, K.F. Tissue Engineering Approaches for Enamel, Dentin, and Pulp Regeneration: An Update. *Stem Cells Int.* **2020**, *2020*, 5734539. [CrossRef] [PubMed]
9. Gong, T.; Heng, B.C.; Lo, E.C.M.; Zhang, C. Current Advance and Future Prospects of Tissue Engineering Approach to Dentin/Pulp Regenerative Therapy. *Stem Cells Int.* **2016**, *2016*, 9204574. [CrossRef] [PubMed]
10. Xie, Z.; Shen, Z.; Zhan, P.; Yang, J.; Huang, Q.; Huang, S.; Chen, L.; Lin, Z. Functional dental pulp regeneration: Basic research and clinical translation. *Int. J. Mol. Sci.* **2021**, *22*, 8991. [CrossRef]

11. Huang, G.T.J.; Liu, J.; Zhu, X.; Yu, Z.; Li, D.; Chen, C.; Azim, A.A. Pulp/Dentin Regeneration: It Should Be Complicated. *J. Endod.* **2020**, *46*, S128–S134. [CrossRef] [PubMed]

12. Bakhtiar, H.; Mazidi, S.A.; Mohammadi Asl, S.; Ellini, M.R.; Moshiri, A.; Nekoofar, M.H.; Dummer, P.M.H. The role of stem cell therapy in regeneration of dentine-pulp complex: A systematic review. *Prog. Biomater.* **2018**, *7*, 249–268. [CrossRef] [PubMed]

13. Shah, R.; Hiremutt, D.; Jajoo, S.; Kamble, A. Dental tissue engineering: Future of regenerative dentistry. *J. Dent. Res. Sci. Dev.* **2016**, *3*, 31. [CrossRef]

14. Kwack, K.H.; Lee, H.W. Clinical Potential of Dental Pulp Stem Cells in Pulp Regeneration: Current Endodontic Progress and Future Perspectives. *Front. Cell Dev. Biol.* **2022**, *10*, 734. [CrossRef] [PubMed]

15. Mitsiadis, T.A.; Orsini, G. Stem Cell-Based Approaches in Dentistry. *Eur. Cells Mater.* **2015**, *30*, 248–257. [CrossRef]

16. Narang, S.; Sehgal, N. Stem cells: A potential regenerative future in dentistry. *Indian J. Hum. Genet.* **2012**, *18*, 150–154. [CrossRef]

17. Nakajima, K.; Kunimatsu, R.; Ando, K.; Hiraki, T.; Rikitake, K.; Tsuka, Y.; Abe, T.; Tanimoto, K. Success rates in isolating mesenchymal stem cells from permanent and deciduous teeth. *Sci. Rep.* **2019**, *9*, 16764. [CrossRef]

18. Shetty, R.M.; Prasad, P.; Shetty, S.; Patil, V.; Ramprasad, V.; Deoghare, A.; Boddun, M. SHED (Stem Cells from Human Exfoliated Deciduous teeth)—A new source of stem cells in dentistry. *Chhattisgarh J. Helath Sci.* **2013**, *1*, 66–68.

19. Rosa, V.; Dubey, N.; Islam, I.; Min, K.S.; Nör, J.E. Pluripotency of Stem Cells from Human Exfoliated Deciduous Teeth for Tissue Engineering. *Stem Cells Int.* **2016**, *2016*, 5957806. [CrossRef] [PubMed]

20. Taguchi, T.; Yanagi, Y.; Yoshimaru, K.; Zhang, X.Y.; Matsuura, T.; Nakayama, K.; Kobayashi, E.; Yamaza, H.; Nonaka, K.; Ohga, S.; et al. Regenerative medicine using stem cells from human exfoliated deciduous teeth (SHED): A promising new treatment in pediatric surgery. *Surg. Today* **2019**, *49*, 316–322. [CrossRef]

21. Jindal, L.; Bhat, N.; Vyas, D.; Thakur, K.; Mehta, S. Stem Cells from Human Exfoliated Deciduous Teeth (SHED)—Turning Useless into Miracle: A Review Article. *Acta Sci. Dent.Sci.* **2019**, *3*, 49–54. [CrossRef]

22. Wang, H.; Zhong, Q.; Yang, T.; Qi, Y.; Fu, M.; Yang, X.; Xiao, L.; Ling, Q.; Liu, S.; Zhao, Y. Comparative characterization of SHED and DPSCs during extended cultivation in vitro. *Mol. Med. Rep.* **2018**, *17*, 6551–6559. [CrossRef]

23. Dong, C.; Lv, Y. Application of collagen scaffold in tissue engineering: Recent advances and new perspectives. *Polymers* **2016**, *8*, 42. [CrossRef] [PubMed]

24. Joseph, N.V. Mesenchymal Stem Cells Seeded Decellularized Tendon Scaffold for Tissue Engineering. *Curr. Stem Cell Res. Ther.* **2021**, *16*, 155–164.

25. Fiorillo, L.; Cervino, G.; Galindo-Moreno, P.; Herford, A.S.; Spagnuolo, G.; Cicciù, M. Growth Factors in Oral Tissue Engineering: New Perspectives and Current Therapeutic Options. *Biomed. Res. Int.* **2021**, *2021*, 8840598. [CrossRef] [PubMed]

26. Duncan, H.F.; Kobayashi, Y.; Shimizu, E. Growth Factors and Cell Homing in Dental Tissue Regeneration. *Curr. Oral Health Rep.* **2018**, *5*, 276–285. [CrossRef]

27. Nosrat, A.; Kim, J.R.; Verma, P.; Chand, P.S. Tissue engineering considerations in dental pulp regeneration. *Iran Endod. J.* **2013**, *9*, 30–39. [PubMed]

28. Siddiqui, Z.; Acevedo-Jake, A.M.; Griffith, A.; Kadincesme, N.; Dabek, K.; Hindi, D.; Kim, K.K.; Kobayashi, Y.; Shimizu, E.; Kumar, V. Cells and material-based strategies for regenerative endodontics. *Bioact. Mater.* **2022**, *14*, 234–249. [CrossRef] [PubMed]

29. Retana-Lobo, C. Dental Pulp Regeneration: Insights from Biological Processes. *Odovtos Int. J. Dent. Sci.* **2017**, *20*, 10–16. [CrossRef]

30. Machla, F.; Angelopoulos, I.; Epple, M.; Chatzinikolaidou, M.; Bakopoulou, A. Biomolecule-Mediated Therapeutics of the Dentin–Pulp Complex: A Systematic Review. *Biomolecules* **2022**, *12*, 285. [CrossRef]

31. Nakashima, M.; Iohara, K.; Murakami, M.; Nakamura, H.; Sato, Y.; Ariji, Y.; Matsushita, K. Pulp regeneration by transplantation of dental pulp stem cells in pulpitis: A pilot clinical study. *Stem Cell Res. Ther.* **2017**, *8*, 1–13. [CrossRef] [PubMed]

32. Chandra Mouli, P.E.; Manoj Kumar, S.; Senthil, B.; Parthiban, S.; Priya, R.; Subha, R. Stem cells in dentistry—A review. *J. Pharm. Sci. Res.* **2012**, *4*, 1872–1876. [CrossRef]

33. Schmalz, G.; Smith, A.J. Pulp development, repair, and regeneration: Challenges of the transition from traditional dentistry to biologically based therapies. *J. Endod.* **2014**, *40* (Suppl. S4), S2–S5. [CrossRef] [PubMed]

34. Saskianti, T.; Ramadhani, R.; Budipramana, E.S.; Pradopo, S.; Suardita, K. Potential Proliferation of Stem Cell from Human Exfoliated Deciduous Teeth (SHED) in Carbonate Apatite and Hydroxyapatite Scaffold. *J. Int. Dent. Med. Res.* **2017**, *10*, 350–353.

35. Kumar, K.P.; Manjunath, S. Regenerative Endodontics: An Update. *J. Int. Acad. Res. Multidiscip.* **2014**, *2*, 139–147.

36. Farzin, A.; Bahrami, N.; Mohamadnia, A.; Mousavi, S.; Gholami, M.; Ai, J.; Moayeri, R.S. Scaffolds in Dental Tissue Engineering: A Review. *Arch. Neurosci.* **2019**, *7*, 1–5. [CrossRef]

37. Cui, D.; Yu, S.; Zhou, X.; Liu, Y.; Gan, L.; Pan, Y.; Zheng, L.; Wan, M. Roles of Dental Mesenchymal Stem Cells in the Management of Immature Necrotic Permanent Teeth. *Front. Cell Dev. Biol.* **2021**, 1030. [CrossRef]

38. Bjørge, I.M.; Kim, S.Y.; Mano, J.F.; Kalionis, B.; Chrzanowski, W. Extracellular vesicles, Exosomes and Shedding Vesicles in Regenerative Medicine—A new paradigm for tissue repair. *Biomater. Sci.* **2017**, *6*, 60–78. [CrossRef]

39. Sreelatha, A.; Nair, U.; Thavarajah, R.; Ranganathan, K. Saliva and dental practice. *J. Dr. NTR Univ. Health Sci.* **2012**, *1*, 72–76. [CrossRef]

40. Wang, S.; Qu, X.; Zhao, R.C. Clinical applications of mesenchymal stem cells. *J. Hematol. Oncol.* **2012**, *5*, 19. [CrossRef]

41. Abdullah, M.F. DPSCs and SHED in Tissue Engineering and Regenerative Medicine. *Open Stem Cell J.* **2013**, *4*, 1–6. [CrossRef]

42. Aljamie, M.; Alessa, L.; Noah, R.; Elsayed, L. Dental Pulp Stem Cells, a New Era in Regenerative Medicine: A Literature Review. *Open J. Stomatol.* **2016**, *6*, 155–163. [CrossRef]

43. Olaru, M.; Sachelarie, L.; Calin, G. Hard dental tissues regeneration—Approaches and challenges. *Materials* **2021**, *14*, 2558. [CrossRef]
44. Romito, A.; Cobellis, G. Pluripotent stem cells: Current understanding and future directions. *Stem Cells Int.* **2016**, *2016*, 9451492. [CrossRef]
45. Obuli Ganesh Kishore, S.; Don, K.R.; Jothi Priya, A. Therapeutic potential of stem cells from human exfoliated deciduous teeth(Shed)—A review. *Indian J. Forensic Med. Toxicol.* **2020**, *14*, 4624–4629. [CrossRef]
46. Mirzaei, H.; Sahebkar, A.; Shiri, L.; Moridikia, A.; Nazari, S.; Nahand, J.S.; Salehi, H.; Stenvang, J.; Masoudifar, A.; Mirzaei, H.R.; et al. Therapeutic application of multipotent stem cells. *J. Cell Physiol.* **2018**, *233*, 2815–2823. [CrossRef] [PubMed]
47. Horst, O.V.; Chavez, M.G.; Jheon, A.H.; Desai, T.; Klein, O.D. Stem Cell and Biomaterials Research in Dental Tissue Engineering and Regeneration. *Dent. Clin. N. Am.* **2012**, *56*, 495–520. [CrossRef] [PubMed]
48. Sohni, A.; Verfaillie, C.M. Mesenchymal stem cells migration homing and tracking. *Stem Cells Int.* **2013**, *2013*, 14–16. [CrossRef]
49. Ma, S.; Xie, N.; Li, W.; Yuan, B.; Shi, Y.; Wang, Y. Immunobiology of mesenchymal stem cells. *Cell Death Differ.* **2014**, *21*, 216–225. [CrossRef]
50. Gao, F.; Chiu, S.M.; Motan, D.A.L.; Zhang, Z.; Chen, L.; Ji, H.L.; Tse, H.F.; Fu, Q.L.; Lian, Q. Mesenchymal stem cells and immunomodulation: Current status and future prospects. *Cell Death Dis.* **2016**, *7*, e2062. [CrossRef]
51. Jacobs, S.A.; Roobrouck, V.D.; Verfaillie, C.M.; Van Gool, S.W. Immunological characteristics of human mesenchymal stem cells and multipotent adult progenitor cells. *Immunol. Cell Biol.* **2013**, *91*, 32–39. [CrossRef] [PubMed]
52. Zhao, Q.; Ren, H.; Han, Z. Mesenchymal stem cells: Immunomodulatory capability and clinical potential in immune diseases. *J. Cell Immunother.* **2016**, *2*, 3–20. [CrossRef]
53. Kim, J.Y.; Kim, M.R.; Kim, S.J. Modulation of osteoblastic/odontoblastic differentiation of adult mesenchymal stem cells through gene introduction: A brief review. *J. Korean Assoc. Oral Maxillofac. Surg.* **2013**, *39*, 55. [CrossRef] [PubMed]
54. Osman, Z.F.; Ahmad, A.; Noordin, K.B.A.A. Naturally derived scaffolds for dental pulp regeneration: A review. *Gulhane Med. J.* **2019**, *61*, 81–88. [CrossRef]
55. Botelho, J.; Cavacas, M.A.; Machado, V.; Mendes, J.J.; Cavacas, M.A.; Machado, V. Dental stem cells: Recent progresses in tissue engineering and regenerative medicine medicine. *Ann. Med.* **2017**, *49*, 644–651. [CrossRef]
56. Feter, Y.; Afiana, N.S.; Chandra, J.N.; Abdullah, K.; Shafira, J.; Sandra, F. Dental Mesenchymal Stem Cell: Its role in tooth development, types, surface antigens and differentiation potential. *Mol. Cell Biomed. Sci.* **2017**, *1*, 50. [CrossRef]
57. Smojver, I.; Katalinić, I.; Bjelica, R.; Gabric, D.; Matisic, V.; Molnar, V.; Primorac, D. Mesenchymal Stem Cells Based Treatment in Dental Medicine: A Narrative Review. *Int. J. Mol. Sci.* **2022**, *23*, 1662. [CrossRef]
58. Anggrarista, K.N.; Cecilia, P.H.N.A.; Saskianti, T.S.M. SHED, PRF, and Chitosan as Three-Dimensional of Tissue Engineering for Dental Pulp Regeneration. *Dent.Hypotheses* **2021**, *12*, 43–46.
59. Mori, G.; Brunetti, G.; Ballini, A.; Benedetto, A.D.; Tarantino, U.; Colucci, S.; Grano, M. Biological characteristics of dental stem cells for tissue engineering. *Key Eng. Mater.* **2013**, *541*, 51–59. [CrossRef]
60. Miura, M.; Gronthos, S.; Zhao, M.; Lu, B.; Fisher, L.W.; Robey, P.G.; Shi, S. SHED: Stem cells from human exfoliated deciduous teeth. *Proc. Natl. Acad. Sci. USA* **2003**, *100*, 5807–5812. [CrossRef] [PubMed]
61. Leyendecker, A., Jr.; Gomes Pinheiro, C.C.; Lazzaretti Fernandes, T.; Franco Bueno, D. The use of human dental pulp stem cells for in vivo bone tissue engineering: A systematic review. *J. Tissue Eng.* **2018**, *9*, 2041731417752766. [CrossRef] [PubMed]
62. Cao, L.; Su, H.; Si, M.; Xu, J.; Chang, X.; Jiajia, L.; Zhai, Y. Tissue Engineering in Stomatology: A Review of Potential Approaches for Oral Disease Treatments. *Front. Bioeng. Biotechnol.* **2021**, *9*, 662418. [CrossRef]
63. Karim, E.; Analysis, F.T.A.C.; Potential, O. A Comparative Analysis of the Osteogenic Potential of Dental Mesenchymal Stem Cells. *Stem Cells Dev.* **2019**, *28*, 1050–1058.
64. Prahasanti, C.; Ulfah, N.; Kusuma, I.I.; Hayati, N. Transforming Growth Factor-β 1 and Runt-related Transcription Factor 2 as Markers of Osteogenesis in Stem Cells from Human Exfoliated Deciduous Teeth Enriched Bone Grafting. *Contemp. Clin. Dent.* **2019**, *9*, 574–576. [CrossRef] [PubMed]
65. Elsayed, I.S.M. Mitigation of the urban heat island of the city of Kuala Lumpur, Malaysia. *Middle East J. Sci. Res.* **2012**, *11*, 1602–1613. [CrossRef]
66. Han, Y.; Zang, L.; Zhang, C.; Dissanayaka, W.L. Guiding Lineage Specific Differention of SHED for Target Tissue/Organ Regeneration. *Curr. Stem Cell Res. Ther.* **2021**, *16*, 518–584. [CrossRef] [PubMed]
67. Esrefoglu, M. Exfoliated Deciduous Teeth Pulp Stem Cells: Data on Experimental and Clinical Potential. *J. Gastroenterol. Hepatol. Res.* **2021**, *10*, 3548–3553. Available online: http://www.ghmet.org/index.php/joghr/article/view/3194 (accessed on 6 August 2022).
68. Khazaei, S.; Khademi, A.; Torabinejad, M.; Nasr Esfahani, M.H.; Khazaei, M.; Razavi, S.M. Improving pulp revascularization outcomes with buccal fat autotransplantation. *J. Tissue Eng. Regen. Med.* **2020**, *14*, 1227–1235. [CrossRef]
69. Vu, H.T.; Han, M.; Lee, J.; Kim, J.S.; Shin, J.S.; Yoon, J.Y.; Park, J.H.; Dashnyam, K.; Knowles, J.C.; Lee, H.H.; et al. Investigating the Effects of Conditioned Media from Stem Cells of Human Exfoliated Deciduous Teeth on Dental Pulp Stem Cells. *Biomedicines.* **2022**, *10*, 906. [CrossRef] [PubMed]
70. de Cara, S.P.H.M.; Origassa, C.S.T.; de Sá Silva, F.; Moreira, M.S.N.A.; de Almeida, D.C.; Pedroni, A.C.F.; Carvalho, G.L.; Cury, D.P.; Camara, N.O.S.; Marques, M.M. Angiogenic properties of dental pulp stem cells conditioned medium on endothelial cells in vitro and in rodent orthotopic dental pulp regeneration. *Heliyon.* **2019**, *5*, e01560. [CrossRef] [PubMed]

71. Bento, L.W.; Zhang, Z.; Imai, A.; Nor, F.; Dong, Z.; Shi, S.; Araujo, F.B.; Nor, J.E. Endothelial differentiation of SHED requires MEK1/ERK signaling. *J. Dent. Res.* **2013**, *92*, 51–57. [CrossRef] [PubMed]
72. Yildirim, S.; Zibandeh, N.; Genc, D.; Ozcan, E.M.; Goker, K.; Akkoc, T. The comparison of the immunologic properties of stem cells isolated from human exfoliated deciduous teeth, dental pulp, and dental follicles. *Stem Cells Int.* **2016**, *2016*, 11–13. [CrossRef]
73. Bhandi, S.; Khatani, A.A.; Sumayli, H.A.; Sabyei, M.Y.; Zailai, A.M.A.; Sumaili, M.A.; Hakami, H.I.; Jafer, M.A.; Vyas, N.; Baeshen, H.A.; et al. Comparative analysis of cytokines and growth factors in the conditioned media of stem cells from the pulp of deciduous, young, and old permanent tooth. *Saudi J. Biol. Sci.* **2021**, *28*, 3559–3565. [CrossRef] [PubMed]
74. Diogenes, A.; Henry, M.A.; Teixeira, F.B.; Hargreaves, K.M. An update on clinical regenerative endodontics. *Br. Dent. J.* **2013**, *215*, 289. [CrossRef]
75. Wu, D.T.; Munguia-Lopez, J.G.; Cho, Y.W.; Ma, X.; Song, V.; Zhu, Z.; Tran, S.D. Polymeric scaffolds for dental, oral, and craniofacial regenerative medicine. *Molecules.* **2021**, *26*, 7043. [CrossRef] [PubMed]
76. Albuquerque, M.T.P.; Valera, M.C.; Nakashima, M.; Nör, J.E.; Bottino, M.C. Tissue-engineering-based strategies for regenerative endodontics. *J. Dent. Res.* **2014**, *93*, 1222–1231. [CrossRef] [PubMed]
77. Gupte, M.J.; Ma, P.X. Nanofibrous scaffolds for dental and craniofacial applications. *J. Dent. Res.* **2012**, *91*, 227–234. [CrossRef] [PubMed]
78. Hagar, M.N.; Yazid, F.; Luchman, N.A.; Hisham, S.; Ariffin, Z. Comparative evaluation of osteogenic differentiation potential of stem cells derived from dental pulp and exfoliated deciduous teeth cultured over granular hydroxyapatite based scaffold. *BMC Oral Health.* **2021**, *21*, 1–13. [CrossRef] [PubMed]
79. Dayı, B.; Sezlev Bilecen, D.; Eröksüz, H.; Yalçın, M.; Hasırcı, V. Evaluation of a collagen-bioaggregate composite scaffold in the repair of sheep pulp tissue. *Eur. Oral Res.* **2021**, *55*, 152–161. [CrossRef] [PubMed]
80. Galler, K.M.; D'Souza, R.N.; Hartgerink, J.D.; Schmalz, G. Scaffolds for dental pulp tissue engineering. *Adv. Dent. Res.* **2011**, *23*, 333–339. [CrossRef] [PubMed]
81. Rosa, V. What and where are the stem cells for Dentistry? *Singap. Dent. J.* **2013**, *34*, 13–18. [CrossRef]
82. Bottino, M.C.; Pankajakshan, D.; Nör, J.E. Advanced Scaffolds for Dental Pulp and Periodontal Regeneration. *Dent. Clin. N. Am.* **2017**, *61*, 689–711. [CrossRef]
83. Rosa, V.; Zhang, Z.; Grande, R.H.M.; Nör, J.E. Dental pulp tissue engineering in full-length human root canals. *J. Dent. Res.* **2013**, *92*, 970–975. [CrossRef] [PubMed]
84. Moussa, D.G.; Aparicio, C. Present and future of tissue engineering scaffolds for dentin-pulp complex regeneration. *J. Tissue Eng. Regen. Med.* **2019**, *13*, 58–75. [CrossRef] [PubMed]
85. Annibali, S.; Cristalli, M.P.; Tonoli, F.; Polimeni, A. Stem cells derived from human exfoliated deciduous teeth: A narrative synthesis of literature. *Eur. Rev. Med. Pharmacol. Sci.* **2014**, *18*, 2863–2881. [PubMed]
86. Xie, F.; He, J.; Chen, Y.; Hu, Z.; Qin, M.; Hui, T. Multi-lineage differentiation and clinical application of stem cells from exfoliated deciduous teeth. *Hum. Cell.* **2020**, *33*, 295–302. [CrossRef] [PubMed]
87. Arany, P.R.; Huang, G.X.; Gadish, O.; Feliz, J.; Weaver, J.C.; Kim, J.; Yuen, W.W.; Mooney, D.J. Multi-lineage MSC differentiation via engineered morphogen fields. *J. Dent. Res.* **2014**, *93*, 1250–1257. [CrossRef] [PubMed]
88. Gupta, S.; Sharma, C.; Dinda, A.K.; Ray, A.K.; Mishra, N.C. Tooth tissue engineering: Potential and piffalls. *J. Biomim. Biomater. Tissue Eng.* **2012**, *12*, 59–81. [CrossRef]
89. y Baena, A.R.; Casasco, A.; Monti, M. Hypes and Hopes of Stem Cell Therapies in Dentistry: A Review. *Stem Cell Rev.Rep.* **2022**, *18*, 1294–1308. [CrossRef] [PubMed]
90. Kerkis, I.; Caplan, A.I. Stem cells in dental pulp of deciduous teeth. *Tissue Eng. Part B Rev.* **2012**, *18*, 129–138. [CrossRef] [PubMed]
91. Hara, K.; Yamada, Y.; Nakamura, S.; Umemura, E.; Ito, K.; Ueda, M. Potential characteristics of stem cells from human exfoliated deciduous teeth compared with bone marrow-derived mesenchymal stem cells for mineralized tissue-forming cell biology. *J. Endod.* **2011**, *37*, 1647–1652. [CrossRef] [PubMed]
92. Koh, B.; Sulaiman, N.; Nursyazwani, S.; Ramli, R.; Yunus, S.S.; Idrus, R.; Arifin, S.H.Z.; Wahab, R.M.A.; Yasid, M.D. Mesenchymal stem cells: A comprehensive methods for odontoblastic induction. *Biol. Proc.Online* **2021**, *23*, 18. [CrossRef] [PubMed]
93. Kim, J.K.; Baker, J.; Nor, J.E.; Hill, E.E. MTor plays an important role in odontoblast differentiation. *J. Endod.* **2011**, *37*, 1081–1085. [CrossRef] [PubMed]
94. Dahake, P.T.; Panpaliya, N.P.; Kale, Y.J.; Dadpe, M.V.; Kendre, S.B.; Bogar, C. Response of stem cells from human exfoliated deciduous teeth (SHED) to three bioinductive materials—An in vitro experimental study. *Saudi Dent. J.* **2020**, *32*, 43–51. [CrossRef] [PubMed]
95. Fujii, H.; Matsubara, K.; Sakai, K.; Ito, M.; Ohno, K.; Ueda, M.; Yamamoto, A. Dopaminergic differentiation of stem cells from human deciduous teeth and their therapeutic benefits for Parkinsonian rats. *Brain Res.* **2015**, *1613*, 59–72. [CrossRef]
96. Nourbakhsh, N.; Soleimani, M.; Taghipour, Z.; Karbalaie, K.; Mousavi, S.B.; Talebi, A.; Nadali, F.; Tanhaei, S.; Kiyani, G.A.; Nematollahi, M.; et al. Induced in vitro differentiation of neural-like cells from human exfoliated deciduous teeth-derived stem cells. *Int. J. Dev. Biol.* **2011**, *55*, 189–195. [CrossRef]
97. Liu, J.; Zhang, Z.Y.; Yu, H.; Yang, A.P.; Hu, P.F.; Liu, Z.; Wang, M. Long noncoding RNA C21orf121/bone morphogenetic protein 2/microRNA-140-5p gene network promotes directed differentiation of stem cells from human exfoliated deciduous teeth to neuronal cells. *J. Cell Biochem.* **2019**, *120*, 1464–1476. [CrossRef]

98. Cordeiro, M.M.; Dong, Z.; Kaneko, T.; Zhang, Z.; Miyazawa, M.; Shi, S.; Smith, A.J.; Nor, J.E. Dental Pulp Tissue Engineering with Stem Cells from Exfoliated Deciduous Teeth. *J. Endod.* **2008**, *34*, 962–969. [CrossRef]

99. Demarco, F.F.; Casagrande, L.; Zhang, Z.; Dong, Z.; Tarquinio, S.B.; Zeitlin, B.D.; Shi, S.; Smith, A.J.; Nor, J.E. Effects of morphogen and scaffold porogen on the differentiation of dental pulp stem cells. *J. Endod.* **2010**, *36*, 1805–1811. [CrossRef]

100. Kodonas, K.; Gogos, C.; Papadimitriou, S.; Kouzi-Koliakou, K.; Tziafas, D. Experimental formation of dentin-like structure in the root canal implant model using cryopreserved swine dental pulp progenitor cells. *J. Endod.* **2012**, *38*, 913–919. [CrossRef]

101. Wang, Y.; Zhao, Y.; Jia, W.; Yang, J.; Ge, L. Preliminary study on dental pulp stem cell-mediated pulp regeneration in canine immature permanent teeth. *J. Endod.* **2013**, *39*, 195–201. [CrossRef] [PubMed]

102. Iohara, K.; Murakami, M.; Nakata, K.; Nakashima, M. Age-dependent decline in dental pulp regeneration after pulpectomy in dogs. *Exp. Gerontol.* **2014**, *52*, 39–45. [CrossRef]

103. Qu, T.; Jing, J.; Jiang, Y.; Tailor, R.J.; Feng, J.Q.; Geiger, B.; Liu, X. Magnesium-containing nanostructured hybrid scaffolds for enhanced dentin regeneration. *Tissue Eng. Part A.* **2014**, *20*, 2422–2433. [CrossRef] [PubMed]

104. Murakami, M.; Hayashi, Y.; Iohara, K.; Osako, Y.; Hirose, Y.; Nakashima, M. Trophic effects and regenerative potential of mobilized mesenchymal stem cells from bone marrow and adipose tissue as alternative cell sources for pulp/dentin regeneration. *Cell Transplant.* **2015**, *24*, 1753–1765. [CrossRef]

105. Kwon, Y.S.; Lee, S.H.; Hwang, Y.C.; Rosa, V.; Lee, K.W.; Min, K.S. Behaviour of human dental pulp cells cultured in a collagen hydrogel scaffold cross-linked with cinnamaldehyde. *Int. Endod. J.* **2017**, *50*, 58–66. [CrossRef]

106. Piva, E.; Tarlé, S.A.; Nör, J.E.; Zou, D.; Hatfield, E.; Guinn, T.; Eubanks, E.J.; Kaigler, D. Dental Pulp Tissue Regeneration Using Dental Pulp Stem Cells Isolated and Expanded in Human Serum. *J. Endod.* **2017**, *43*, 568–574. [CrossRef]

107. Widbiller, M.; Driesen, R.B.; Eidt, A.; Lambrichts, I.; Hiller, K.; Buchalla, W.; Schmalz, G.; Galle, K. Cell Homing for Pulp Tissue Engineering with Endogenous Dentin Matrix Proteins. *J. Endod.* **2018**, *44*, 956–962.e2. [CrossRef] [PubMed]

108. Chang, C.C.; Lin, T.A.; Wu, S.Y.; Lin, C.P.; Chang, H.H. Regeneration of Tooth with Allogenous, Autoclaved Treated Dentin Matrix with Dental Pulpal Stem Cells: An In Vivo Study. *J. Endod.* **2020**, *46*, 1256–1264. [CrossRef]

109. Chen, H.; Fu, H.; Wu, X.; Duan, Y.; Zhang, S.; Hu, H.; Liao, Y.; Wang, T.; Yang, Y.; Chen, G.; et al. Regeneration of pulpo-dentinal-like complex by a group of unique multipotent CD24a+ stem cells. *Sci. Adv.* **2020**, *6*, 1–15. [CrossRef]

110. Jang, J.H.; Moon, J.H.; Kim, S.G.; Kim, S.Y. Pulp regeneration with hemostatic matrices as a scaffold in an immature tooth minipig model. *Sci. Rep.* **2020**, *10*, 12536. [CrossRef]

111. Gl, S.P.; Ramalingam, S.; Udhayakumar, Y. Human dental pulp stem cells and its applications in regenerative medicine—A literature review. *J.Glob. Oral Health* **2019**, *1*, 59–67. [CrossRef]

112. Cooper, P.R.; Holder, M.J.; Smith, A.J. Inflammation and regeneration in the dentin-pulp complex: A double-edged sword. *J. Endod.* **2014**, *40* (Suppl. S4), S46–S51. [CrossRef] [PubMed]

113. Janebodin, K.; Chavanachat, R.; Hays, A. Silencing VEGFR-2 Hampers Odontoblastic Differentiation of Dental Pulp Stem Cells. *Front. Cell Dev. Biol.* **2021**, *9*, 1–14. [CrossRef]

114. Hu, L.; Liu, Y.; Wang, S. Stem cell based tooth and periodontal regeneration. *Oral Dis.* **2018**, *24*, 696–705. [CrossRef]

115. Morotomi, T.; Washio, A.; Kitamura, C. Current and future options for dental pulp therapy. *Jpn. Dent. Sci. Rev.* **2019**, *55*, 5–11. [CrossRef] [PubMed]

116. Malik, Z.; Roth, D.M.; Eaton, F.; Theodor, J.M.; Graf, D. Mesenchymal Bmp7 Controls Onset of Tooth Mineralization: A Novel Way to Regulate Molar Cusp Shape. *Front. Physiol.* **2020**, *11*, 1–13. [CrossRef]

117. Vera, C.; Tapia, V.; Vega, M.; Romero, C. Role of nerve growth factor and its TRKA receptor in normal ovarian and epithelial ovarian cancer angiogenesis. *J.Ovarian Res.* **2014**, *7*, 1–8. [CrossRef]

118. Wang, H.; Wang, R.; Thrimawithana, T.; Little, P.J.; Xu, J.; Feng, Z.; Zheng, W. The Nerve Growth Factor Signaling and Its Potential as Therapeutic Target for Glaucoma. *Biomed. Res. Int.* **2014**, *2014*, 759473. [CrossRef] [PubMed]

119. Zha, K.; Yang, Y.; Tian, G.; Sun, Z.; Yang, Z.; Li, X.; Sui, X.; Liu, S.; Zhao, J.; Guo, Q. Nerve growth factor (NGF) and NGF receptors in mesenchymal stem/stromal cells: Impact on potential therapies. *Stem Cells Transl. Med.* **2021**, *10*, 1008–1020. [CrossRef]

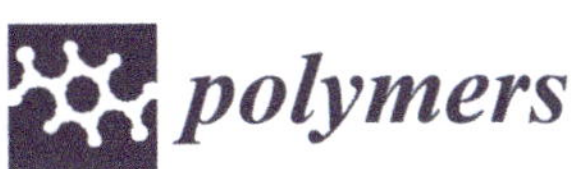

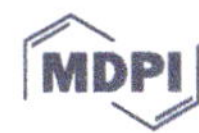

Article

Identification and Characterization of Fibronectin-Binding Peptides in Gelatin

Yuying Liu [1,2], Jianping Gao [1,2], Lin Liu [3], Jiyao Kang [1], Xi Luo [1], Yingjun Kong [1] and Guifeng Zhang [1,2,*]

1   State Key Laboratory of Biochemical Engineering, Institute of Process Engineering, Chinese Academy of Sciences, Beijing 100190, China
2   School of Chemical and Engineering, University of Chinese Academy of Sciences, Beijing 100049, China
3   Library of Shandong Agricultural University, Tai'an 271018, China
*   Correspondence: gfzhang@ipe.ac.cn

Abstract: Collagen and fibronectin (FN) are important components in the extracellular matrix (ECM). Collagen-FN binding belongs to protein-protein interaction and plays a key role in regulating cell behaviors. In this study, FN-binding peptides were isolated from gelatin (degraded collagen) using affinity chromatography, and the amino acid sequences were determined using HPLC-MS. The results indicated that all FN-binding peptides contained GPAG or GPPG. Matrix-assisted laser desorption/ionization time-of-flight mass spectrometry (MALDI-TOF MS) and dual-polarization interferometry (DPI) were used to analyze the effects of hydroxylation polypeptide on FN binding activity. DPI analysis indicated that peptides with molecular weight (MW) between 2 kDa and 30 kDa showed higher FN-binding activity, indicating MW range played an important role in the interaction between FN and peptides. Finally, two peptides with similar sequences except for hydroxylation of prolines were synthesized. The FN-binding properties of the synthesized peptides were determined by MALDI-TOF MS. For peptide, GAPGADGP*AGAPGTP*GPQGIAGQR, hydroxylation of P8 and P15 is necessary for FN-binding. For peptide, GPPGPMGPPGLAGPPGESGR, the FN-binding process is independent of proline hydroxylation. Thus, FN-binding properties are proline-hydroxylation dependent.

Keywords: collagen; gelatin; fibronectin-binding; peptides; HPLC-MS

Citation: Liu, Y.; Gao, J.; Liu, L.; Kang, J.; Luo, X.; Kong, Y.; Zhang, G. Identification and Characterization of Fibronectin-Binding Peptides in Gelatin. *Polymers* **2022**, *14*, 3757. https://doi.org/10.3390/polym14183757

Academic Editors: Nunzia Gallo, Marta Madaghiele, Alessandra Quarta and Amilcare Barca

Received: 6 August 2022
Accepted: 5 September 2022
Published: 8 September 2022

Publisher's Note: MDPI stays neutral with regard to jurisdictional claims in published maps and institutional affiliations.

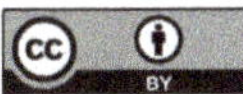

Copyright: © 2022 by the authors. Licensee MDPI, Basel, Switzerland. This article is an open access article distributed under the terms and conditions of the Creative Commons Attribution (CC BY) license (https://creativecommons.org/licenses/by/4.0/).

1. Introduction

Collagen and fibronectin (FN) play a vital role in the extracellular matrix (ECM). Collagen is a biopolymer synthesized by animal cells, due to its special physiological function and high nutritional value, it is widely used in healthcare, cosmetics, and medical materials. It could prevent cardiovascular and cerebrovascular diseases and can lower blood pressure [1–3]. Collagen could interact with FN [4], but gelatin and denatured collagen have stronger binding activities than collagen [5]. In the ECM, the conjugation has important biological significance. The binding of collagen to FN could cause a conformational change in FN, leading to various biological responses, such as attachment to the cell surface to promote cell migration and wound repair, as well as differences in integrin receptor binding [6]. However, the absence of collagen in cultured primary fibroblasts will affect the arrangement of FN in the ECM [7]. Consequently, the study of collagen and FN binding sites is key to some relevant biological interactions.

FN, a 450 kDa glycoprotein, is composed of three modules (F1, F2, and F3). In the binding of FN and collagen, it is known that the 42 kDa fragment near the N-terminal of FN, 6F1-1F2-2F2-7F1-8F1-9F1 (n denotes the nth type in the nomenclature nFX) [8], is the collagen-binding domain. The F2 module plays a pivotal role in the interaction, but almost all the modules in the 42-kDa fragment are important [9].

In collagen, the specific FN-binding sites have not yet been identified. The binding activity is influenced by many factors, including the molecular weight (MW) and the hydroxylation modification of collagen. Hydroxyproline is a unique amino acid of collagen, and the content of hydroxyproline differs with age and gender [10,11]. Therefore, hydroxyproline plays a critical role in collagen-FN binding. Due to the stronger binding activity of gelatin, undoubtedly, MW contributes to the binding because the modest MW radically exposed more FN-binding sites in denatured collagen than in collagen. However, these factors have yet to be thoroughly studied. In 1978, Kleinman discovered α1-CB7, digested by CNBr and purified by ion exchange chromatography, in residues 757–791, and the author identified this as the classic FN-binding region [12]. In Dessau's study, FN could bind to collagen type I, II, III, IV, and V in vitro, as there is a binding site in every helix of collagen. Positions 643–819 in the α1 chain contain an FN-binding site, and a domain homologous to the binding site in residues 693–1101 of the α2 chain was identified by fluorescence chromatography [13]. Gao separated two non-triple helical regions of collagen by FN-sepharose affinity chromatography, size exclusion high-performance liquid chromatography (HPLC), and enzyme-linked immunosorbent assay (ELISA) [14]. In addition, CNBr cleaved collagen α1(II) to obtain CB10 (position 550–900), CB11 (100–400), CB8 (400–550), CB9.7 (900–1000), and CB12 (0–100). In these fragments, CB10 and CB12 had binding activity, as detected by fluorescence polarization, and the activity of CB8 was weaker. Furthermore, α2(I)-CB4 and CB5, which were homologous to CB10 and CB12, respectively, were active in FN binding [15]. More recent research suggested that there were at least fourteen distinct sites in collagen type I to interact with FN: five on each of the α1 chains and four on the α2 chain, using fluorescence anisotropy [16]. However, all the above-mentioned studies used CNBr to cleave collagen and analyzed the binding activity of the cleaved fragments to FN, without specific binding site analysis. These fragments comprised a longer region, and the MW range was broad (from several thousand to tens of thousands). The binding sites were still uncertain. Furthermore, the detection and analysis methods almost used fluorescence chromatography.

High-performance liquid chromatography/tandem mass spectrometry (HPLC-MS) has been successfully applied to the analysis of the digested peptides in collagens or post-translational modification residues of peptides. Dual-polarization interferometry (DPI) has been employed for the analysis of protein-protein/small molecule interactions, protein conformational changes in the solid interface, and protein-solid interface interactions [17]. In this paper, the interaction of peptides and FN was analyzed by HPLC-MS/MS in combination with DPI, and key factors of the binding were investigated. Specifically, bovine gelatin was digested by trypsin after passing through the FN affinity column. The sequence of the separated peptides was analyzed, and the hydroxylation modification position of proline was determined by HPLC-MS/MS. Then, the sequences were synthesized, including hydroxylation modification, and the interaction with FN was detected via MALDI-TOF MS. In addition, the effect of the MW was analyzed by DPI.

2. Materials and Methods

2.1. Materials

Bovine gelatin (G9382, type B) and human FN were purchased from Sigma-Aldrich (St. Louis, MO, USA). Trypsin (sequencing grade) was obtained from Promega (Madison, WI, USA). Trifluoroacetic acid (TFA) and acetonitrile (ACN) were purchased from Fisher Scientific (Fair Lawn, JN, USA). α-Cyano-4-hydroxycinnamic acid (CHCA) was purchased from Bruker (Billerica, MA, USA). 3-Aminopropyltriethoxysilane (APTES) was purchased from Alfa Aesar (Haverhill, MA, USA). An unmodified Anachip was purchased from Farfield (Sensors Ltd., Salford, UK). The four synthesized peptides were purified by Beijing Scilight Biotechnology Led. Co. (Beijing, China).

2.2. Methods

2.2.1. Preparation of FN Sepharose Affinity Media

Sepharose 4FF (National Engineering Research Center for Biotechnology, Beijing, China) was activated by 1,4-butanediol diglycidyl ether. Human FN (1 mg/mL) was coupled to 3 mL of activated sepharose for 24 h at 37 °C. Active groups were blocked with ethanolamine for 4 h at 37 °C. Then, the sepharose was washed alternatively with buffer solutions at pH 8.0 and pH 4.0. The matrix was filled in the column (1.0 cm × 4.0 cm) to prepare FN-affinity column. The same method was also used to prepare the micro-FN-affinity column (100 µL).

2.2.2. Tryptic Digestion

Twenty milligrams of bovine gelatin were dissolved in 5 mL of ultrapure water. Two times the volume of ethanol was added, and the mixture was kept at 4 °C for 30 min. The gelatin solution was centrifuged at 10,000 r/min for 10 min to precipitate the gelatin. The high MW peptides of the precipitate were recovered in trypsin resuspension buffer (pH 8.0), and 1:50 (w/w) trypsin solution (1 µg/µL in trypsin resuspension buffer, pH 8.0) was added. The mixture was incubated at 37 °C for 12 h.

2.2.3. FN Affinity Chromatography [9,14,17]

The digest was loaded onto the FN-affinity column and stabilized in 20 mM PBS equilibrium buffer (pH = 7.4). The column was washed in equilibrium buffer, and peptides were eluted with 3 M urea in equilibrium buffer. The eluted peptides were desalted by Sephadex G-25 (GE Healthcare, Chicago, IL, USA) and concentrated. The obtained peptides were referred to as sample 1.

The undigested gelatin was separated in the same way, and the isolated peptides were digested by trypsin at 37 °C for 12 h. The obtained peptides were referred to as sample 2.

2.2.4. MALDI-TOF MS Analysis

The MW ranges of samples 1 and 2 were determined using MALDI-TOF-MS (autoflex III smartbeam, Bruker, Bremen, Germany) [18]. The samples were mixed in the ratio 1:1 with the α-cyano-4-hydroxycinnamic acid matrix (5 mg/mL in 50% ACN containing 0.1% TFA), and the samples were spotted on the MALDI target. The mass scan range was set from m/z 600 to 10,000. A mass scan was performed in the positive ion mode and linear detector.

The synthesized peptides were loaded onto the micro-FN-affinity column, followed by the washing solution. The eluted peptides were also analyzed by MALDI-TOF MS.

2.2.5. HPLC-MS Analysis

The separated peptides in samples 1 and 2 were analyzed by HPLC-MS [19]. The HPLC-MS system consisted of an Agilent 1100 HPLC and MS (LCQ DecaXP, Thermo Electron, San Jose, CA, USA). The samples were loaded onto an Agilent Zorbax SB C18 column (2.1 mm × 150 mm, 5 µm). Mobile phase A was water (containing 0.1% TFA), and mobile phase B was ACN (containing 0.1% TFA). The HPLC gradient was 5–40% B from 0 to 50 min; 40–80% B from 50 to 80 min. The flow rate was 0.2 mL/min. The outlet of the column was introduced into the ion source of an electrospray ionization mass spectrometer. The spray voltage was 4.5 kV, and the capillary was kept at 300 °C. The data acquisition consisted of three scan events: an MS scan, followed by one zoom scan to determine the charge state of the ion, and an MS/MS scan to generate an MS/MS spectrum. The MS scan range was from m/z 400 to 2000. The zoom scan and tandem mass spectrometry (MS/MS) functions were performed in data-dependent mode. Dynamic exclusion was adopted to one count and a 0.5 min exclusion duration unit. The collision energy value was installed to 35%.

2.2.6. Database Searching and Data Processing

Sequence information from MS/MS data was processed using the Turbo SEQUEST algorithm in Bioworks 3.2 software (Thermo Electron, San Jose, CA, USA). A database was created by extracting bovine type I collagen entries from the Swiss-Prot/TrEMBL database (http://www.expasy.org, accessed on 15 July 2020). The database searches and SEQUEST criteria were based on a previously published method [19].

2.2.7. Surface Modification of DPI Chip

The unmodified DPI sensor chip (AnaChip™, Farfield Sensors Ltd., Manchester, UK) was successively cleaned by ultrasonication in ethanol, acetone, and ultrapure water for 5 min. Then, the chip was immersed in piranha solution (7:3 sulfuric acid to hydrogen peroxide) at 90 °C for 2 h, rinsed in ultrapure water, and dried. APTES was added to anhydrous toluene to create solution concentrations of 0.001 mol/L APTES. The chip was placed in the APTES solution to react for 30 min, followed by ultrasonication in anhydrous toluene. The chip was dried by nitrogen stream. Finally, an amine-functionalized surface formed on the chip [20].

2.2.8. DPI Analysis and Data Processing [17,20]

The modified chip was installed in an AnaLight® Bio200 dual-polarization interferometer (Farfield Sensors Ltd., Salford, UK). The laser beam (λ = 632.8 nm) with two orthogonal polarizations passed through the chip. When the protein was loaded on the chip surface, the upper sensing waveguide was changed, and the lower reference waveguide of the chip was of no influence, causing the laser to produce an evanescent field change. This resulted in a shift of the interference fringes. Subsequently, the change in transverse magnetic (TM) and transverse electric (TE) phases was used to calculate the refractive index and thickness, respectively, via the Maxwell equation. Tris-HCl buffer (pH 7.4, including the 0.1 M NaCl) flowed over the chip surface. The instrument was calibrated with ethanol and H_2O prior to the experiment. To prepare the chip, 100 μg/mL FN was injected, followed by the sealing agent. Then, the peptides samples were injected, and the surface dimensions and densities were measured. The data were automatically analyzed by AnaLight DAQ.

3. Results and Discussion

3.1. Separation of Peptides through FN Affinity Chromatography

Due to the affinity of FN with gelatin, peptides in gelatin were separated by affinity chromatography, in which affinity media was prepared by coupling FN on agarose media. The sample was precipitated by ethanol and then was dissolved with PBS buffer (pH = 7.4) before adding to the separating column. The affinity chromatography results were shown in Figure 1. Fragments of nonspecific adsorption were removed by washing the column with 20 mM PBS buffer (pH 7.4), and the binding peptides were eluted with 3 M urea [21]. The elution peak with the high concentration of salt would affect the mass spectrometric detection. The peptide fraction was desalted with SephadexG-25(10 mL) (Figure 2). Figure 1 illustrated that not all the peptides from the digested gelatin could bind to the FN, and only a few containing special sequences could bind to the N-terminal 42 kDa region of FN. We inferred that the special sequences may play an important role in FN-affinity. In Figure 2, it could be seen that the MW range of the separated peptides changed. The main peaks were distributed in 6–8 mL, which were some peptides with larger MW.

3.2. MALDI-TOF MS Analysis of the MW Range

The MW range of the two separated samples was analyzed using MALDI-TOF MS. The mass spectra in Figures 3 and 4 showed that the MW range of both samples was from approximately 1000 to less than 6000 Da but was mainly distributed between 2000 and 3000 Da. In Figure 3, the analysis for sample 1 indicated that the separated peptides were degraded into the lower MW range, and the sequences could be analyzed by HPLC-MS. The analysis of sample 2 in Figure 4 indicated that the lower MW peptides of the digested gelatin could also bind to FN alone.

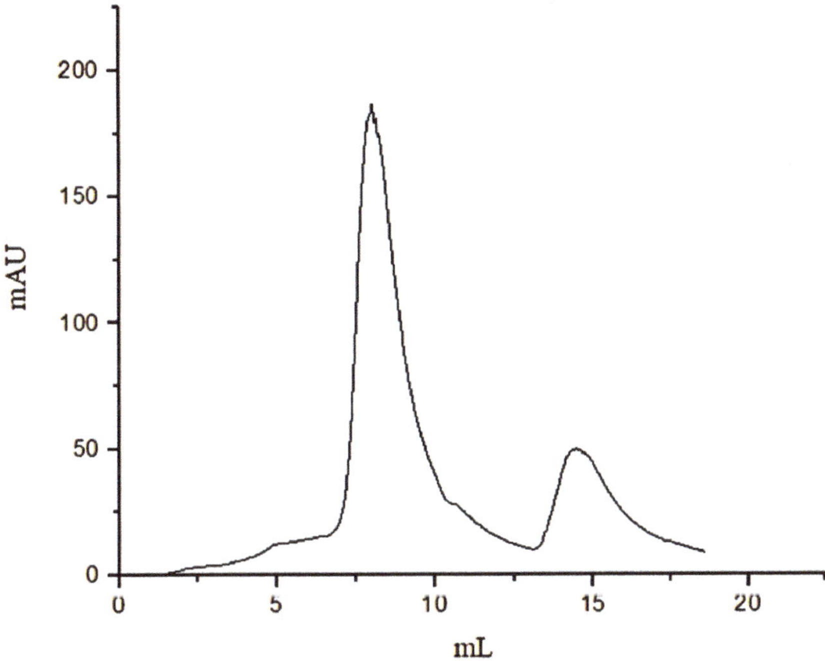

Figure 1. Affinity chromatography of separation peptides in the gelatin.

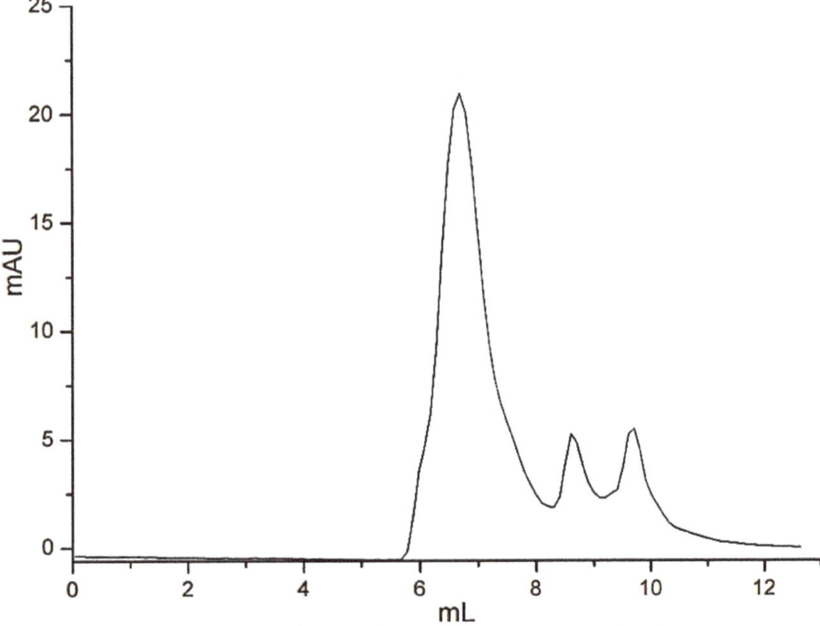

Figure 2. Gel filtration chromatograms of the desalinated peptide fraction.

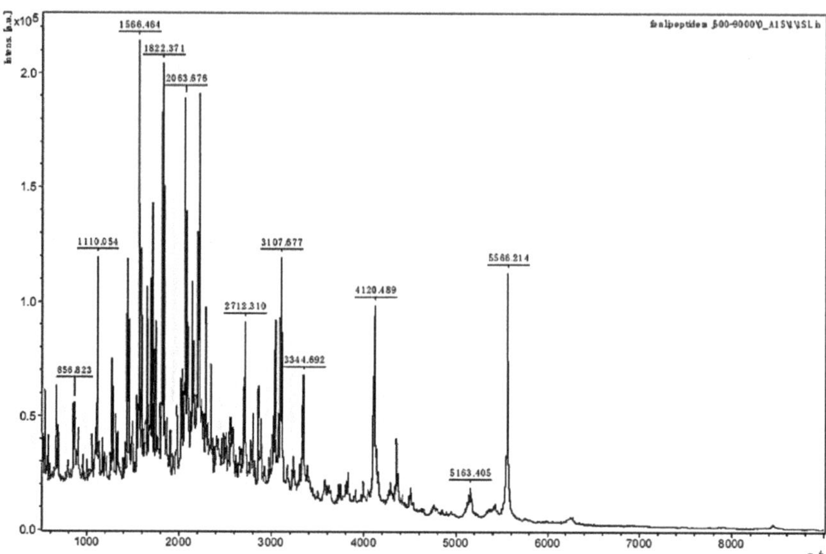

Figure 3. MALDI-TOF MS mass spectra of sample 1.

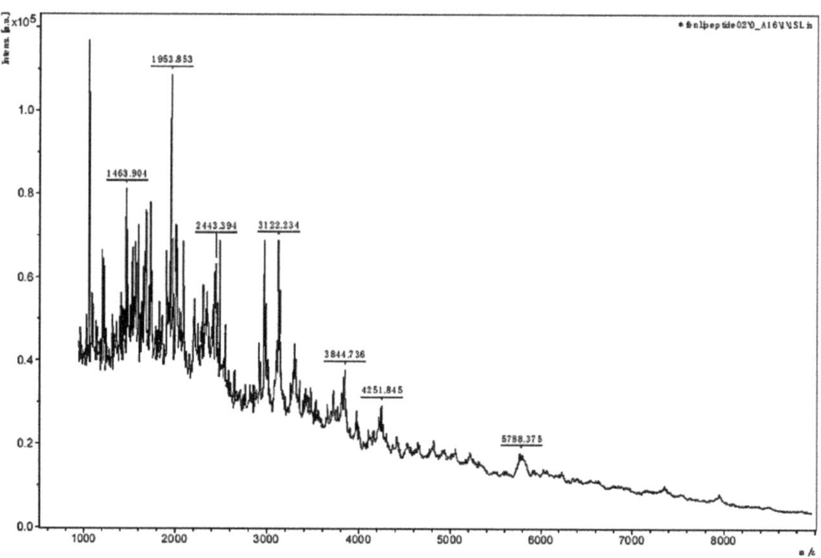

Figure 4. MALDI-TOF MS mass spectra of sample 2.

3.3. HPLC-MS Analysis of the Peptide Sequences

Bovine gelatin, the separated gelatin (not digested), sample 1, and sample 2 were analyzed by HPLC-MS, and the corresponding chromatograms are shown in Figure 5. The similarity of the traces in Figure 5A,B indicated that gelatin contains many peptides that could bind to FN. In contrast to Figure 5B–D, the retention time in Figure 5C,D was much shorter than that in Figure 5B, further indicating that the larger peptides in the gelatin were degraded into smaller peptides. Database searching and software analysis (2.2.6) of the mass spectra shown in Figure 5C,D were performed, and the results are listed in Table 1. Thirteen varieties of peptides were found in both samples 1 and 2. Sample 1 was obtained by tryptic digestion of gelatin followed by FN affinity column separation, while sample 2 was obtained by FN affinity column separation of gelation followed by tryptic digestion. The identified peptides in sample 2 consisted of shorter sequences that could directly bind to FN, and so do the extended sequences before tryptic digestion. Therefore, the region of the FN-binding sites could be narrowed to these sequences, including GPAG and GPPG, which were repeated in one sequence. The hydroxylation modification degree of proline in the repeated GPAG and GPPG sequences was not high. In the reported literature, the Y position of G-X-Y in the FN-binding region had lower hydroxyproline content and stronger hydrophobicity, causing the collagen helix expansion to expose the active FN-binding site [22]. Consequently, the active sites of FN-binding might exist in GPAG and GPPG. Ingham K.C. found that type I collagen contains at least 14 cryptic FN binding sites of similar affinity [16].

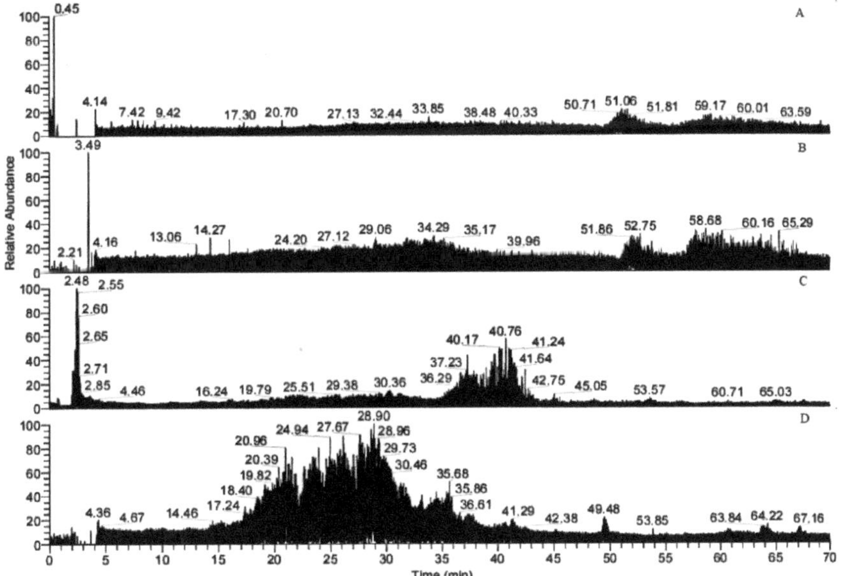

Figure 5. Total ion chromatograms of the bovine gelatins digested at 37 °C for 12 h. (**A**) Bovine gelatin; (**B**) separated gelatin before sample 1 was digested; (**C**) sample 1; (**D**) sample 2.

Table 1. Peptides in samples 1 and 2 identified from database searching.

Number	*m/z*	Position	Sequence
1	1590.82	α1.586–603	GLTGPIGPP*GPAGAP*GDK
2	2089.02	α1.757–780	GAPGADGP*AGAPGTP*GPQGIAGQR
3	1816.88	α1.817–836	GPP*GPMGPPGLAGPP*GESGR
4	1560.81	α1.889–906	GETGPAGPAGPIGPVGAR
5	868.47	α2.102–111	VGAP*GPAGAR
6	1287.64	α2.328–341	GFP*GSP*GNIGPAGK
7	1427.74	α2.451–465	GIP*GEFGLPGP*AGAR
8	1580.77	α2.469–486	GPP*GESGAAGPTGPIGSR
9	1845.92	α2.672–692	TGPP*GP*SGISGPP*GPPGP*AGK
10	1492.70	α2.708–723	SGETGASGPP*GFVGEK
11	2115.13	α2.760–783	GLP*GVAGSVGEPGP*LGIAGPPGAR
12	1580.79	α2.856–873	GEP*GP*AGAVGP*AGAVGP*R
13	895.46	α2.931–941	GPAGPSGPAGK

Then, the sequence RGEP*GPP*GPAG (*indicated the hydroxylation modification of the proline) and GAPG (n = 39, n represents the number of repeats in the chain), GPAG (n = 61), GARG (n = 19), and GERG (n =19) were synthesized, but they failed to bind FN. The moderate hydroxylation modification of proline might play an important role in recognition by FN. Furthermore, the shorter synthesized peptides, which contained FN-binding sites, failed to bind FN, indicating that the combined action of other residues was clearly required for full affinity.

The specific "GPPG" sequences in different peptides are highlighted in red. The specific "GPAG" sequences in different peptides are marked with underlines.

In the study by Kleinman H. K., α1-CB7, a type I collagen, was digested with cyanogen bromide and was identified as the classic fragment of the FN-binding [12]. The fragment lies within residues 757–791 of the α1 chain and contains the vertebrate collagenase (MMP-1) cleavage site of residues 775–776. In our research, m/z 1043.31 in Table 1 was doubly charged in the zoom scan, and the ion corresponded to the sequence, GAPGADGP*AGAPGTP*GPQGIAGQR, in the region of α1.757–780. The sequence belonged to α1-CB7 and contained the cleavage site Q-G#I-A (# represents the bond cleaved) of MMP-1 [23]. This suggested that the fragment, which independently interacted with FN in the domain of α1.757–791, could reduce to the sequence, GPQGIAGQR, in the region of α1.772–780. In addition, the sequence, GP*AG, might be another binding site. The sequence GLP*GVAGSVGEPGP*LGIAGPPGAR in the region of α2.760–783 corresponded to m/z 1058.07 (doubly charged) in Table 1, and it contained the cleavage site L-G#I-A. As a result, we inferred that in addition to the collagenase cleavage site, GPAG and GPPG were also binding sites of FN, but the excessive hydroxylation modification of the proline in the sequence GPPG weakened the adhesion to FN.

Studies showed that both α1.552–819 and 643–932 exhibit high FN-binding activity [13]. In Table 1, the peptides numbered 1–4 belonged to the region (Figure 6). The retention time of m/z 796.8, 1042.3, 908.9, and 780.9 with two charges was 29.46, 38.34, 30.25, and 30.18 min, respectively. In addition, m/z 793, a double charge, originated from the sequence GANGAP*GIAGAP*GFP*GAR in Figure 7. The result was consistent with that reported by Fietzek et al., in which α1-CB8 and α1.124–402 could bind to FN [24]. The region of α1.220–237 shortened the binding region of α1-CB8 and made the binding site more obvious.

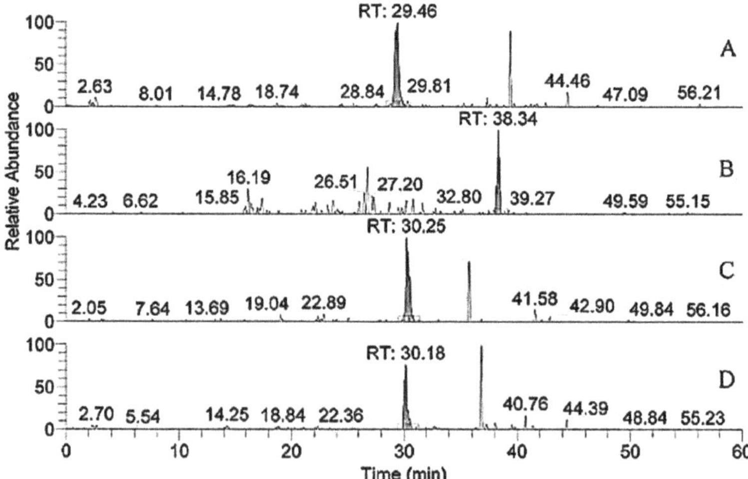

Figure 6. Extracted ion chromatogram of the peptides, numbers 1–4, in Table 1. (**A**) m/z 796.8; (**B**) m/z 1042.3; (**C**) m/z 908.9; (**D**) m/z 780.9.

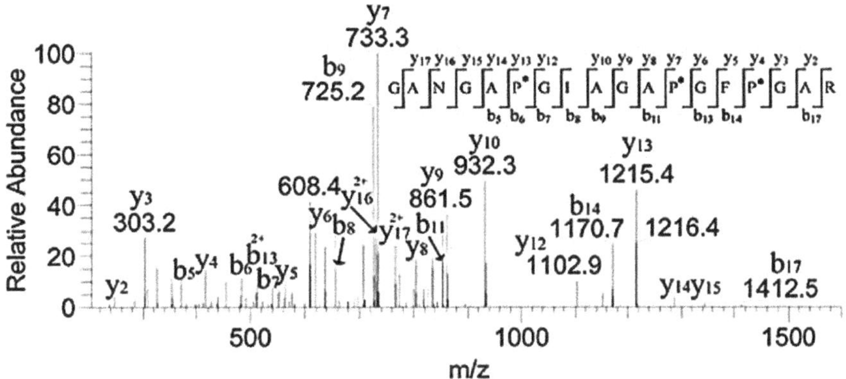

Figure 7. MS/MS spectrum of *m/z* 793.6 corresponding to the sequence GAN-GAP*GIAGAP*GFP*GAR. "*" indicated the hydroxylation modification of the proline.

Our research identified some binding peptides from the α2 chain. Guidry C. digested collagen I and II using CNBr and found that both CB4 from α2(I) homologous with CB10 from α1(II) and CB5 from α2(I) homologous with CB12 from α1(II) exhibited FN-binding activity. CB4 and CB5 were located in the regions of α2(I).0–300 and 693–1011, but the binding activity of CB4 was weaker than that of CB5 [15]. Table 1 showed that the peptides of regions α2.102–111, α2.708–723, α2.856–873, and α2.931–941 were included in the binding region. This further suggested that the bound region could cut down these sequences. They contained the same peptide sequences of GPAG and GPPG. Therefore, GPAG or GPPG was the binding site of FN. Moreover, this is the first report on these sequences in α1.91–99, α2.328–341, α2.451–465, α2.469–486, and α2.672–692 (Table 1) and their binding with FN. For example, the sequence GFSGLDGAK corresponded to *m/z* 851.4, and the matched b and y ions were shown in Figure 8.

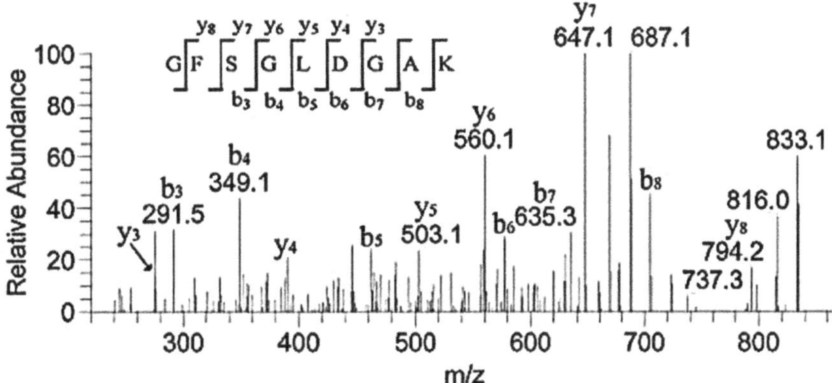

Figure 8. MS/MS spectrum of *m/z* 851.4 corresponding to the sequence GFSGLDGAK.

3.4. DPI Analysis of the Effect of MW on FN Binding

After FN was immobilized on the chip, the 1, 3, and 10 kDa peptides and bovine gelatin were, respectively, injected into the two channels of DPI and reacted with immobilized FN. The MW range of bovine gelatin was 1.4–33 kDa, as determined by gel filtration chromatography. The adsorption conditions of these samples were shown in Figures 9–11, including the real-time profile (A) and the resolved layer thickness-mass (B).

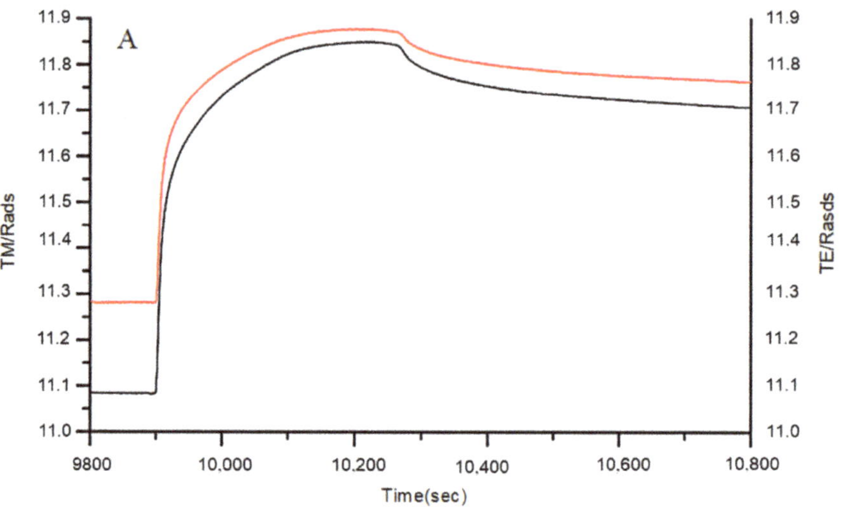

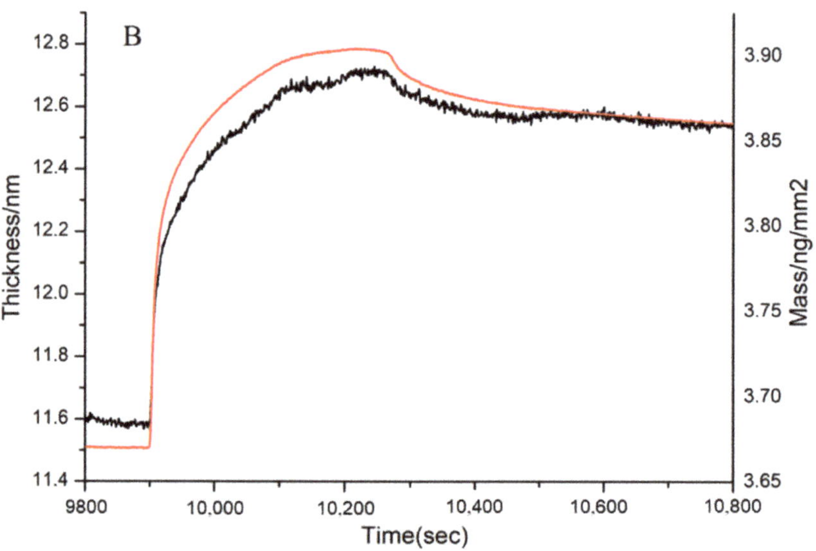

Figure 9. Adsorption of gelatin to immobilized FN on the chip surface as shown by (**A**) the measured TM (black line) and TE (red line) phase changes, and (**B**) the resolved layer thickness (black line) and mass (red line).

In Figure 9B, the thickness increased from 11.60 nm to 12.55 nm, and the mass increased from 3.68 to 3.86 ng/mm^2. The obvious increases in thickness and mass demonstrated that gelatin of MW range 1.4–33 kDa interacted with the immobilized FN. Certainly, not the entirety of the MW range (1.4–33 kDa) could bind to FN; thus, 1, 3, and 10 kDa peptides were further analyzed.

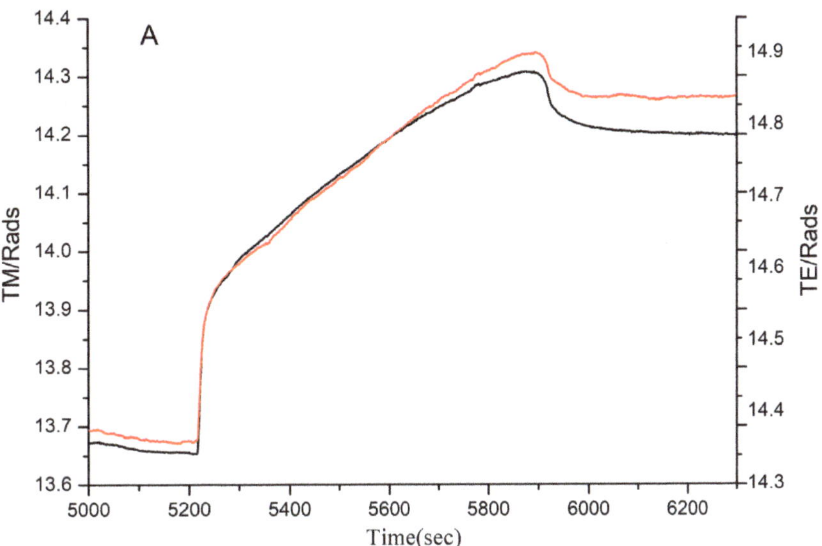

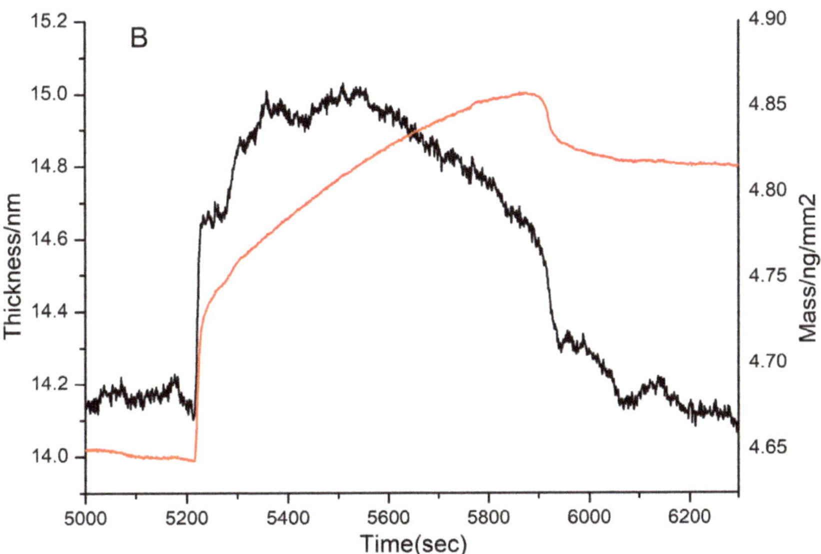

Figure 10. Adsorption of 3 kDa sample to immobilized FN on the chip surface as shown by (**A**) the measured TM (black line) and TE (red line) phase changes and (**B**) the resolved layer thickness (black line) and mass (red line).

According to DPI data analysis, the 1 kDa sample failed to bind FN (Figure not shown). Although the thickness did not increase significantly, there was a significant increase in the mass in the 3 kDa sample (Figure 10). This proved that the 3 kDa sample bound to FN.

Similarly, the mass and thickness of the 10 kDa sample indicated that it could interact with FN (Figure 11).

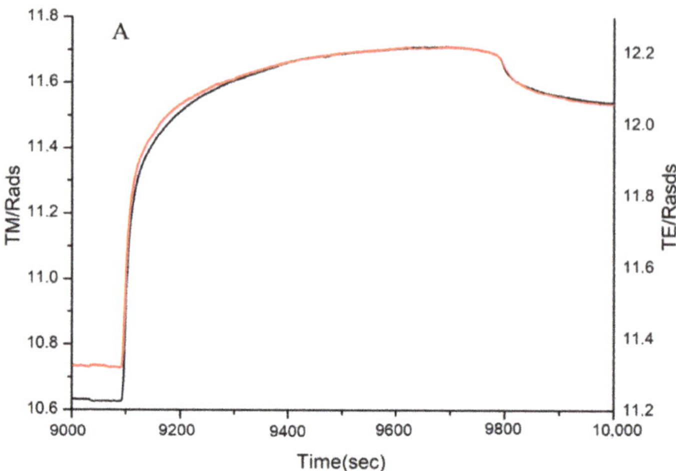

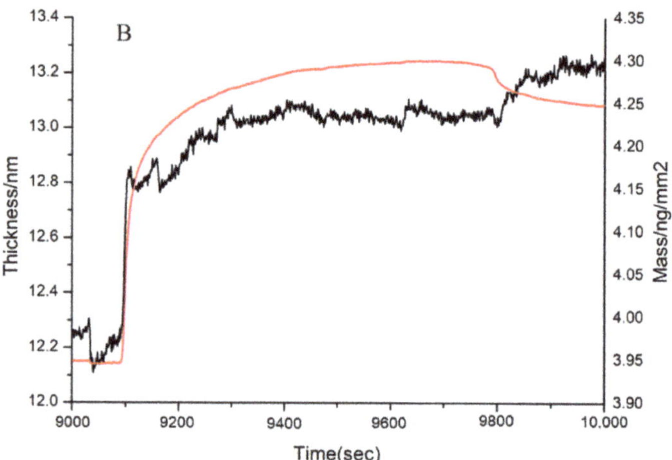

Figure 11. Adsorption of 10 kDa sample to immobilized FN on the chip surface, as shown by (**A**) the measured TM (black line) and TE (red line) phase changes and (**B**) the resolved layer thickness (black line) and mass (red line).

It is known that the FN-binding activity of collagen is lower than that of gelatin [5]. Our study suggested that the peptides lower than 1 kDa did not readily bind to FN. Thus, the bigger MW of peptides, the better the FN-binding activity. In other words, there was stronger binding activity in the suitable MW range of peptides, because a modest MW might radically expose more FN-binding sites than collagen. In this paper, peptides in the range of 2–30 kDa exhibited better affinity to FN. Therefore, the MW plays an important role in the interaction between FN and peptides.

3.5. MALDI-TOF MS Analysis of the Effect of Hydroxylation Modification on FN Binding

The sequence and MW of the four synthesized peptides were listed in Table 2. They were the peptides of FN-binding in Table 1 and contained two non-hydroxylation (1 and 3) and two hydroxylation modifications (2 and 4). In order to investigate the effect of hydroxylation modification on FN binding, peptides 1 and 2, and peptides 3 and 4, were, respectively, mixed in a 1:1 mass ratio and separately named GIA and GPP. The two mixed samples were separately loaded onto the micro affinity column. The column was eluted until the washing solution did not include the sample by MALDI-TOF MS, following the elution solution analyzed. Figures 12 and 13 showed the MALDI-TOF mass spectra of the two samples' elution.

Table 2. Sequence and molecular weight of the four synthesized peptides.

No.	Mixed Sample Name	No hyp Modification	Molecular Weight
1	GIA	GAPGADGPAGAPGTPGPQGIAGQR	2058.08
2		GAPGADGP*AGAPGTP*GPQGIAGQR	2089.47
3	GPP	GPPGPMGPPGLAGPPGESGR	1784.53
4		GPP*GPMGPPGLAGPP*GESGR	1816.36

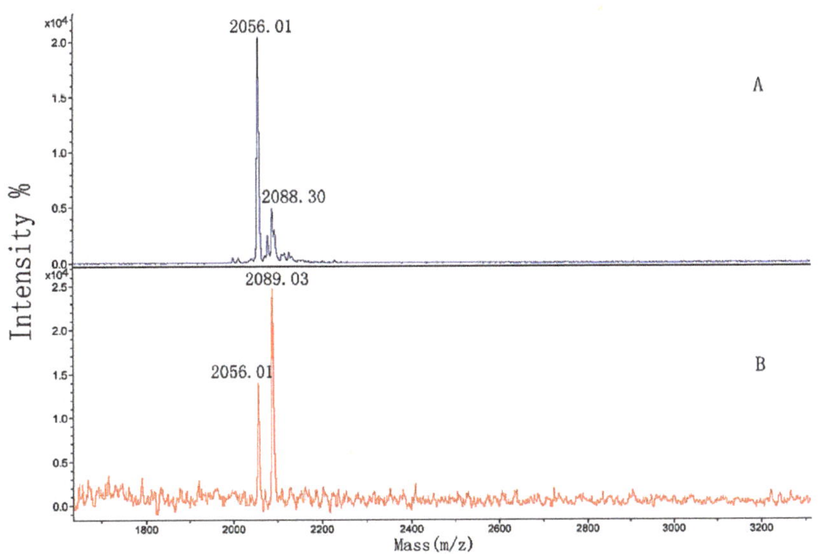

Figure 12. MALDI-TOF MS spectra of (**A**) GIA sample and (**B**) the elution solution.

In Figure 12A, m/z 2056.01 and 2088.30 were produced by peptides 1 and 2 from Table 2, respectively, and m/z 2078.19 was m/z 2056.01 + Na$^+$. The figure showed that the washing solution no longer included the GIA sample after the column was fully washed (Figure not shown). By comparing Figure 12A,B, the larger peak area of peptide 1 developed into smaller than that of peptide 2. The differences between the spectra indicated that the hydroxylation modification of peptide 2 led to stronger binding activity than the non-hydroxylation of peptide 1. Again, the appropriate position and amount of hydroxyproline in the sequence of peptide 2 had a significant influence on the binding activity.

In comparison with Figure 13A, the peak areas in Figure 13B did not significantly change. We hypothesized that the amount of proline in the sequence of peptide 3 was so high that slight hydroxylation modifications might influence the binding, or even inhibit it.

Interestingly, all four synthesized peptides could interact with FN, and it was incorrect to infer that only the sequences with hydroxylation modification could bind to FN. The addition of the binding was also attributed to the position and amount of hydroxyproline, both of which are essential.

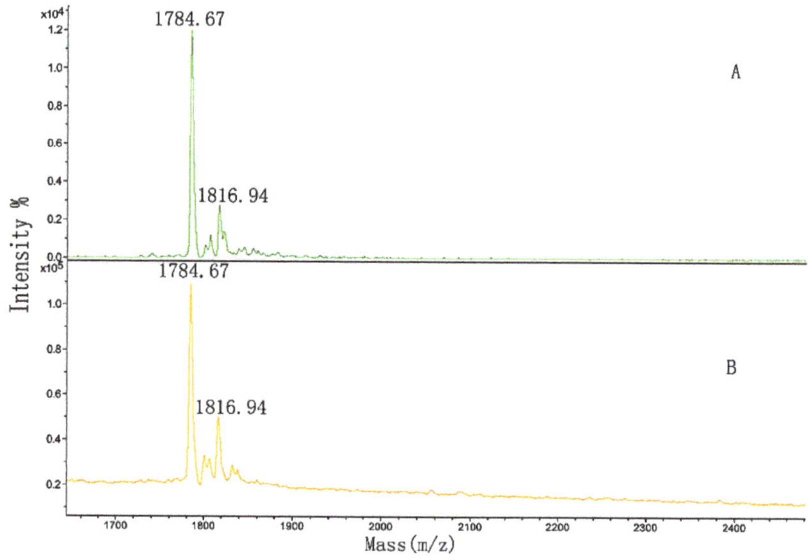

Figure 13. MALDI-TOF MS spectra of (**A**) GPP sample and (**B**) the elution solution.

4. Conclusions

Affinity chromatography was used to isolate peptides that could bind to FN, and the amino acid sequence of peptides was determined by HPLC-MS. MALDI-TOF MS and DPI were used to analyze the effects of MW and hydroxylation modification of peptides on FN binding activity.

The sequences of peptides that could bind FN all contained GPAG or GPPG; thus, they may be regarded as the core sequences of FN binding peptides. The MW of these peptides was mainly distributed in the range of 1000–2000 Da, and the FN-binding regions in peptide sequences were identified. These peptides, with MW between 1000 and 2000 Da, are also more easily absorbed by the human body, providing a foundation for the development of new functional health products.

DPI was used to measure the adsorption thickness and mass of peptides with different MW ranges on a chip with immobilized FN. Peptides with MW below 1 kDa did not readily bind to FN, while peptides with MW between 2 and 30 kDa were more likely to bind to FN. The result indicates that peptides with moderate MW exert greater binding activity, where more FN binding sites are exposed in the peptide sequence. Therefore, the MW range plays an important role in the interaction between FN and peptides.

Two different sequences of peptides (including hydroxylated and unmodified peptides) were synthesized, and the amount of hydroxylated and unhydroxylated peptides was mixed. MALDI-TOF MS was used to measure the influence of hydroxylated modification on FN binding, and all four synthetic polypeptides could bind to FN. However, the location and amount of hydroxylation modification play a key role in binding strength.

In this paper, bio-enzymatic hydrolysis technology was used to degrade gelatin, and combined with mass spectrometry analysis, the core sequence of FN binding in peptides was identified at the molecular level. The FN binding domain of the peptide sequence was shortened, providing a strategy for new raw materials and a basis for the study of functional factors of functional food. In this paper, DPI and MALDI-TOF MS were used for the first time to analyze the dynamic binding process of peptides to FN online, and the influence of various factors on the binding was discussed. The results provide a new technical method of analysis, as well as a theoretical basis for studying the binding characteristics of peptides to FN.

Author Contributions: Conceptualization, G.Z.; methodology, G.Z., J.G., L.L., J.K. and Y.K.; formal analysis, J.G., L.L. and Y.L.; writing—original draft preparation, L.L. and Y.L.; writing—review and editing, Y.L.; supervision, G.Z. and X.L. All authors have read and agreed to the published version of the manuscript.

Funding: This work was supported by the National Key Technology R&D Programs of China (Grant No. 2021YFC2400804), the Open Funding Project of the State Key Laboratory of Biochemical Engineering (Grant No. 2021KF-04), and the Independent Research Project of the State Key Laboratory of Biochemical Engineering (Grant No. 2021ZZ-03).

Institutional Review Board Statement: Not applicable.

Informed Consent Statement: Not applicable.

Data Availability Statement: The data presented in this study are available on request from the corresponding author.

Conflicts of Interest: The authors declare no conflict of interest.

References

1. León-López, A.; Morales-Pealoza, A.; Martínez-Juárez, V.M.; Vargas-Torres, A.; Zeugolis, D.I.; Aguirre-Álvarez, G. Hydrolyzed Collagen—Sources and Applications. *Molecules* **2019**, *24*, 4031. [CrossRef] [PubMed]
2. Sionkowska, A.; Adamiak, K.; Musiał, K.; Gadomska, M. Collagen Based Materials in Cosmetic Applications: A Review. *Materials* **2020**, *13*, 4217. [CrossRef]
3. Jafari, H.; Lista, A.; Siekapen, M.M.; Ghaffari-Bohlouli, P.; Nie, L.; Alimoradi, H.; Shavandi, A. Fish Collagen: Extraction, Characterization, and Applications for Biomaterials Engineering. *Polymers* **2020**, *12*, 2230. [CrossRef] [PubMed]
4. A Bocquier, A.; Potts, J.R.; Pickford, A.; Campbell, I.D. Solution structure of a pair of modules from the gelatin-binding domain of fibronectin. *Structure* **1999**, *7*, 1451–1460. [CrossRef]
5. Hynes, R.O. *Fibronectin*; Springer: New York, NY, USA, 1990.
6. Garcıa, A.J.; Vega, M.D.; Boettiger, D. Modulation of Cell Proliferation and Differentiation through Substrate-dependent Changes in Fibronectin Conformation. *Mol. Biol. Cell* **1999**, *10*, 785–798. [CrossRef] [PubMed]
7. Sabatelli, P.; Bonaldo, P.; Lattanzi, G.; Braghetta, P.; Bergamin, N.; Capanni, C.; Mattioli, E.; Columbaro, M.; Ognibene, A.; Pepe, G.; et al. Collagen VI deficiency affects the organization of fibronectin in the extracellular matrix of cultured fibroblasts. *Matrix Biol.* **2001**, *20*, 475–486. [CrossRef]
8. Potts, J.R.; Campbell, I.D. Structure and function of fibronectin modules. *Matrix Biol.* **1996**, *15*, 313–320. [CrossRef]
9. Pagett, A.; Campbell, I.D.; Pickford, A.R. Gelatin binding to the 6F11F22F2 fragment of fibronectin is independent of module-module interactions. *Biochemistry* **2005**, *44*, 14682–14687. [CrossRef] [PubMed]
10. Brüel, A.; Oxlund, H. Changes in biomechanical properties, composition of collagen and elastin, and advanced glycation endproducts of the rat aorta in relation to age. *Atherosclerosis* **1996**, *127*, 155–165. [CrossRef]
11. Rotter, N.; Tobias, G.; Lebl, M.; Roy, A.K.; Hansen, M.C.; A Vacanti, C.; Bonassar, L.J. Age-related changes in the composition and mechanical properties of human nasal cartilage. *Arch. Biochem. Biophys.* **2002**, *403*, 132–140. [CrossRef]
12. Kleinman, H.; McGoodwin, E.; Martin, G.; Klebe, R.; Fietzek, P.; Woolley, D. Localization of the binding site for cell attachment in the alpha1(I) chain of collagen. *J. Biol. Chem.* **1978**, *253*, 5642–5646. [CrossRef]
13. Dessau, W.; Adelmann, B.C.; Timpl, R. Identification of the sites in collagen α-chains that bind serum anti-gelatin factor (cold-insoluble globulin). *Biochem. J.* **1978**, *169*, 55–59. [CrossRef]
14. Gao, X.; Groves, M.J. Fibronectin-binding peptides. I. Isolation and characterization of two unique fibronectin-binding peptides from gelatin. *Eur. J. Pharm. Biopharm.* **1998**, *45*, 275–284. [CrossRef]
15. Guidry, C.; Miller, E.J.; Hook, M. A second fibronectin-binding region is present in collagen a chains. *J. Biol. Chem.* **1990**, *31*, 19230–19236. [CrossRef]
16. Ingham, K.; Brew, S.; Migliorini, M. Type I collagen contains at least 14 cryptic fibronectin binding sites of similar affinity. *Arch. Biochem. Biophys.* **2002**, *407*, 217–223. [CrossRef]
17. Swann, M.J.; Peel, L.L.; Carrington, S.; Freeman, N.J. Dual-polarization interferometry: An analytical technique to measure changes in protein structure in real time, to determine the stoichiometry of binding events, and to differentiate between specific and nonspecific interactions. *Anal. Biochem.* **2004**, *329*, 190–198. [CrossRef]
18. Kumar, R.; Sripriya, R.; Balaji, S.; Kumar, M.S.; Sehgal, P. Physical characterization of succinylated type I collagen by Raman spectra and MALDI-TOF/MS and in vitro evaluation for biomedical applications. *J. Mol. Struct.* **2011**, *994*, 117–124. [CrossRef]

19. Zhang, G.; Liu, T.; Wang, Q.; Chen, L.; Lei, J.; Luo, J.; Ma, G.; Su, Z. Mass spectrometric detection of marker peptides in tryptic digests of gelatin: A new method to differentiate between bovine and porcine gelatin. *Food Hydrocoll.* **2009**, *23*, 2001–2007. [CrossRef]
20. Sheu, B.C.; Lin, Y.H.; Lin, C.C.; Yuan, A.S.; Chang, W.; Wu, J.H.; Tsai, J.C.; Lin, S. Significance of the pH-induced conformational changes in the structure of C-reactive protein measured by dual polarization interferometry. *Biosens. Bioelectron.* **2010**, *26*, 822–827. [CrossRef]
21. Patel, S.; Chaffotte, A.F.; Goubard, F.; Pauthe, E. Urea-Induced Sequential Unfolding of Fibronectin: A Fluorescence Spectroscopy and Circular Dichroism Study. *Biochemistry* **2004**, *43*, 1724–1735. [CrossRef] [PubMed]
22. Dzamba, B.J.; Wu, H.; Jaenisch, R.; Peters, D.M. Fibronectin binding site in type I collagen regulates fibronectin fibril formation. *J. Cell Biol.* **1993**, *121*, 1165–1172. [CrossRef] [PubMed]
23. Chung, L.; Dinakarpandian, D.; Yoshida, N.; Lauer-Fields, J.L.; Fields, G.B.; Visse, R.; Nagase, H. Collagenase unwinds triple-helical collagen prior to peptide bond hydrolysis. *EMBO J.* **2004**, *23*, 3020–3030. [CrossRef] [PubMed]
24. Fietzek, P.P.; Kühn, K. The primary structure of collagen. *Int. Rev. Connect. Tissue Res.* **1976**, *7*, 1–60.

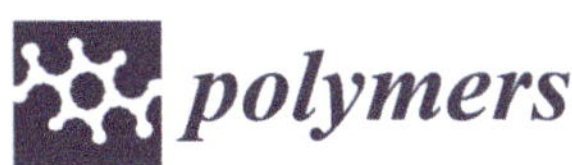

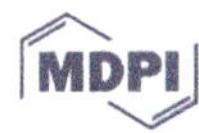

Article

Tailored Polyelectrolyte Multilayer Systems by Variation of Polyelectrolyte Composition and EDC/NHS Cross-Linking: Controlled Drug Release vs. Drug Reservoir Capabilities and Cellular Response for Improved Osseointegration

Johanna Ludolph [1], Holger Rothe [1], Uwe Schirmer [1], Katharina Möbus [1], Christina Behrens [2], Henning Schliephake [2] and Klaus Liefeith [1,*]

1   Institute for Bioprocessing and Analytical Measurement Techniques e.V., 37308 Heilbad Heiligenstadt, Germany

2   Department of Oral and Maxillofacial Surgery, Georg-August-University, 37073 Göttingen, Germany

*   Correspondence: klaus.liefeith@iba-heiligenstadt.de

Citation: Ludolph, J.; Rothe, H.; Schirmer, U.; Möbus, K.; Behrens, C.; Schliephake, H.; Liefeith, K. Tailored Polyelectrolyte Multilayer Systems by Variation of Polyelectrolyte Composition and EDC/NHS Cross-Linking: Controlled Drug Release vs. Drug Reservoir Capabilities and Cellular Response for Improved Osseointegration. *Polymers* **2022**, *14*, 4315. https://doi.org/10.3390/polym14204315

Academic Editors: Nunzia Gallo, Marta Madaghiele, Alessandra Quarta and Amilcare Barca

Received: 8 September 2022
Accepted: 10 October 2022
Published: 14 October 2022

Publisher's Note: MDPI stays neutral with regard to jurisdictional claims in published maps and institutional affiliations.

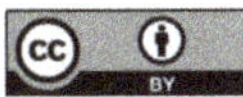

Copyright: © 2022 by the authors. Licensee MDPI, Basel, Switzerland. This article is an open access article distributed under the terms and conditions of the Creative Commons Attribution (CC BY) license (https://creativecommons.org/licenses/by/4.0/).

Abstract: Polyelectrolyte multilayers (PEM) are versatile tools used to investigate fundamental interactions between material-related parameters and the resulting performance in stem cell differentiation, respectively, in bone tissue engineering. In the present study, we investigate the suitability of PEMs with a varying collagen content for use as drug carriers for the human bone morphogenetic protein 2 (rhBMP-2). We use three different PEM systems consisting either of the positively charged poly-L-lysine or the glycoprotein collagen type I and the negatively charged glycosaminoglycan heparin. For a specific modification of the loading capacity and the release kinetics, the PEMs were stepwise cross-linked before loading with cytokine. We demonstrate the possibility of immobilizing significant amounts of rhBMP-2 in all multilayer systems and to specifically tune its release via cross-linking. Furthermore, we prove that the drug release of rhBMP-2 plays only a minor role in the differentiation of osteoprogenitor cells. We find a significantly higher influence of the immobilized rhBMP-2 within the collagen-rich coatings that obviously represent an excellent mimicry of the native extracellular matrix. The cytokine immobilized in its bioactive form was able to achieve an increase in orders of magnitude both in the early stages of differentiation and in late calcification compared to the unloaded layers.

Keywords: polyelectrolyte multilayer; collagen; cross-linking; bone tissue engineering; drug release; drug reservoir; BMP-2; osteogenic differentiation

1. Introduction

The layer-by-layer (LbL) coating strategy via polyelectrolytes is a powerful and simple technique to modify and functionalize nearly any kind of surfaces like membranes, discs, hollow tubes, capsules or nanoparticles independently whether they are made of polymers, glasses, ceramics or metals. Moreover, the LbL method has proven to be simple, flexible, effective, inexpensive and reproducible. In other words, the method imposes no restrictions on the size or shape of the substrate and does not require harsh process conditions during the coating process. In this way, an enormous field of applications has emerged over the years, for example in regenerative medicine, as a drug delivery vehicle or as a bioactive coating to render medical implants or prostheses, such as cardiovascular devices, joint prostheses or bone replacement, respectively, making bone augmentation materials more bioactive [1–4]. Notably, even hydrogels can be modified with polyelectrolyte multilayers (PEM) to enhance cell adhesion, which could be an option especially for synthetic hydrogels with less bioactivity [5]. In addition, the first studies have been published recently in which even native cells were coated with PEM films [6].

From a physico-chemical point of view, polyelectrolytes are polymers that dispose of numerous ionizable groups. In polar solvents, this group starts to dissociate in dependence of the pH, so that these molecules are then electrically charged. Negatively charged polymers are called polyanions and positively charged molecules are called polycations. Special polyelectrolytes that have both positive and negative charges are called polyampholytes or betaines [7].

In the early 1990s, Decher et al. introduced the LbL technique, which is based on the self-assembly of alternating charged polyelectrolytes. Now it is a powerful alternative to self-assembled monolayers or Langmuir–Blodgett deposition. The driving force of the layer formation is the ionic attraction between the opposite charges and the release of counterions [8]. The polyelectrolyte multilayer formation is a complex balance between electrostatic interactions, non-electrostatic interactions and a gain in entropy as the main driving factor [9,10].

It can be ascertained that the original assembly technique for the fabrication of LbL films has not much changed since its seminal introduction by G. Decher. The most extended protocol is the alternated dipping of flat macroscopic substrates into solutions of polyanions and polycations, including the corresponding rinsing cycles between the different dipping steps [11–13].

A polyelectrolyte multilayer consists of a predetermined number of double layers, created from alternating the deposition of polyanions and polycations. Such coatings should have certain key features, like biocompatibility, biodegradability and environmental benignity. The physical, chemical and biological properties of PEMs are defined by the used polyelectrolytes and their molecular composition and conformation, the coating architecture, the fabrication process and the possible post-fabrication treatments where required [14].

Exemplarily, in conventional prosthetics, PEMs are used for the modification of implants for bone augmentation or replacement to improve osseointegration or as drug reservoir, e.g., to release antibiotics to prevent implant-associated infections [15,16]. As mentioned above, the application for PEMs is of special importance in the field of TE. In this area, the LbL technique is often used to mimic the natural extracellular matrix for a better tissue integration and biofunctionality. The ECM consists mainly of glycosaminoglycans (GAGs) like chondroitin sulfate, heparin and hyaluronic acid and fibrillary glycoproteins like collagen, fibronectin and laminin. The use of such natural ECM molecules can help to improve the integration of implants by establishing an ECM-analogue microenvironment.

GAGs are linear and polar polysaccharides, which interact more or less intensely with water molecules [17]. Heparin is a highly sulfated GAG in the ECM and is often used to establish drug carrier systems because it has a high binding capacity for cytokines and growth factors. Collagen is the most common ECM component. It has a defined 3D structure with numerous cell-binding sites. Poly-L-lysin (PLL) is a positively charged polyelectrolyte and often used in PEM films to improve the cell adhesion capability and biocompatibility of surfaces due to the Coulomb interaction. In this study, we have investigated PEMs composed of PLL, heparin and collagen in view of their effect on MC3T3 cell differentiation. MC3T3 pre-osteoblasts represent an established model for in vitro osteoblast differentiation and ECM signaling.

In the last decade, the influence of substrate stiffness on the behavior of biological systems is increasingly becoming the focus of many research activities. Therefore, PEMs are often cross-linked after their assembly to modulate the mechanical properties. A detailed overview of different cross-linking strategies is given in the excellent review of Ghiorghita (2019) [18]. The most common method is cross-linking via EDC (1-ethyl-3-[3-dimethylaminopropyl] carbodiimide hydrochloride) and NHS for PEMs with appropriate functional groups, such as amine and carboxyl groups in aqueous solutions. Cross-linkers like EDC are used to couple carboxyl and amine groups in order to get amide bonds [19]. Ren and coworkers showed that an increase in the EDC concentration is directly proportional to the mechanical stiffness of a $(PLL/PA)_{12}$ PEM. They generated PEMs that showed Young's moduli from 3 kPa for native films, 100 kPa for low cross-linked films to

400 kPa for highly cross-linked films. Obviously, a higher cross-linker concentration also enhances the myoblast adhesion on the stiffest PEMs and well-defined focal adhesions were observed [20]. Schneider et al. (2007) cross-linked a PLL/HA and a CHI/HA PEM with EDC/NHS. The cross-linked film was about 10 times stiffer than the native non-cross-linked counterpart (native PLL/HA 20 kPa, cross-linked PLL/HA 250 kPa; native CHI/HA 15 kPa, cross-linked CHI/HA 159 kPa). For EDC and NHS concentrations of 70 mg/mL, respectively, 22 mg/mL were employed in a 0.15 M NaCl solution at a pH of 4.5 in order to deposit a thin film for 18 h at 4 °C [21].

For cross-linking PEM films made of collagen, it should be mentioned that the EDC/NHS chemistry can change the structure of the collagen while cross-linking. This may lead to a change in the cell adhesion behavior. The group of Cameron et al. observed a decreasing cell adhesion with an increasing EDC/NHS concentration for cross-linking [22,23]. The reason is that EDC inhibits the cation-dependent cell adhesion to collagen, because the binding sites for the collagen binding integrins $\alpha_1\beta_1$, $\alpha_2\beta_1$, $\alpha_{10}\beta_1$ and $\alpha_{11}\beta_1$ are changed [22].

A possible alternative to cross-link PEMs is given by the use of glutaraldehyde (GA). The amine groups react with the GA and form an imide bond, resulting in a cross-linked PEM. This method was successful used in the field of environmental technology to cross-link PEMs on membranes for water treatment facilities or to improve the stability of PEM microcapsules for pharmacological purposes [19,24,25]. Another option of an increasing importance seems to be the use of genipin to cross-link PEMs. Genipin is a natural cross-linking agent which is found in plants, and it has been quite efficient in protein cross-linking. It can be an interesting alternative for cross-linking with EDC or glutaraldehyde, which often changes the physicochemical properties of the PEM film while cross-linking. In tissue engineering, genipin has shown beneficial effects like the control of inflammation or the enhancement of fibroblastic cell attachment [26]. Chaubaroux et al. (2012) assembled a film of collagen and alginate cross-linked with genipin to stabilize the film at physiological pH values. Compared to films cross-linked with glutaraldehyde, the genipin cross-linked film shows the same structure as a non-cross-linked film. They also observed a satisfying degree of proliferation of HUVECs. The cells grow more confluently and a better spreading behavior was observed on genipin cross-linked films in comparison with a glutaraldehyde cross-linked film [26].

It is well known that growth factors like hBMP-2 can be sequestered within the ECM by means of binding to the protein moieties or to charged glycosaminoglycans, for example, to establish growth factor gradients or to build up a growth factor reservoir for later use. Among the many advantages of LbL assembly are the mild aqueous fabrication conditions and the associated possibility of incorporating cytokines or growth factors without the risk of destabilizing these compounds. This circumstance, along with the potential multivalent charge interactions between the ionized groups of the polyelectrolytes and the charged drugs, renders PEMs as a versatile technology platform to immobilize bioactive agents.

These components can be loaded as direct building blocks during the assembly process or by post-diffusion into the final multilayer system. The subsequent release is controlled by the molecular structure and the charge of the different polyelectrolytes [17], leading to a more or less defined permeability of the polyelectrolyte multilayer in dependence of an external stimuli such as the pH, ionic strength, temperature, etc. [18]. The study of Dash et al. (2010) gives an overview of the mathematical models used to describe the release kinetics of drug delivery systems [27]. The most commonly used kinetic models for PEM films are based on Fick's law of diffusion and the well-known algorithms of Korsmeyer–Peppas and Higuchi [28].

In bone tissue engineering, BMPs play an important role. The molecular weight of hBMP-2 is 32 kDa and the isoelectric point is given with a pH value of 8.5. In solutions with lower pH values, it is slightly positively charged and can therefore also be electrostatically incorporated into PEMs. BMP-2 is a cytokine and a growth factor and, as such, it is involved in bone healing and different phases of bone repair as a kind of osseous inductor [29].

It should be noted that the clinical dose for therapeutical purposes is relatively high, ranging from 0.1 to 0.5 mg BMP-2/kg body weight [30]. BMPs have a conserved binding site with a specific affinity for sulfated glycosaminoglycans, which renders GAGs as a promising BMP-2 delivery tool. Especially, heparin has a high dissociation constant K_d of 20 nM for BMP-2 and can also enhance the BMP-2 activity [30]. An N-terminal sequence of approximately 13 amino acid residues mediates the binding of the cytokine to heparin [31].

Numerous studies were published which show the positive effect of hBMP-2 in the process of bone formation after drug release. MacDonald et al. (2011) have fabricated a special PEM made of Poly2, a synthetic, intrinsically tunable cationic polymer, and chondroitin sulfate to be able to functionalize 3D scaffolds based on a polycaprolactone/β-tricalcium phosphate (PCL/BTCP) co-polymer blend. The BMP-2 was introduced directly in the coating process. Subsequently, the following tetralayers were obtained: [Poly2/chondroitin sulfate/BMP-2/chondroitin sulfate]$_n$, where n is the repeating unit of the tetralayer ($n = 100$). The films show distinct release profiles. A linear release is observed for the first 2 days, where 80% of the BMP-2 is released. In the additional 2 weeks, the last 20% are slowly released. In total, the scaffolds released around 11 mg of BMP-2. The bioactivity of the coating was tested in vitro with MC3T3 E1 subclone 4 pre-osteoblasts and in vivo with sixteen 350–400 g male Sprague Dawley rats. The experiments show a significantly better bone formation for coatings that contain BMP-2 [32]. Guillot and coworkers (2016) investigated the osseointegration of titanium implants (Ti-6Al-4V) and poly(etheretherketone) (PEEK) implants coated with a PEM film which was loaded with BMP-2. The PEM consist of 24 double layers of poly-L-lysine and hyaluronic acid. To enhance the PEM film adhesion on the implant, a Polyethyleneimine layer was introduced at first. After the multilayer generation, the films were cross-linked with EDC/NHS. The coated implants were incubated with 100 μg/mL BMP-2 for 90 min at 37 °C. Uncoated and coated (total dose of 9.3 μg BMP-2) screw implants were inserted in the femoral condyles of rabbits and the osseointegration was compared after 4 and 8 weeks. Surprisingly, the bone-to-implant contact and the bone area around the implant were significantly lower for the coated implants than for the uncoated implants. This impressive study shows that it is important to choose a proper dose of the growth factor, otherwise localized and temporary bone impairment can appear [33].

As already mentioned, both the absolute amount and the release time/kinetic represents an important aspect of drug release. Thus, numerous works have been performed to try to develop biomimetic delivery systems that control the localization, the release time and the kinetics as well as the spatial and temporal release patterns [34]. The goal is to achieve a long-term delivery system that releases the drug component precisely when the cells remodulate the PEM system.

In this context, an intensive scientific debate is taking place about the preference of physiological drug reservoir systems vs. a drug release system. Most release systems start with an initial burst release where almost 80% of the loaded drug is released in the first few hours. However, the adhesion and healing process in vivo takes a significantly longer time. Furthermore, the burst release of cytokines can lead to a very high concentration in the tissue and subsequent tissue inflammation and ectopic ossification [30,33]. Therefore, a drug reservoir, which releases the cytokine just when the cells remodulate the artificial matrix, seems to be extremely attractive.

In this study, we investigated three different polyelectrolyte multilayer systems consisting of PLL, heparin and collagen. The amount of collagen in the layer systems was variable. Each layer system was gradually cross-linked by EDC/NHS chemistry to generate polyelectrolyte multilayers with a different stiffness and defined release kinetics. The PEMs were loaded with hBMP-2 and the total amount in the coating as well as the release as a function of time and in dependence of PEM composition and a degree of cross-linking was investigated. The experiments aim to comparatively quantify the balance between hBMP-2 release and hBMP-2 sequestering within the PEM in terms of bioavailability and the effect on osteoprogenitor cell differentiation.

2. Materials and Methods

2.1. Coating and Cross-Linking

Chemicals and reagents were used without further purification, unless stated otherwise. PEM films were assembled from poly-L-lysine (Sigma-Aldrich GmbH, Taufkirchen, Germany, P2636, PLL, 30–70 kDa), heparin (Sigma-Aldrich GmbH, Taufkirchen, Germany, H3393, Hep, from porcine intestinal mucosa) and collagen (ibidi GmbH, Gräfelfing, Germany, 50202, rat tail collagen type I). The polyelectrolytes for PLL–Hep films were dissolved in a Na-acetate buffer (20 mM, pH 4.5) at a concentration of 1 mg/mL. For the deposition of Col-Hep multilayers, the polyelectrolytes were dissolved in 5 mM Acetate (pH 3.5) at a concentration of 1 mg/mL. The film construction was performed automatically by employing a dipping robot (DR3, Riegler & Kirstein GmbH, Potsdam, Germany). Briefly, the cleaned substrates were first dipped into the polycation solution (PLL) and left to adsorb for 5 min. After that, the samples were washed three times in double-distilled water to rinse the surface from the unbound polyelectrolyte. Subsequently, (Hep) was deposited in the same manner. For the (Col-Hep) film construction, the substrate was dipped for 30 min into the solved polyelectrolyte. The rinsing steps here were the same as described for the (PLL-Hep) films. Each cycle was repeated until the desired number was reached of double layers and film architecture. All samples were rinsed in double-distilled water and air dried in a gentle stream of pressurized air. Figure 1 illustrates the coating architecture of the three investigated multilayer systems.

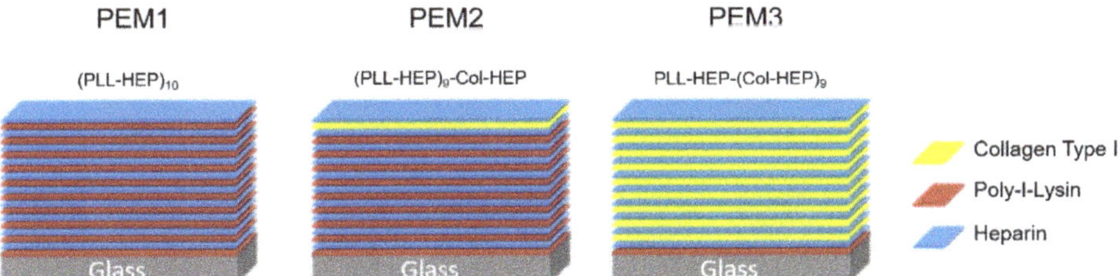

Figure 1. Architecture of the investigated LbL coatings.

The cross-linking was done using EDC/NHS chemistry at five different EDC concentration levels (0, 5, 25, 100 and 200 mg/mL) in order to obtain peptide bonds within the polyelectrolyte multilayers between the carboxylic groups of the poly-anion (heparin) and the amine groups of the poly-cations (poly-L-lysin; collagen). The EDC stock solution (400 mg/mL) was prepared in ice cold 0.15 M of NaCl with a pH value of 5, and from this the solution was further diluted in separate volumes until the two-fold target concentration was reached. Finally, these two-fold pre-dilutions were further mixed in an equal volume with a 22 mg/mL NHS solution. Each cross-linking reaction was done in 1 mL EDC/NHS-solution in 24-well plates. All working steps were performed on ice with pre-cooled buffer and all samples were incubated over night at 4 °C. After the cross-linking, all samples were rinsed three times with 0.15 M NaCl, pH 8 at room temperature. Between each washing step, the samples were incubated for 1 h. Finally, the samples were rinsed with water and allowed to dry in air at room temperature. For sterilization the samples were placed for 30 min under UV light.

2.2. Loading of BMP-2

For the loading of the cytokine in the PEM films, the BMP-2 (PeproTech Germany, Hamburg, Germany) was diluted to a final concentration of 75 µg/mL. The loading was performed in a 24-well plate, where in each well a coated glass disc was placed. An aliquot of 200 µL of the BMP-2 solution was added to each sample per well and incubated over night at 4 °C. The cytokine solution was replaced and the samples were rinsed three times with double-distilled water for 5 min. The samples were then air-dried and stored at 4 °C until further use.

2.3. Release Kinetic

All coated glass discs were placed into a 24-well plate and incubated with 400 μL of DMEM with 1% Penicillin/Streptomycin at 37 °C and 5% CO_2. The medium was collected and replaced by a fresh medium after 1 h, 2 h, 4 h, 6 h, 8 h, 10 h, 24 h, 48 h, 96 h and 192 h.

There are some advanced approaches that can be used to model the loading quantities in polyelectrolyte multilayers, e.g., based on ellipsometry data [35]. In the present study, however, both the release and the loading quantities were high enough to realize the quantification directly via a commercial fluorescence kit. The initial loading capacity as well as the release of rhBMP-2 were measured using a Human/Murine/Rat BMP-2 Standard TMB ELISA Development Kit (PeproTech Germany, Hamburg, Germany), according to the manufacturer's instructions. The loading amount was calculated by a measurement of the growth factor concentration of the loading solution before and after the incubation. All measurements were done in triplicate on three samples, respectively.

2.4. Cell Culture Tests

Mouse fibroblasts MC3T3 cells were obtained from Leibniz Institute DSMZ (Leibniz Institute DSMZ German Collection of Microorganisms and Cell Cultures GmbH, Braunschweig, Germany) and cultured in a proliferation medium, which consisted of α-MEM with 10% FBS and 1% Penicillin/Streptomycin (all the medium components were obtained from PAN-Biotech, Aidenbach, Germany). The cells were subcultured prior to reaching a 70–80% confluence. For the differentiation into osteoblasts, the culture medium was changed to a differentiation medium, which consisted of α-MEM, 10% FBS, 1% Penicillin/Streptomycin and additionally 10 mM of β-Glycerolphosphate and 0.05 mM of ascorbic acid (Sigma Aldrich GmbH, Taufkirchen, Germany).

2.5. Proliferation Assay—XTT

For the analysis of proliferation and the viability of the MC3T3 cells on different coatings, an XTT assay was employed. This is a colorimetric assay using XTT (2,3-Bis-(2-Methoxy-4-Nitro-5-Sulfophenyl)-2*H*-Tetrazolium-5-Carboxanilide), a yellow tetrazolium salt, which is reduced in the presence of an electron coupling reagent (5-Methylphenazinium-methasulfat, PMS) to an orange formazan dye by metabolically active cells. The formazan salt is soluble in aqueous solutions and can be directly quantified using a spectrophotometer. For the assay, the MC3T3 cells were cultured with a proliferation medium on the coated discs in 24-well plates. At the sample points, the culture medium was replaced by a 300 μL fresh proliferation medium, then 150 μL of XTT solution (1 mg/mL XTT in RPMI medium and XX mg/mL Electron coupling reagent) were added and incubated at 37 °C for 4 h. After the incubation period, the absorbance of the supernatant was measured using an ELISA plate spectrometer at a wavelength of 405 nm. The cells were washed twice in PBS and then further cultivated in a proliferation medium.

2.6. ALP Assay

The cells were seeded at a density of 10,000 cells/cm^2 on the samples in 24-well plates. The alkaline phosphatase (ALP) activity is a marker for early osteogenic differentiation. To measure the ALP activity, the cells were washed twice with PBS and then lysed with a lysis buffer (50 mM Tris-HCl pH 8.0, 150 mM NaCl, 1% Triton X-100, 100 μg/mL PMSF) for 30 min on ice. One capsule of phosphatase substrate (Sigma Aldrich GmbH, Taufkirchen, Germany) was dissolved in 25 mL of ddH$_2$O and then mixed in equal parts with an alkaline buffer (Sigma Aldrich GmbH, Taufkirchen, Germany).

An aliquot of 10 μL of each sample was added to a 96-well plate on ice. The plate was placed to a Thermoblock at 37 °C and 100 μL of the phosphatase solution was added. After

15 min of incubation, the reaction was stopped with 100 µL of 0.5 M NaOH. The absorbance at 405 nm was analyzed with an ELISA reader. For the standard curve, a Nitrophenol solution (Sigma Aldrich GmbH, Taufkirchen, Germany) was diluted with 0.02 M NaOH and used to calculate the units of the enzyme activity.

2.7. Matrix Calcification—Alizarin Red S Assay

The calcium deposition and matrix calcification are later markers of osteogenic differentiation and can be analyzed with an Alizarin Red Assay. The cells were seeded at a density of 10,000 cells/cm^2 on samples in 24-well plates and incubated for 28 days at 37 °C. Then they were washed twice with PBS and fixed with 4% PFA for 60 min. A staining solution was prepared with 2% Alizarin Red S in ddH$_2$O at a pH of 4.2. A volume of 200 µL of staining solution was added to each sample and incubated for 45 min in the dark. The samples were washed four times with ddH$_2$O for 5 min. For destaining, the samples were incubated with 10% acetic acid for 30 min. The absorbance was analyzed at 405 nm with an ELISA reader.

2.8. Microscopy

The cells on the samples were rinsed twice with PBS and then were fixed with 4% PFA for 20 min. The cells were stained with Phalloidin590 (MoBiTec GmbH, Göttingen, Germany) and Hoechst33258 (Thermo Fisher Scientific GmbH, Bremen, Germany) according to the manufacturer's instruction and analyzed with a Confocal Laser Scanning Microscope (Carl Zeiss Microscopy GmbH, Oberkochen, Germany).

2.9. Statistical Analysis

All the results are shown as mean values $\pm$ standard deviation. The results of a one-way ANOVA test can be found in the Appendix A.

3. Results and Discussion

We examined three different layer systems based on the three different polymers: heparin (Hep), poly-L-lysin (PLL) and collagen (Col). The polyelectrolyte multilayers were built up using the LbL technique until a final film architecture consisting of ten double layers was achieved. PEM1 consists of ten double layers (PLL-Hep)$_{10}$. PEM2 has nearly the same structure as PEM1, however, in the last double layer, PLL was replaced by collagen (PLL-Hep)$_9$-(Col-Hep)$_1$. For the PEM3 system, this replacement strategy was continued for all double layers except for the first double layer, where a strong polycation is needed to guarantee a stable adhesion on the substrate. Thus, the final PEM3 structure is given with the following coating sequence (PLL-Hep)$_1$-(Col-Hep)$_9$.

For further information, these three layer systems were thoroughly investigated by the means of a specifically adapted spectrum of the physicochemical methods in order to obtain precise data on the multilayer architecture and morphology. A detailed presentation and discussion of the results with special attention to the most important factors of influence such as the stiffness, layer thickness, zetapotential, roughness parameter and the intrinsic and extrinsic charge compensation, respectively, has already been published by the authors [33]. Table 1 summarizes the relevant data on the respective physicochemical investigations.

Table 1. Summarized results from physicochemical investigations as published and discussed in detail in [36].

	EDC	Roughness (AFM)				Thickness (Ellipsometry)		Amid-I (FTIR)		Young's Modulus (AFM)		Wettability (CA H_2O)	
	mg/mL	Sa [nm]	SD	Sdr [%]	SD	d [nm]	SD	Abs.	SD	E [kPa]	SD	CA [°]	SD
PEM1	0	0.68	0.10	0.01	0.00	70.07	3.75	0.24	0.03	-	-	28.07	2.20
	5	1.41	0.37	0.07	0.04	51.00	9.24	0.35	0.06	-	-	19.74	3.72
	25	1.38	0.10	0.04	0.01	42.37	16.21	0.37	0.06	-	-	14.60	4.50
	100	2.03	0.10	0.09	0.01	59.07	5.25	0.59	0.19	-	-	7.69	5.37
	200	3.61	1.21	0.32	0.21	61.33	11.56	0.78	0.38	-	-	46.96	0.99
PEM2	0	4.60	3.64	0.33	0.29	116.25	1.06	0.38	0.07	30.29	4.944	20.48	7.40
	5	1.90	0.21	0.10	0.02	115.95	0.92	0.52	0.07	279.8	66.7	10.27	7.96
	25	1.21	0.20	0.03	0.01	140.15	50.70	0.48	0.03	302	145.4	11.44	5.52
	100	7.14	1.91	0.38	0.19	117.30	14.42	0.59	0.06	248.2	131.2	12.81	3.62
	200	5.68	0.45	0.41	0.03	97.20	19.87	0.75	0.10	640.8	138.3	20.85	13.97
PEM3	0	7.32	2.88	0.26	0.07	227.00	111.72	0.88	0.19	19.6	5.302	20.48	8.40
	5	5.71	0.78	0.23	0.04	249.03	84.68	1.71	0.34	116.7	104.7	14.62	3.02
	25	5.63	0.59	0.26	0.03	327.50	44.55	1.45	0.39	245.1	103.6	15.14	6.34
	100	5.11	0.74	0.29	0.03	292.90	4.20	2.12	0.55	475.3	189.1	45.96	1.32
	200	2.09	0.39	0.16	0.04	233.90	73.54	3.36	1.12	600.7	88.95	50.62	3.23

As can be seen, the layer composition and the post-cross-linking hardly shows a clear influence on the wettability of the layer systems. The water contact angle is below 30° in the very hydrophilic range. Only highly cross-linked coatings (200 mg/mL EDC/NHS with PEM-1; 100 mg/mL and 200 mg/mL EDC/NHS with PEM-3) particularly show a slight increase in the water contact angle to 40° to 50°. However, clear trends cannot be derived from the wettability, which is why a significant influence of the wetting on the release or the binding behavior of the cytokine can be excluded.

The same applies to the roughness determined by AFM. Since the specific surface of the layer systems is relevant for a release of the cytokine, the Sdr value was determined in addition to the Ra value. Slight trends are recognizable from the results. With increasing the cross-linking, the roughness of the PEM-1 and PEM-2 systems increases slightly. This trend is not observed for the PEM-3 system. However, the changes in the specific surface area for all layer systems are below 1%, so an influence of the roughness on the release behavior is very unlikely.

The FT-IR measurements show an increase in the amide-I bands, which demonstrates the successful cross-linking of the coatings using EDC/NHS. For the PEM-2 and PEM-3 coating systems, an expected stiffening due to cross-linking could also be demonstrated. The PEM-I system produces a layer thickness that is too low to reliably determine data on the stiffness using AFM, as an influence of the substrate material cannot be ruled out.

Nevertheless, due to the cross-linking and the resulting compacting of the layer systems, both a reduction in the loading capacity and a delay in the release can be expected.

3.1. Loading Capacity and Release Kinetics

The different PEM systems were loaded with rhBMP-2 and the release of the cytokine was observed over 192 h. The amount of released rhBMP-2 was measured by an ELISA and the results were accumulated for each time point.

Figure 2 shows the resulting release profiles for each PEM system. Especially for the coatings PEM1 and PEM2, a release of the cytokine can be observed mainly within the first 48 h. The collagen-rich system PEM3 shows a burst release within the first 10 h.

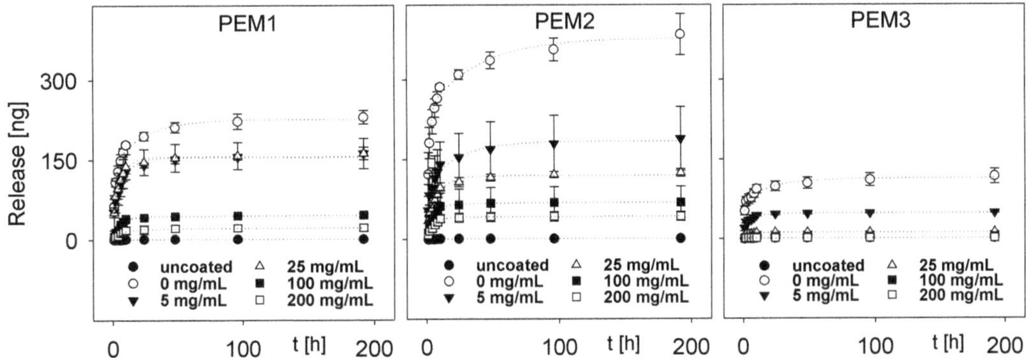

Figure 2. Release kinetics of the three coatings in dependence of the degree of cross-linking, dotted lines are to guide the eyes.

As expected, the multilayer films PEM1 and PEM2 show very similar release characteristics due to the comparable layer architecture. Both multilayers consist of a backbone of nine PLL–HEP double layers and in contrast to PEM1, PLL was substituted by collagen within the top layer of PEM2. A detailed consideration shows a slightly increased release of rhBMP-2 from the PEM2 system in comparison to the PEM1 system. Probably, this effect could be explained by the higher layer thickness of the coating. As we have shown elsewhere, the substitution of PLL by collagen results in a sudden increase in the coating thickness, which is a result of an incomplete charge compensation by the weak poly-cation collagen [36].

Apparently, this change in the layer architecture may lead to a slightly looser, open-porous layer architecture and a decrease in layer stiffness, which enables a higher release.

A completely different release behavior was observed for the PEM3 multilayer. The release of rhBMP-2 was significantly decreased. In addition to the simple quantitative effect caused by the thickness difference, it can be assumed that, caused by the weak cationic character of collagen, heparin is much more freely available within the PEM3 multilayer, which can act as a kind of drug reservoir for rhBMP-2. Consequently, this (i) increases the total loading capacity of the polyelectrolyte multilayer and (ii) inhibits the release due to the high binding capability of heparin. For a better comparability, the total release and the absolute amount of the initial rhBMP-2 loading are shown in Figure 3. It is remarkable that the total release is more than one order of magnitude lower than the initial loading of the coatings with cytokine. In percentage terms, the release amounts for PEM-1 range from ~4% for the not cross-linked coatings down to ~1% for the highest degree of cross-linking. The PEM-2 system shows a respective percentage release between ~5% down to ~1.5%, while the PEM-3 system shows a significant lower percentage release of ~1.3% down to almost zero.

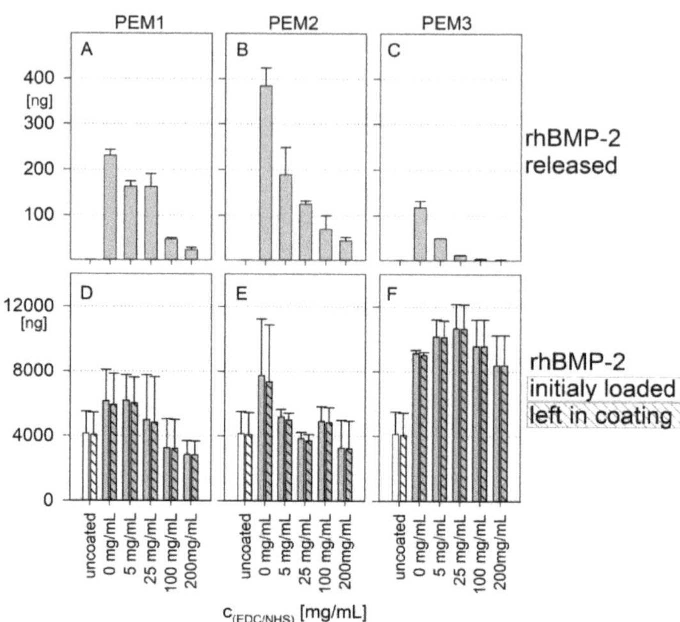

$c_{(EDC/NHS)}$ [mg/mL]

Figure 3. (**A–C**): Amount of the released rhBMP-2 after 192 h; (**D–F**): amount of rhBMP-2 initially loaded (clear bars) and left in coatings (hatched bars) in dependence of the degree of cross-linking. Results of a one-way ANOVA test can be found in the Appendix A in Figures A1 and A2.

Furthermore, it becomes clear that the loading capacity of the coatings (Figure 3D–F) is only slightly influenced by the cross-linking. Instead, it can be inferred that the loading capacity of the coatings is primarily determined by the coating architecture. With that in mind, it is important to mention that the PEM3 multilayer, which is composed of heparin and collagen, shows a loading capacity of around 8000 ng rhBMP-2, whereas the multilayers PEM1 and PEM2, which have a backbone consisting predominantly of PLL–HEP, show a significantly reduced loading capacity of around 4000 ng.

Obviously, drug delivery can also be targeted by a defined variation of the degree of cross-linking. A higher cross-linking of the multilayer films initially leads to a higher stiffness of the coatings and causes a significant inhibition of the release of BMP-2 [36]. This observation is particularly true for the PEM3 multilayer, as could be shown by the near zero order release kinetic for higher degrees of cross-linking (Figure 3C).

A similar phenomenon was observed by Crouzier et al. in 2009 who investigated PEM systems containing poly-L-lysine as cationic and hyaluronic acid as anionic polyelectrolytes. The authors incorporated BMP-2 in the layer and determined also a low initial release of the cytokine. The BMP-2 remains predominately in the layer and is still available for the cells in its bioactive form [37].

Nevertheless, numerous studies were focused on GAG-based PEMs as drug delivery system for cytokines and growth factors, especially with heparin and BMP-2. These investigations were usually carried out with the aim to establish a controlled and localized or site-specific drug delivery over a long period of time [17,38]. Introducing ECM-analogue polyelectrolytes like hydrogels or heparin leads to an additional protective function for cytokines, especially BMP-2, and can slow down the release rate. In hyaluronic acid hydrogel particles which are decorated with heparin, the loading capacity and the release of BMP-2 is strongly influenced by the heparin. The heparin changed the initial burst phase of the cytokine release to a near zero order release kinetic [39]. Ao et al. (2020) observed that the incorporation of heparin in a fibrin glue/fibronectin hydrogel significantly decreased the release of BMP-2 and prevented, effectively, the initial burst release. Additionally, the heparin cannot only influence the release kinetic, it also inhibits the in vivo-degradation of the cytokine by proteases [40,41]. In addition, it has been noted in the literature that tricalcium phosphate/hydroxyapatite bone substitutes coated with collagen type I and/or heparin show a higher loading capacity for BMP-2 and a different release pattern when the coating contains heparin. Thus, as might be expected, after 14 days, there is still BMP-2 bound in the layer system. For the samples made with collagen alone, almost all BMP-2 was released [42]. This can be explained by the enormous binding capacity of heparin which is also described for other cytokines and growth factors [43]. As demonstrated in this study, all the investigated PEMs contain heparin as a polyanion in each of the 10 double layers. So, this can be an indication of the observed low release of the BMP-2, insofar as the heparin binds the cytokine extremely stable and slows down the release kinetic. In this context, Laub et al. (2007) show the limited binding capacity of BMP-2 and other members of the TGF-β family to different collagen types [44]. Therefore, the high binding capacity of our multilayer systems is probably not mediated by the collagen, but rather through the heparin. An explanation, as to why the PEM3 system could be loaded with much more BMP-2 than the other two systems but releases less BMP-2, is the layer buildup. PEM3 is significantly thicker than PEM1 and PEM2 and shows an exponential growth because of the decreased intrinsic charge compensation and the open network structure, respectively, of the increased chain mobility within the PEM3 system. Beside the simple quantitative effect, it can be assumed that due to the weak cationic character of collagen, much more sulfate groups of heparin are available for the interaction with BMP-2 [45]. Hence, heparin is available much more freely within the PEM3 system, which then can act as a drug reservoir for BMP-2. This, consequently, increases the total loading capacity of the polyelectrolyte multilayer.

In this study, we observed the release under physiological conditions. Correspondingly, a conventional DMEM medium with a pH of 7.4 was used for all of the release experiments. Other studies have shown that the pH of the release medium influences the release of cytokines. Salvi et al. (2016) adsorbed around 2 $\mu g/cm^2$ BMP-2 directly on anodized titanium covered with $(PMAA/PLH)_5$. The release behavior was investigated in dependence of the pH value. The PEMs prepared at the lowest pH (pH = 4) show the highest BMP-2 release over 25 days. If the pH becomes more alkalic, the release decreases, reaching a minimum of around pH 6 and 7. This may reflect the fact that the change in the release kinetic results from changes in the internal structure of the PEM and the pH during preparation [46].

In any event, the investigated PEM systems here obviously serve much better as a drug reservoir than as a release system. This has, of course, some important consequences. For example, the incorporated drug is strongly bound in the matrix and is not delivered through diffusion caused by the concentration gradients in the media or the body fluids. In vivo cells adhere at the matrix and begin to modulate the cellular microenvironment, respectively, built up by their own ECM. This inevitably leads to a situation where the access to the cytokines is coupled to the rate of matrix degradation until the PEMs are fully degraded. In other words, in the case for bone regeneration, the BMP-2 is probably available for the entire bone healing process. Another fact is that BMP-2 delivery being higher than the clinically relevant doses might be associated with numerous complications, for instance tissue inflammation and abnormal or ectopic ossification. These complications result from the high doses which are needed to overcome short half-life and rapid clearance of the cytokine in vivo [30]. Thus, it can be speculated that a tailor-made PEM which serves primarily as a kind of BMP-2 drug reservoir is more advantageous than any burst release system. Hettiaratchi et al. (2020) investigated the positive effect of a drug reservoir for BMP-2 based on heparin microparticles [30].

3.2. Cell Response

To prove the cytocompatibility and suitability of the PEMs as a coating system for the better integration of implants in bone tissue, the PEMs were seeded with MC3T3-E1 cells, a mouse osteoblasts progenitor cell line, and the cell response was investigated thoroughly. The cell viability was measured by an XTT assay over a time period of 14 days.

Figure 4 show the measured absorption in the XTT assay for the time points 3 and 7 days without BMP-2 and with BMP-2 stimulation, relative to an uncoated tissue culture polystyrene reference (TCPS).

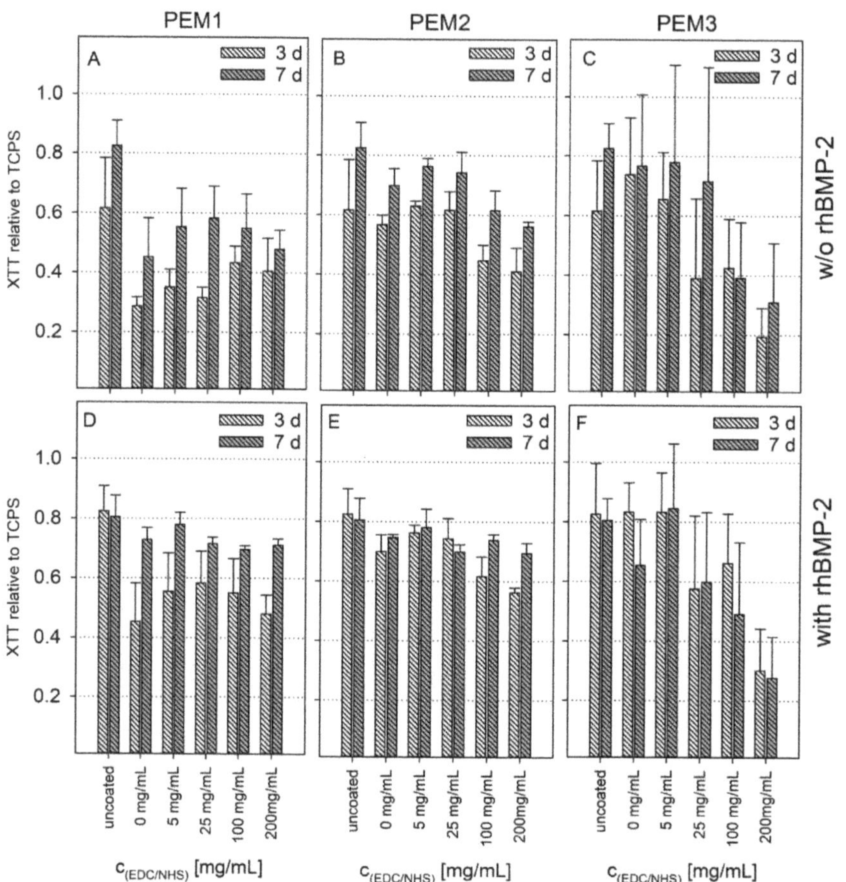

Figure 4. Absorbance in XTT assay relative to TCPS after 3 and 7 days on different cross-linked PEMs without BMP-2 (**A–C**) or loaded with BMP-2 (**D–F**). Error bars represent standard deviations of three independent experiments with three technical replicates each. Results of a one-way ANOVA test can be found in the Appendix A in Figures A3 and A4.

As shown in Figure 4A, the coating of PLL–HEP initially inhibits the cell viability at early time points. This effect can be explained by the reduced initial adhesion and proliferation of the cells on the relatively soft multilayers, as we have shown recently [36]. Cross-linking here results in a stiffening of the coating and thus an increased proliferation at EDC/NHS concentrations >100 mg/mL. The incorporation of a collagen top layer immediately leads to an increase in the viability of approximately 50% (Figure 4B). Strikingly, the cross-linking of the PEM2 coatings has negative effects above a certain concentration of EDC/NHS, which is particularly evident in the collagen-rich PEM3 system (Figure 4C).

On this background, it must be considered that cell binding to collagen is mediated by integrin binding sites. In the case of collagen, it is mainly the binding motif GFOGER on the helical collagen fiber which comes into play [23]. The EDC/NHS cross-linking chemistry obviously affects this binding site, because it forms amide bonds between primary amines and adjacent carboxylic groups. Thus, carboxylic groups which were modulated by the EDC/NHS cross-linking chemistry are no longer available as a bioactive group within the integrin binding motif. Indeed, this can result in a reduction in cell proliferation on EDC/NHS cross-linked collagen films [22]. This explanation is supported by the fact that cross-linking of the PEM2 coatings above an EDC/NHS concentration of 100 mg/mL causes a reduction in the viability, approximating the values of the corresponding PEM1 system, which has a similar coating architecture but does not contain the top collagen layer (Figure 4A,B).

However, for the non-cross-linked PEMs or the PEMs having a low degree of cross-linking, a positive effect on the cell viability was observed by introducing collagen type I.

BMP-2 loading generally leads to a slight but not significant increase in cell viability and partially compensates for the negative effects of cross-linking. Nevertheless, the influence of BMP-2 on the proliferation is weak, which is not surprising since BMP-2 is not a proliferation but a differentiation promoter.

3.3. Differentiation of MC3T3 into Bone Cells

3.3.1. Early Differentiation

The cells were cultured on different cross-linked PEMs loaded or non-loaded with BMP-2. After 7 days, the ALP activity was measured (Figure 5).

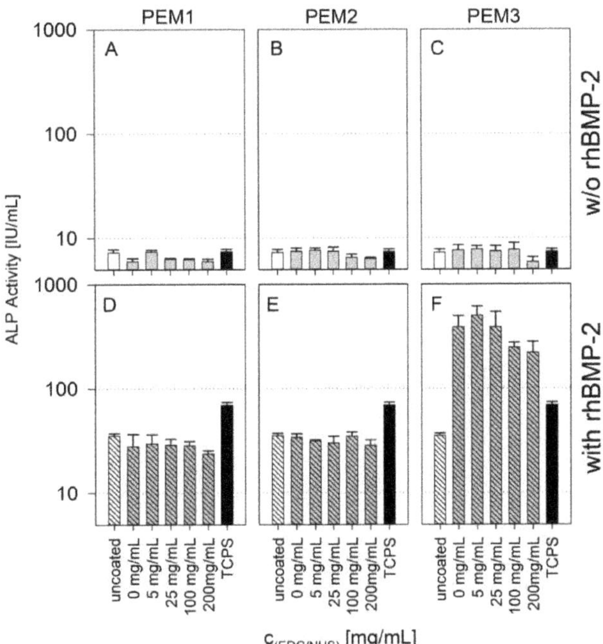

Figure 5. Results of ALP activity measurements after 7 days of cultivation in logarithmic scale; (**A–C**) without BMP-2; (**D–F**) with BMP-2. Results of a one-way ANOVA test can be found in the Appendix A in Figure A5.

The presence of BMP-2 leads to an increase in ALP activity of about one order of magnitude for PEM1 and PEM2 as well as for uncoated glass and TCPS.

This is a relevant finding since the uncoated glass surface and the TCPS surface also shows this increase. The ALP activity was measured after 7 days, at a time when no release of BMP-2 was measurable on either the PEM coatings or the references.

However, the non-cross-linked coatings of the PEM1 and PEM2 systems show higher amounts of immobilized BMP-2 compared to the uncoated reference (Figures 3D and 5). This means that the additional amount of cytokine immobilized in the PEM1 and PEM2 coating is obviously not bioavailable.

The PEM3 system shows a 10-fold increase in ALP activity compared to the PEM1 and PEM2 systems. There is a slight decrease in activity at high EDC/NHS concentrations, but this can be attributed to the already discussed reduced availability of binding motifs in the cross-linked collagen. Nevertheless, this increase in one magnitude of order can only be explained by the bioactive availability of the cytokine immobilized within the multilayer. The coating of heparin and collagen is apparently able to incorporate rhBMP-2 in its bioactive form. This observation was not made for PEM coatings containing less or no type I collagen.

3.3.2. Late Differentiation

As osteogenesis progresses, the ECM acts, to an increasing extent, as a template for mineralization processes and more and more calcium is deposited to build up a calcified bone structure. Calcium deposition is a late marker of osteogenic differentiation. This process can be monitored with an Alizarin Red S Assay. The red dye Alizarin Red S binds to the calcium depositions in the matrix and can be removed with acetic acid. The more calcium that is incorporated in the matrix, the more dye that is released. Usually, this can be quantified by simple absorption measurements.

The results of the calcification by the Alizarin Red assay support the conclusions made on the basis of the ALP activity results (Figure 6). Both PEM1 and PEM2 coatings show no enhanced calcification after 21 days due to BMP-2 loading, whereas the PEM3 coatings show an enhancement of one order of magnitude.

Keeping in mind that the used MC3T3-E1 cell line is a specifically sensitive cell line to investigate surface-related effects on calcification, it can be stated that the late cell differentiation is strictly dependent on the bioavailability of immobilized BMP-2. This finding is in a good accordance with other studies which investigated the differentiation behavior of MC3T3-E1 cells on GAG/BMP-2-containing coatings [32,40].

Another effect shown by the results is the trend that PEM3 shows as a function of cross-linking. In both cases, with or without BMP-2 loading, an obvious correlation between the cross-linking and the ARS assay is evident. This effect might have mechanical reasons, as the cross-linked coatings show a drastic increased layer stiffness [36]. Nevertheless, it suggests that the immobilized rhBMP-2 cytokine plays a major key role concerning the observed differentiation behavior. These findings are supported by some other publications which focused on related topics [4,47,48].

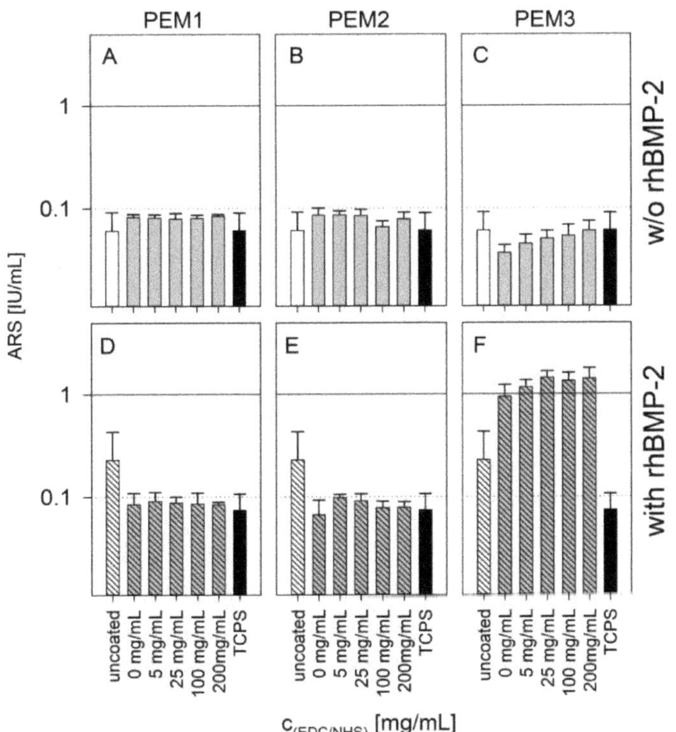

Figure 6. Absorbance of ARS assay on different cross-linked PEMs unloaded (**A–C**) or loaded with BMP-2 (**D–F**) after 21 days of cultivation in logarithmic scale. Error bars represent standard deviations of three independent experiments with three technical replicates each. Results of a one-way ANOVA test can be found in the Appendix A in Figure A6.

4. Conclusions

The aim of this study was to investigate the performance of three LbL films with different multilayer compositions and architectures, regarding their suitability as drug reservoirs, respectively, and drug release systems. The investigations essentially focused on the effect of rhBMP-2 in bone contact. For this purpose, PEM systems were constructed on the basis of poly-L-lysine, a relatively strong poly-cation and heparin, a GAG of the ECM as well as collagen type I, a glycoprotein and one of the main components of the osteoid ECM. By gradually cross-linking the layers, we were also able to vary the stiffness of the multilayer films and, consequently, the release kinetics of rhBMP-2.

We found that a minor part of the incorporated rhBMP-2 was released from the coatings. Furthermore, the release occurred mainly within the first 48 h. We were able to confirm the hypothesis, that the release can be adjusted in a defined way by means of a cross-linking of the multilayers. In cell biological experiments, we referred to the differentiation of the osteoprogenitor cell line MC3T3-E1, however, we were able to demonstrate that neither the amount nor the kinetics of the release plays the primary role in osteogenic differentiation. Rather, BMP-2 immobilized in collagen-rich films was found to be highly bioactive. An impressive increase in ALP activity by two orders of magnitude after 7 d and an increase in calcification by one order of magnitude after 21 d were observed.

It must be concluded that polyelectrolyte multilayers made on the basis of heparin and collagen type I represent an excellent artificial ECM mimicry and a promising approach for the development of therapeutic options in bone regeneration and implantology.

Author Contributions: Conceptualization, K.L. and H.S.; funding acquisition, K.L. and H.S.; methodology, J.L., K.M., U.S. and H.R.; investigation, J.L., K.M., U.S. and H.R.; resources, K.L.; data curation, J.L. and H.R.; writing—original draft preparation, J.L.; writing—review and editing, H.R., K.L., U.S., H.S. and C.B.; visualization, H.R.; supervision, J.L.; project administration, J.L. All authors have read and agreed to the published version of the manuscript.

Funding: This work has been funded by grants from the German Research Foundation (DFG) SCHL 168-12/1 and LI 916/18-1.

Institutional Review Board Statement: Not applicable.

Informed Consent Statement: Not applicable.

Data Availability Statement: The data presented in this study are available on request from the corresponding author.

Acknowledgments: We kindly thank Martina Lackner, Anika Hartleib and Juliane Papra for their technical and experimental support.

Conflicts of Interest: The authors declare no conflict of interest.

Appendix A

ANOVA Figure 3A-C Release	EDC	B33 — 0	PEM1 — 0	5	25	100	200	PEM2 — 0	5	25	100	200	PEM3 — 0	5	25	100
B33	0															
PEM1	0	***														
PEM1	5	***	**													
PEM1	25	***	**	n.s.												
PEM1	100	**	***	***	***											
PEM1	200	*	***	***	***	n.s.										
PEM2	0	***	***	***	***	***	***									
PEM2	5	***	n.s.	n.s.	n.s.	***	***	***								
PEM2	25	**	***	n.s.	n.s.	**	***	***	**							
PEM2	100	*	***	***	***	n.s.	n.s.	***	***	n.s.						
PEM2	200	*	***	***	***	n.s.	n.s.	***	***	**	n.s.					
PEM3	0	**	***	n.s.	n.s.	**	***	***	**	n.s.	n.s.	**				
PEM3	5	*	***	***	***	n.s.	n.s.	***	***	**	n.s.	n.s.	**			
PEM3	25	n.s.	***	***	***	n.s.	n.s.	***	***	***	n.s.	n.s.	***	n.s.		
PEM3	100	n.s.	***	***	***	n.s.	n.s.	***	***	***	**	n.s.	***	n.s.	n.s.	
PEM3	200	n.s.	***	***	***	n.s.	n.s.	***	***	***	**	n.s.	***	n.s.	n.s.	n.s.

Figure A1. Results of one-way ANOVA for data related to Figure 3A–C; n.s.: not significant; *: $p < 0.1$; **: $p < 0.05$; ***: $p < 0.001$.

ANOVA Figure 3D - F Immobilized	EDC	B33	PEM1					PEM2					PEM3			
		0	0	5	25	100	200	0	5	25	100	200	0	5	25	100
B33	0															
PEM1	0	n.s.														
	5	n.s.	n.s.													
	25	n.s.	n.s.	n.s.												
	100	n.s.	n.s.	n.s.	n.s.											
	200	n.s.	n.s.	n.s.	n.s.	n.s.										
PEM2	0	n.s.	n.s.	n.s.	n.s.	n.s.	n.s.									
	5	n.s.	n.s.	n.s.	n.s.	n.s.	n.s.	n.s.								
	25	n.s.	n.s.	n.s.	n.s.	n.s.	n.s.	n.s.	n.s.							
	100	n.s.	n.s.	n.s.	n.s.	n.s.	n.s.	n.s.	n.s.	n.s.						
	200	n.s.	n.s.	n.s.	n.s.	n.s.	n.s.	n.s.	n.s.	n.s.	n.s.					
PEM3	0	n.s.	n.s.	n.s.	n.s.	**	**	n.s.	n.s.	*	n.s.	**				
	5	**	n.s.	n.s.	*	**	***	n.s.	*	**	*	**	n.s.			
	25	**	n.s.	n.s.	**	***	***	n.s.	**	**	**	***	n.s.	n.s.		
	100	**	n.s.	n.s.	n.s.	**	**	n.s.	n.s.	**	n.s.	**	n.s.	n.s.	n.s.	
	200	n.s.	n.s.	n.s.	n.s.	*	**	n.s.	n.s.	n.s.	n.s.	*	n.s.	n.s.	n.s.	n.s.

Figure A2. Results of one-way ANOVA for data related to Figure 3D–F; n.s.: not significant; *: $p < 0.1$; **. $p < 0.05$, ***. $p < 0.001$.

			with BMP2																w/o BMP2														
ANOVA Figure 4:			**B33**	**TCPS**	**PEM1**					**PEM2**					**PEM3**					**B33**	**TCPS**	**PEM1**					**PEM2**					**PEM3**			
XTT 3 d		**EDC**	0	0	0	5	25	100	200	0	5	25	100	200	0	5	25	100	200	0	0	0	5	25	100	200	0	5	25	100	200	0	5	25	100
with BMP2	B33	0																																
	TCPS	0	n.s.																															
	PEM1	0	n.s.	*																														
		5	n.s.	n.s.	n.s.																													
		25	n.s.	n.s.	n.s.	n.s.																												
		100	n.s.	n.s.	n.s.	n.s.	n.s.																											
		200	n.s.	n.s.	n.s.	n.s.	n.s.	n.s.																										
	PEM2	0	n.s.	n.s.	n.s.	n.s.	n.s.	n.s.	n.s.																									
		5	n.s.	n.s.	n.s.	n.s.	n.s.	n.s.	n.s.	n.s.																								
		25	n.s.	n.s.	n.s.	n.s.	n.s.	n.s.	n.s.	n.s.	n.s.																							
		100	n.s.	n.s.	n.s.	n.s.	n.s.	n.s.	n.s.	n.s.	n.s.	n.s.																						
		200	n.s.	n.s.	n.s.	n.s.	n.s.	n.s.	n.s.	n.s.	n.s.	n.s.	n.s.																					
	PEM3	0	n.s.	n.s.	n.s.	n.s.	n.s.	n.s.	n.s.	n.s.	n.s.	n.s.	n.s.	n.s.																				
		5	n.s.	n.s.	n.s.	n.s.	n.s.	n.s.	n.s.	n.s.	n.s.	n.s.	n.s.	n.s.	n.s.																			
		25	n.s.	n.s.	n.s.	n.s.	n.s.	n.s.	n.s.	n.s.	n.s.	n.s.	n.s.	n.s.	n.s.	n.s.																		
		100	n.s.	**	n.s.	n.s.	n.s.	n.s.	n.s.	n.s.	n.s.	n.s.	n.s.	n.s.	n.s.	n.s.	n.s.																	
		200	n.s.	**	n.s.	n.s.	n.s.	n.s.	n.s.	n.s.	n.s.	n.s.	n.s.	n.s.	n.s.	n.s.	n.s.	n.s.																
w/o BMP2	B33	0	n.s.	n.s.	n.s.	n.s.	n.s.	n.s.	n.s.	n.s.	n.s.	n.s.	n.s.	n.s.	n.s.	n.s.	n.s.	n.s.	n.s.															
	TCPS	0	n.s.	n.s.	***	***	**	***	***	*	n.s.	n.s.	**	**	n.s.	n.s.	*	***	***	n.s.														
	PEM1	0	n.s.	**	n.s.	n.s.	n.s.	n.s.	n.s.	n.s.	n.s.	n.s.	n.s.	n.s.	n.s.	n.s.	n.s.	n.s.	n.s.	n.s.	***													
		5	n.s.	*	n.s.	n.s.	n.s.	n.s.	n.s.	n.s.	n.s.	n.s.	n.s.	n.s.	n.s.	n.s.	n.s.	n.s.	n.s.	n.s.	***	n.s.												
		25	n.s.	**	n.s.	n.s.	n.s.	n.s.	n.s.	n.s.	n.s.	n.s.	n.s.	n.s.	n.s.	n.s.	n.s.	n.s.	n.s.	n.s.	***	n.s.	n.s.											
		100	n.s.	n.s.	n.s.	n.s.	n.s.	n.s.	n.s.	n.s.	n.s.	n.s.	n.s.	n.s.	n.s.	n.s.	n.s.	n.s.	n.s.	n.s.	***	n.s.	n.s.	n.s.										
		200	n.s.	n.s.	n.s.	n.s.	n.s.	n.s.	n.s.	n.s.	n.s.	n.s.	n.s.	n.s.	n.s.	n.s.	n.s.	n.s.	n.s.	n.s.	***	n.s.	n.s.	n.s.	n.s.									
	PEM2	0	n.s.	n.s.	n.s.	n.s.	n.s.	n.s.	n.s.	n.s.	n.s.	n.s.	n.s.	n.s.	n.s.	n.s.	n.s.	n.s.	n.s.	n.s.	*	n.s.	n.s.	n.s.	n.s.	n.s.								
		5	n.s.	n.s.	n.s.	n.s.	n.s.	n.s.	n.s.	n.s.	n.s.	n.s.	n.s.	n.s.	n.s.	n.s.	n.s.	n.s.	n.s.	n.s.	n.s.	n.s.	n.s.	n.s.	n.s.	n.s.	n.s.							
		25	n.s.	n.s.	n.s.	n.s.	n.s.	n.s.	n.s.	n.s.	n.s.	n.s.	n.s.	n.s.	n.s.	n.s.	n.s.	n.s.	n.s.	n.s.	n.s.	n.s.	n.s.	n.s.	n.s.	n.s.	n.s.	n.s.						
		100	n.s.	n.s.	n.s.	n.s.	n.s.	n.s.	n.s.	n.s.	n.s.	n.s.	n.s.	n.s.	n.s.	n.s.	n.s.	n.s.	n.s.	n.s.	**	n.s.	n.s.	n.s.	n.s.	n.s.	n.s.	n.s.	n.s.					
		200	n.s.	n.s.	n.s.	n.s.	n.s.	n.s.	n.s.	n.s.	n.s.	n.s.	n.s.	n.s.	n.s.	n.s.	n.s.	n.s.	n.s.	n.s.	***	n.s.	n.s.	n.s.	n.s.	n.s.	n.s.	n.s.	n.s.	n.s.				
	PEM3	0	n.s.	n.s.	n.s.	n.s.	n.s.	n.s.	n.s.	n.s.	n.s.	n.s.	n.s.	n.s.	n.s.	n.s.	n.s.	n.s.	n.s.	**	n.s.	n.s.	*	n.s.	n.s.	n.s.	n.s.	n.s.	n.s.	n.s.	n.s.			
		5	n.s.	n.s.	n.s.	n.s.	n.s.	n.s.	n.s.	n.s.	n.s.	n.s.	n.s.	n.s.	n.s.	n.s.	n.s.	n.s.	n.s.	n.s.	n.s.	n.s.	n.s.	n.s.	n.s.	n.s.	n.s.	n.s.	n.s.	n.s.	n.s.	n.s.		
		25	n.s.	n.s.	n.s.	n.s.	n.s.	n.s.	n.s.	n.s.	n.s.	n.s.	n.s.	n.s.	n.s.	n.s.	n.s.	n.s.	n.s.	n.s.	***	n.s.	n.s.	n.s.	n.s.	n.s.	n.s.	n.s.	n.s.	n.s.	n.s.	n.s.	n.s.	
		100	n.s.	n.s.	n.s.	n.s.	n.s.	n.s.	n.s.	n.s.	n.s.	n.s.	n.s.	n.s.	n.s.	n.s.	n.s.	n.s.	n.s.	n.s.	***	n.s.	n.s.	n.s.	n.s.	n.s.	n.s.	n.s.	n.s.	n.s.	n.s.	n.s.	n.s.	n.s.
		200	**	***	n.s.	n.s.	n.s.	n.s.	n.s.	n.s.	n.s.	n.s.	n.s.	n.s.	n.s.	n.s.	n.s.	n.s.	n.s.	n.s.	***	n.s.	n.s.	n.s.	n.s.	n.s.	n.s.	*	n.s.	n.s.	n.s.	**	**	n.s.	n.s.

Figure A3. Results of one-way ANOVA for data related to Figure 4 (3 d); n.s.: not significant; *: $p < 0.1$; **: $p < 0.05$; ***: $p < 0.001$.

| ANOVA Figure 4: | | | with BMP2 | | | | | | | | | | | | | | | | w/o BMP2 | | | | | | | | | | | | | | | |
| XTT 7 d | | | B33 | TCPS | PEM1 | | | | | PEM2 | | | | | PEM3 | | | | | B33 | TCPS | PEM1 | | | | | PEM2 | | | | | PEM3 | | | |
		EDC	0	0	0	5	25	100	200	0	5	25	100	200	0	5	25	100	200	0	0	0	5	25	100	200	0	5	25	100	200	0	5	25	100
with BMP2	B33	0																																	
	TCPS	0	n.s.																																
	PEM1	0	n.s.	n.s.																															
		5	n.s.	n.s.	n.s.																														
		25	n.s.	n.s.	n.s.	n.s.																													
		100	n.s.	n.s.	n.s.	n.s.	n.s.																												
		200	n.s.	n.s.	n.s.	n.s.	n.s.	n.s.																											
	PEM2	0	n.s.	n.s.	n.s.	n.s.	n.s.	n.s.	n.s.																										
		5	n.s.	n.s.	n.s.	n.s.	n.s.	n.s.	n.s.	n.s.																									
		25	n.s.	n.s.	n.s.	n.s.	n.s.	n.s.	n.s.	n.s.	n.s.																								
		100	n.s.	n.s.	n.s.	n.s.	n.s.	n.s.	n.s.	n.s.	n.s.	n.s.																							
		200	n.s.	n.s.	n.s.	n.s.	n.s.	n.s.	n.s.	n.s.	n.s.	n.s.	n.s.																						
	PEM3	0	n.s.	n.s.	n.s.	n.s.	n.s.	n.s.	n.s.	n.s.	n.s.	n.s.	n.s.	n.s.																					
		5	n.s.	n.s.	n.s.	n.s.	n.s.	n.s.	n.s.	n.s.	n.s.	n.s.	n.s.	n.s.	n.s.																				
		25	n.s.	**	n.s.	n.s.	n.s.	n.s.	n.s.	n.s.	n.s.	n.s.	n.s.	n.s.	n.s.	n.s.																			
		100	n.s.	***	n.s.	n.s.	n.s.	n.s.	n.s.	n.s.	n.s.	n.s.	n.s.	n.s.	n.s.	n.s.	n.s.																		
		200	***	***	**	***	**	**	**	**	***	**	**	**	*	***	n.s.	n.s.																	
w/o BMP2	B33	0	n.s.	n.s.	n.s.	n.s.	n.s.	n.s.	n.s.	n.s.	n.s.	n.s.	n.s.	n.s.	n.s.	n.s.	n.s.	n.s.	***																
	TCPS	0	n.s.	n.s.	n.s.	n.s.	n.s.	n.s.	n.s.	n.s.	n.s.	n.s.	n.s.	n.s.	n.s.	n.s.	n.s.	**	***	***															
	PEM1	0	**	***	n.s.	**	n.s.	n.s.	n.s.	*	**	n.s.	*	n.s.	n.s.	**	n.s.	n.s.	n.s.	**	***														
		5	n.s.	n.s.	n.s.	n.s.	n.s.	n.s.	n.s.	n.s.	n.s.	n.s.	n.s.	n.s.	n.s.	n.s.	n.s.	n.s.	n.s.	n.s.	*	n.s.													
		25	n.s.	*	n.s.	n.s.	n.s.	n.s.	n.s.	n.s.	n.s.	n.s.	n.s.	n.s.	n.s.	n.s.	n.s.	n.s.	n.s.	n.s.	**	n.s.	n.s.												
		100	n.s.	*	n.s.	n.s.	n.s.	n.s.	n.s.	n.s.	n.s.	n.s.	n.s.	n.s.	n.s.	n.s.	n.s.	n.s.	n.s.	n.s.	**	n.s.	n.s.	n.s.											
		200	n.s.	n.s.	n.s.	n.s.	n.s.	n.s.	n.s.	n.s.	n.s.	n.s.	n.s.	n.s.	n.s.	n.s.	n.s.	n.s.	n.s.	n.s.	*	n.s.	n.s.	n.s.	n.s.										
	PEM2	0	n.s.	***	n.s.	n.s.	n.s.	n.s.	n.s.	n.s.	n.s.	n.s.	n.s.	n.s.	n.s.	*	n.s.	n.s.	n.s.	*	***	n.s.	n.s.	n.s.	n.s.	n.s.									
		5	n.s.	n.s.	n.s.	n.s.	n.s.	n.s.	n.s.	n.s.	n.s.	n.s.	n.s.	n.s.	n.s.	n.s.	n.s.	n.s.	**	n.s.	n.s.	n.s.	n.s.	n.s.	n.s.	n.s.	n.s.								
		25	n.s.	n.s.	n.s.	n.s.	n.s.	n.s.	n.s.	n.s.	n.s.	n.s.	n.s.	n.s.	n.s.	n.s.	n.s.	n.s.	*	n.s.	n.s.	n.s.	n.s.	n.s.	n.s.	n.s.	n.s.	n.s.							
		100	n.s.	n.s.	n.s.	n.s.	n.s.	n.s.	n.s.	n.s.	n.s.	n.s.	n.s.	n.s.	n.s.	n.s.	n.s.	n.s.	**	n.s.	n.s.	n.s.	n.s.	n.s.	n.s.	n.s.	n.s.	n.s.	n.s.						
		200	n.s.	n.s.	n.s.	n.s.	n.s.	n.s.	n.s.	n.s.	n.s.	n.s.	n.s.	n.s.	n.s.	n.s.	n.s.	n.s.	*	n.s.	n.s.	n.s.	n.s.	n.s.	n.s.	n.s.	n.s.	n.s.	n.s.	n.s.					
	PEM3	0	n.s.	n.s.	n.s.	n.s.	n.s.	n.s.	n.s.	n.s.	n.s.	n.s.	n.s.	n.s.	n.s.	n.s.	n.s.	n.s.	***	n.s.	n.s.	***	n.s.	n.s.	n.s.	n.s.	*	n.s.	n.s.	n.s.	n.s.				
		5	n.s.	n.s.	n.s.	n.s.	n.s.	n.s.	n.s.	n.s.	n.s.	n.s.	n.s.	n.s.	n.s.	n.s.	n.s.	n.s.	***	n.s.	n.s.	***	n.s.	n.s.	n.s.	n.s.	*	n.s.	n.s.	n.s.	n.s.	n.s.			
		25	n.s.	**	n.s.	n.s.	n.s.	n.s.	n.s.	n.s.	n.s.	n.s.	n.s.	n.s.	n.s.	n.s.	n.s.	n.s.	n.s.	n.s.	**	n.s.	n.s.	n.s.	n.s.	n.s.	n.s.	n.s.	n.s.	n.s.	n.s.	n.s.	n.s.		
		100	n.s.	n.s.	n.s.	n.s.	n.s.	n.s.	n.s.	n.s.	n.s.	n.s.	n.s.	n.s.	n.s.	n.s.	n.s.	n.s.	**	n.s.	n.s.	n.s.	n.s.	n.s.	n.s.	n.s.	n.s.	n.s.	n.s.	n.s.	n.s.	n.s.	n.s.	n.s.	
		200	***	***	**	**	**	*	**	**	**	**	**	*	n.s.	***	n.s.	n.s.	n.s.	***	***	n.s.	n.s.	n.s.	n.s.	n.s.	n.s.	*	n.s.	*	n.s.	***	***	n.s.	n.s.

Figure A4. Results of one-way ANOVA for data related to Figure 4 (7 d); n.s.: not significant; *: $p < 0.1$; **: $p < 0.05$; ***: $p < 0.001$.

The table below reproduces the figure. Column headers combine BMP2 condition, material and EDC concentration. "w" = with BMP2; "wo" = w/o BMP2. Each data column header is written as condition·material·EDC (e.g. `w·PEM1·25` = with BMP2, PEM1, EDC 25). Empty cells are blank (lower-triangular matrix).

ANOVA Figure 5: ALP	Material	EDC	w·B33·0	w·TCPS·0	w·PEM1·0	w·PEM1·5	w·PEM1·25	w·PEM1·100	w·PEM1·200	w·PEM2·0	w·PEM2·5	w·PEM2·25	w·PEM2·100	w·PEM2·200	w·PEM3·0	w·PEM3·5	w·PEM3·25	w·PEM3·100	w·PEM3·200	wo·B33·0	wo·TCPS·0	wo·PEM1·0	wo·PEM1·5	wo·PEM1·25	wo·PEM1·100	wo·PEM1·200	wo·PEM2·0	wo·PEM2·5	wo·PEM2·25	wo·PEM2·100	wo·PEM2·200	wo·PEM3·0	wo·PEM3·5	wo·PEM3·25	wo·PEM3·100
with BMP2	B33	0																																	
	TCPS	0	n.s.																																
	PEM1	0	n.s.	n.s.																															
	PEM1	5	n.s.	n.s.	n.s.																														
	PEM1	25	n.s.	n.s.	n.s.	n.s.																													
	PEM1	100	n.s.	n.s.	n.s.	n.s.	n.s.																												
	PEM1	200	n.s.	n.s.	n.s.	n.s.	n.s.	n.s.																											
	PEM2	0	n.s.	n.s.	n.s.	n.s.	n.s.	n.s.	n.s.																										
	PEM2	5	n.s.	n.s.	n.s.	n.s.	n.s.	n.s.	n.s.	n.s.																									
	PEM2	25	n.s.	n.s.	n.s.	n.s.	n.s.	n.s.	n.s.	n.s.	n.s.																								
	PEM2	100	n.s.	n.s.	n.s.	n.s.	n.s.	n.s.	n.s.	n.s.	n.s.	n.s.																							
	PEM2	200	n.s.	n.s.	n.s.	n.s.	n.s.	n.s.	n.s.	n.s.	n.s.	n.s.	n.s.																						
	PEM3	0	***	***	***	***	***	***	***	***	***	***	***	***																					
	PEM3	5	***	***	***	***	***	***	***	***	***	***	***	***	n.s.																				
	PEM3	25	***	***	***	***	***	***	***	***	***	***	***	***	n.s.	n.s.																			
	PEM3	100	***	***	***	***	***	***	***	***	***	***	***	***	**	***	**																		
	PEM3	200	***	**	***	***	***	***	***	***	***	***	***	***	***	***	***	n.s.																	
w/o BMP2	B33	0	n.s.	n.s.	n.s.	n.s.	n.s.	n.s.	n.s.	n.s.	n.s.	n.s.	n.s.	n.s.	***	***	***	***	***																
	TCPS	0	n.s.	n.s.	n.s.	n.s.	n.s.	n.s.	n.s.	n.s.	n.s.	n.s.	n.s.	n.s.	***	***	***	***	***	n.s.															
	PEM1	0	n.s.	n.s.	n.s.	n.s.	n.s.	n.s.	n.s.	n.s.	n.s.	n.s.	n.s.	n.s.	***	***	***	***	***	n.s.	n.s.														
	PEM1	5	n.s.	n.s.	n.s.	n.s.	n.s.	n.s.	n.s.	n.s.	n.s.	n.s.	n.s.	n.s.	***	***	***	***	***	n.s.	n.s.	n.s.													
	PEM1	25	n.s.	n.s.	n.s.	n.s.	n.s.	n.s.	n.s.	n.s.	n.s.	n.s.	n.s.	n.s.	***	***	***	***	***	n.s.	n.s.	n.s.	n.s.												
	PEM1	100	n.s.	n.s.	n.s.	n.s.	n.s.	n.s.	n.s.	n.s.	n.s.	n.s.	n.s.	n.s.	***	***	***	***	***	n.s.	n.s.	n.s.	n.s.	n.s.											
	PEM1	200	n.s.	n.s.	n.s.	n.s.	n.s.	n.s.	n.s.	n.s.	n.s.	n.s.	n.s.	n.s.	***	***	***	***	***	n.s.	n.s.	n.s.	n.s.	n.s.	n.s.										
	PEM2	0	n.s.	n.s.	n.s.	n.s.	n.s.	n.s.	n.s.	n.s.	n.s.	n.s.	n.s.	n.s.	***	***	***	***	***	n.s.	n.s.	n.s.	n.s.	n.s.	n.s.	n.s.									
	PEM2	5	n.s.	n.s.	n.s.	n.s.	n.s.	n.s.	n.s.	n.s.	n.s.	n.s.	n.s.	n.s.	***	***	***	***	***	n.s.	n.s.	n.s.	n.s.	n.s.	n.s.	n.s.	n.s.								
	PEM2	25	n.s.	n.s.	n.s.	n.s.	n.s.	n.s.	n.s.	n.s.	n.s.	n.s.	n.s.	n.s.	***	***	***	***	***	n.s.	n.s.	n.s.	n.s.	n.s.	n.s.	n.s.	n.s.	n.s.							
	PEM2	100	n.s.	n.s.	n.s.	n.s.	n.s.	n.s.	n.s.	n.s.	n.s.	n.s.	n.s.	n.s.	***	***	***	***	***	n.s.	n.s.	n.s.	n.s.	n.s.	n.s.	n.s.	n.s.	n.s.	n.s.						
	PEM2	200	n.s.	n.s.	n.s.	n.s.	n.s.	n.s.	n.s.	n.s.	n.s.	n.s.	n.s.	n.s.	***	***	***	***	***	n.s.	n.s.	n.s.	n.s.	n.s.	n.s.	n.s.	n.s.	n.s.	n.s.	n.s.					
	PEM3	0	n.s.	n.s.	n.s.	n.s.	n.s.	n.s.	n.s.	n.s.	n.s.	n.s.	n.s.	n.s.	***	***	***	***	***	n.s.	n.s.	n.s.	n.s.	n.s.	n.s.	n.s.	n.s.	n.s.	n.s.	n.s.	n.s.				
	PEM3	5	n.s.	n.s.	n.s.	n.s.	n.s.	n.s.	n.s.	n.s.	n.s.	n.s.	n.s.	n.s.	***	***	***	***	***	n.s.	n.s.	n.s.	n.s.	n.s.	n.s.	n.s.	n.s.	n.s.	n.s.	n.s.	n.s.	n.s.			
	PEM3	25	n.s.	n.s.	n.s.	n.s.	n.s.	n.s.	n.s.	n.s.	n.s.	n.s.	n.s.	n.s.	***	***	***	***	***	n.s.	n.s.	n.s.	n.s.	n.s.	n.s.	n.s.	n.s.	n.s.	n.s.	n.s.	n.s.	n.s.	n.s.		
	PEM3	100	n.s.	n.s.	n.s.	n.s.	n.s.	n.s.	n.s.	n.s.	n.s.	n.s.	n.s.	n.s.	***	***	***	***	***	n.s.	n.s.	n.s.	n.s.	n.s.	n.s.	n.s.	n.s.	n.s.	n.s.	n.s.	n.s.	n.s.	n.s.	n.s.	
	PEM3	200	n.s.	n.s.	n.s.	n.s.	n.s.	n.s.	n.s.	n.s.	n.s.	n.s.	n.s.	n.s.	***	***	***	***	***	n.s.	n.s.	n.s.	n.s.	n.s.	n.s.	n.s.	n.s.	n.s.	n.s.	n.s.	n.s.	n.s.	n.s.	n.s.	n.s.

Figure A5. Results of one-way ANOVA for data related to Figure 5; n.s.: not significant; *: $p < 0.1$; **: $p < 0.05$; ***: $p < 0.001$.

ANOVA Figure 6: ARS			with BMP2																w/o BMP2															
			B33	TCPS	PEM1					PEM2					PEM3					B33	TCPS	PEM1					PEM2					PEM3			
		EDC	0	0	0	5	25	100	200	0	5	25	100	200	0	5	25	100	200	0	0	0	5	25	100	200	0	5	25	100	200	0	5	25	100
with BMP2	B33	0																																	
	TCPS	0	n.s.																																
	PEM1	0	n.s.	n.s.																															
		5	n.s.	n.s.	n.s.																														
		25	n.s.	n.s.	n.s.	n.s.																													
		100	n.s.	n.s.	n.s.	n.s.	n.s.																												
		200	n.s.	n.s.	n.s.	n.s.	n.s.	n.s.																											
	PEM2	0	n.s.	n.s.	n.s.	n.s.	n.s.	n.s.	n.s.																										
		5	n.s.	n.s.	n.s.	n.s.	n.s.	n.s.	n.s.	n.s.																									
		25	n.s.	n.s.	n.s.	n.s.	n.s.	n.s.	n.s.	n.s.	n.s.																								
		100	n.s.	n.s.	n.s.	n.s.	n.s.	n.s.	n.s.	n.s.	n.s.	n.s.																							
		200	n.s.	n.s.	n.s.	n.s.	n.s.	n.s.	n.s.	n.s.	n.s.	n.s.	n.s.																						
	PEM3	0	***	***	***	***	***	***	***	***	***	***	***	***																				
		5	***	***	***	***	***	***	***	***	***	***	***	***	n.s.																			
		25	***	***	***	***	***	***	***	***	***	***	***	***	***	n.s.																		
		100	***	***	***	***	***	***	***	***	***	***	***	***	**	n.s.	n.s.																	
		200	***	***	***	***	***	***	***	***	***	***	***	***	***	n.s.	n.s.	n.s.																
w/o BMP2	B33	0	n.s.	n.s.	n.s.	n.s.	n.s.	n.s.	n.s.	n.s.	n.s.	n.s.	n.s.	n.s.	***	***	***	***	***															
	TCPS	0	n.s.	n.s.	n.s.	n.s.	n.s.	n.s.	n.s.	n.s.	n.s.	n.s.	n.s.	n.s.	***	***	***	***	***	n.s.														
	PEM1	0	n.s.	n.s.	n.s.	n.s.	n.s.	n.s.	n.s.	n.s.	n.s.	n.s.	n.s.	n.s.	***	***	***	***	***	n.s.	n.s.													
		5	n.s.	n.s.	n.s.	n.s.	n.s.	n.s.	n.s.	n.s.	n.s.	n.s.	n.s.	n.s.	***	***	***	***	***	n.s.	n.s.	n.s.												
		25	n.s.	n.s.	n.s.	n.s.	n.s.	n.s.	n.s.	n.s.	n.s.	n.s.	n.s.	n.s.	***	***	***	***	***	n.s.	n.s.	n.s.	n.s.											
		100	n.s.	n.s.	n.s.	n.s.	n.s.	n.s.	n.s.	n.s.	n.s.	n.s.	n.s.	n.s.	***	***	***	***	***	n.s.	n.s.	n.s.	n.s.	n.s.										
		200	n.s.	n.s.	n.s.	n.s.	n.s.	n.s.	n.s.	n.s.	n.s.	n.s.	n.s.	n.s.	***	***	***	***	***	n.s.	n.s.	n.s.	n.s.	n.s.	n.s.									
	PEM2	0	n.s.	n.s.	n.s.	n.s.	n.s.	n.s.	n.s.	n.s.	n.s.	n.s.	n.s.	n.s.	***	***	***	***	***	n.s.	n.s.	n.s.	n.s.	n.s.	n.s.	n.s.								
		5	n.s.	n.s.	n.s.	n.s.	n.s.	n.s.	n.s.	n.s.	n.s.	n.s.	n.s.	n.s.	***	***	***	***	***	n.s.	n.s.	n.s.	n.s.	n.s.	n.s.	n.s.	n.s.							
		25	n.s.	n.s.	n.s.	n.s.	n.s.	n.s.	n.s.	n.s.	n.s.	n.s.	n.s.	n.s.	***	***	***	***	***	n.s.	n.s.	n.s.	n.s.	n.s.	n.s.	n.s.	n.s.	n.s.						
		100	n.s.	n.s.	n.s.	n.s.	n.s.	n.s.	n.s.	n.s.	n.s.	n.s.	n.s.	n.s.	***	***	***	***	***	n.s.	n.s.	n.s.	n.s.	n.s.	n.s.	n.s.	n.s.	n.s.	n.s.					
		200	n.s.	n.s.	n.s.	n.s.	n.s.	n.s.	n.s.	n.s.	n.s.	n.s.	n.s.	n.s.	***	***	***	***	***	n.s.	n.s.	n.s.	n.s.	n.s.	n.s.	n.s.	n.s.	n.s.	n.s.	n.s.				
	PEM3	0	n.s.	n.s.	n.s.	n.s.	n.s.	n.s.	n.s.	n.s.	n.s.	n.s.	n.s.	n.s.	***	***	***	***	***	n.s.	n.s.	n.s.	n.s.	n.s.	n.s.	n.s.	n.s.	n.s.	n.s.	n.s.	n.s.			
		5	n.s.	n.s.	n.s.	n.s.	n.s.	n.s.	n.s.	n.s.	n.s.	n.s.	n.s.	n.s.	***	***	***	***	***	n.s.	n.s.	n.s.	n.s.	n.s.	n.s.	n.s.	n.s.	n.s.	n.s.	n.s.	n.s.	n.s.		
		25	n.s.	n.s.	n.s.	n.s.	n.s.	n.s.	n.s.	n.s.	n.s.	n.s.	n.s.	n.s.	***	***	***	***	***	n.s.	n.s.	n.s.	n.s.	n.s.	n.s.	n.s.	n.s.	n.s.	n.s.	n.s.	n.s.	n.s.	n.s.	
		100	n.s.	n.s.	n.s.	n.s.	n.s.	n.s.	n.s.	n.s.	n.s.	n.s.	n.s.	n.s.	***	***	***	***	***	n.s.	n.s.	n.s.	n.s.	n.s.	n.s.	n.s.	n.s.	n.s.	n.s.	n.s.	n.s.	n.s.	n.s.	n.s.
		200	n.s.	n.s.	n.s.	n.s.	n.s.	n.s.	n.s.	n.s.	n.s.	n.s.	n.s.	n.s.	***	***	***	***	***	n.s.	n.s.	n.s.	n.s.	n.s.	n.s.	n.s.	n.s.	n.s.	n.s.	n.s.	n.s.	n.s.	n.s.	n.s.

Figure A6. Results of one-way ANOVA for data related to Figure 6; n.s.: not significant; *: $p < 0.1$; **: $p < 0.05$; ***: $p < 0.001$.

References

1. Boura, C.; Muller, S.; Vautier, D.; Dumas, D.; Schaaf, P.; Claude Voegel, J.; Francois Stoltz, J.; Menu, P. Endothelial cell–interactions with polyelectrolyte multilayer films. *Biomaterials* **2005**, *26*, 4568–4575. [CrossRef] [PubMed]
2. Boura, C.; Muller, S.; Voegel, J.C.; Schaaf, P.; Stoltz, J.F.; Menu, P. Influence of polyelectrolyte multilayer films on the ICAM-1 expression of endothelial cells. *Cell Biochem. Biophys.* **2006**, *44*, 223–231. [CrossRef]
3. Martinez, J.S.; Kelly, K.D.; Ghoussoub, Y.E.; Delgado, J.D.; Keller, T.C., III; Schlenoff, J.B. Cell resistant zwitterionic polyelectrolyte coating promotes bacterial attachment: An adhesion contradiction. *Biomater. Sci.* **2016**, *4*, 689–698. [CrossRef] [PubMed]
4. Silva, J.M.; Reis, R.L.; Mano, J.F. Biomimetic Extracellular Environment Based on Natural Origin Polyelectrolyte Multilayers. *Small* **2016**, *12*, 4308–4342. [CrossRef] [PubMed]
5. Yamanlar, S.; Sant, S.; Boudou, T.; Picart, C.; Khademhosseini, A. Surface functionalization of hyaluronic acid hydrogels by polyelectrolyte multilayer films. *Biomaterials* **2011**, *32*, 5590–5599. [CrossRef]
6. Fakhrullin, R.F.; Zamaleeva, A.I.; Minullina, R.T.; Konnova, S.A.; Paunov, V.N. Cyborg cells: Functionalisation of living cells with polymers and nanomaterials. *Chem. Soc. Rev.* **2012**, *41*, 4189–4206. [CrossRef] [PubMed]
7. Barrat, J.-L.; Joanny, J.-F. Theory of Polyelectrolyte Solutions. *Adv. Chem. Phys.* **1996**, *94*, 1–66.
8. Decher, G.; Hong, J.D.; Schmitt, J. Buildup of ultrathin multilayer films by a self-assembly process: III. Consecutively alternating adsorption of anionic and cationic polyelectrolytes on charged surfaces. *Thin Solid Films* **1992**, *210/211*, 831–835. [CrossRef]
9. Klitzing, R.V. Internal structure of polyelectrolyte multilayer assemblies. *Phys. Chem. Chem. Phys.* **2006**, *8*, 5012–5033. [CrossRef]
10. Zhang, S.; Xing, M.; Li, B. Biomimetic Layer-by-Layer Self-Assembly of Nanofilms, Nanocoatings, and 3D Scaffolds for Tissue Engineering. *Int. J. Mol. Sci.* **2018**, *19*, 1641. [CrossRef]
11. Costa, R.R.; Mano, J.F. Polyelectrolyte multilayered assemblies in biomedical technologies. *Chem. Soc. Rev.* **2014**, *43*, 3453–3479. [CrossRef] [PubMed]
12. Guzman, E.; Mateos-Maroto, A.; Ruano, M.; Ortega, F.; Rubio, R.G. Layer-by-Layer polyelectrolyte assemblies for encapsulation and release of active compounds. *Adv. Colloid Interface Sci.* **2017**, *249*, 290–307. [CrossRef] [PubMed]
13. Pahal, S.; Gakhar, R.; Raichur, A.M.; Varma, M.M. Polyelectrolyte multilayers for bio-applications: Recent advancements. *IET Nanobiotechnology* **2017**, *11*, 903–908. [CrossRef] [PubMed]
14. Zhong, Y.; Whittington, C.F.; Haynie, D.T. Stimulated release of small molecules from polyelectrolyte multilayer nanocoatings. *Chem. Commun.* **2007**, *14*, 1415–1417. [CrossRef] [PubMed]
15. Dash, P.; Thirumurugan, S.; Hu, C.-C.; Wu, C.-J.; Shih, S.-J.; Chung, R.-J. Preparation and characterization of polyelectrolyte multilayer coatings on 316L stainless steel for antibacterial and bone regeneration applications. *Surf. Coat. Technol.* **2022**, *435*, 128254. [CrossRef]
16. Kuo, Y.J.; Chen, C.H.; Dash, P.; Lin, Y.C.; Hsu, C.W.; Shih, S.J.; Chung, R.J. Angiogenesis, Osseointegration, and Antibacterial Applications of Polyelectrolyte Multilayer Coatings Incorporated With Silver/Strontium Containing Mesoporous Bioactive Glass on 316L Stainless Steel. *Front. Bioeng. Biotechnol.* **2022**, *10*, 818137. [CrossRef] [PubMed]
17. Hachim, D.; Whittaker, T.E.; Kim, H.; Stevens, M.M. Glycosaminoglycan-based biomaterials for growth factor and cytokine delivery: Making the right choices. *J. Control Release* **2019**, *313*, 131–147. [CrossRef]
18. Ghiorghita, C.A.; Bucatariu, F.; Dragan, E.S. Influence of cross-linking in loading/release applications of polyelectrolyte multilayer assemblies. A review. *Mater. Sci. Eng. C Mater. Biol. Appl.* **2019**, *105*, 110050. [CrossRef] [PubMed]
19. Detzel, C.J.; Larkin, A.L.; Rajagopalan, P. Polyelectrolyte multilayers in tissue engineering. *Tissue Eng. Part B Rev.* **2011**, *17*, 101–113. [CrossRef]
20. Ren, K.; Crouzier, T.; Roy, C.; Picart, C. Polyelectrolyte multilayer films of controlled stiffness modulate myoblast cells differentiation. *Adv. Funct. Mater.* **2008**, *18*, 1378–1389. [CrossRef]
21. Schneider, A.; Vodouhe, C.; Richert, L.; Francius, G.; Le Guen, E.; Schaaf, P.; Voegel, J.C.; Frisch, B.; Picart, C. Multifunctional polyelectrolyte multilayer films: Combining mechanical resistance, biodegradability, and bioactivity. *Biomacromolecules* **2007**, *8*, 139–145. [CrossRef] [PubMed]
22. Bax, D.V.; Davidenko, N.; Hamaia, S.W.; Farndale, R.W.; Best, S.M.; Cameron, R.E. Impact of UV- and carbodiimide-based crosslinking on the integrin-binding properties of collagen-based materials. *Acta Biomater.* **2019**, *100*, 280–291. [CrossRef] [PubMed]
23. Pawelec, K.M.; Best, S.M.; Cameron, R.E. Collagen: A network for regenerative medicine. *J. Mater. Chem. B* **2016**, *4*, 6484–6496. [CrossRef] [PubMed]
24. Cho, K.L.; Hill, A.J.; Caruso, F.; Kentish, S.E. Chlorine resistant glutaraldehyde crosslinked polyelectrolyte multilayer membranes for desalination. *Adv. Mater.* **2015**, *27*, 2791–2796. [CrossRef] [PubMed]
25. Jiang, B.; Defusco, E.; Li, B. Polypeptide multilayer film co-delivers oppositely-charged drug molecules in sustained manners. *Biomacromolecules* **2010**, *11*, 3630–3637. [CrossRef]
26. Chaubaroux, C.; Vrana, E.; Debry, C.; Schaaf, P.; Senger, B.; Voegel, J.C.; Haikel, Y.; Ringwald, C.; Hemmerle, J.; Lavalle, P.; et al. Collagen-based fibrillar multilayer films cross-linked by a natural agent. *Biomacromolecules* **2012**, *13*, 2128–2135. [CrossRef] [PubMed]
27. Dash, S.; Murthy, P.N.; Nath, L.; Chowdhury, P. Kinetic modeling on drug release from controlled drug delivery systems. *Acta Pol. Pharm.-Drug Res.* **2010**, *67*, 217–223.
28. Singhvi, G.; Singh, M. Review: In-Vitro Drug Release Characterization Models. *IJPSR* **2011**, *2*, 77–84.

29. Bouyer, M.; Guillot, R.; Lavaud, J.; Plettinx, C.; Olivier, C.; Curry, V.; Boutonnat, J.; Coll, J.L.; Peyrin, F.; Josserand, V.; et al. Surface delivery of tunable doses of BMP-2 from an adaptable polymeric scaffold induces volumetric bone regeneration. *Biomaterials* **2016**, *104*, 168–181. [CrossRef]
30. Hettiaratchi, M.H.; Krishnan, L.; Rouse, T.; Chou, C.; McDevitt, T.C.; Gullberg, D. Heparin-mediated delivery of bone morphogenetic protein-2 improves spatial localization of bone regeneration. *Sci. Adv.* **2020**, *6*, eaay1240. [CrossRef]
31. Ruppert, R.; Hoffmann, E.; Sebald, W. Human bone morphogenetic protein 2 contains a heparin-binding site which modifies its biological activity. *Eur. J. Biochem.* **1996**, *237*, 295–302. [CrossRef] [PubMed]
32. Macdonald, M.L.; Samuel, R.E.; Shah, N.J.; Padera, R.F.; Beben, Y.M.; Hammond, P.T. Tissue integration of growth factor-eluting layer-by-layer polyelectrolyte multilayer coated implants. *Biomaterials* **2011**, *32*, 1446–1453. [CrossRef] [PubMed]
33. Guillot, R.; Pignot-Paintrand, I.; Lavaud, J.; Decambron, A.; Bourgeois, E.; Josserand, V.; Logeart-Avramoglou, D.; Viguier, E.; Picart, C. Assessment of a polyelectrolyte multilayer film coating loaded with BMP-2 on titanium and PEEK implants in the rabbit femoral condyle. *Acta Biomater.* **2016**, *36*, 310–322. [CrossRef] [PubMed]
34. Oliveira, E.R.; Nie, L.; Podstawczyk, D.; Allahbakhsh, A.; Ratnayake, J.; Brasil, D.L.; Shavandi, A. Advances in Growth Factor Delivery for Bone Tissue Engineering. *Int. J. Mol. Sci.* **2021**, *22*, 903. [CrossRef] [PubMed]
35. Kostruba, A.; Stetsyshyn, Y.; Mayevska, S.; Yakovlev, M.; Vankevych, P.; Nastishin, Y.; Kravets, V. Composition, thickness and properties of grafted copolymer brush coatings determined by ellipsometry: Calculation and prediction. *Soft Matter* **2018**, *14*, 1016–1025. [CrossRef]
36. Schirmer, U.; Ludolph, J.; Rothe, H.; Hauptmann, N.; Behrens, C.; Bittrich, E.; Schliephake, H.; Liefeith, K. Tailored Polyelectrolyte Multilayer Systems by Variation of Polyelectrolyte Composition and EDC/NHS Cross-Linking: Physicochemical Characterization and In Vitro Evaluation. *Nanomaterials* **2022**, *12*, 2054. [CrossRef] [PubMed]
37. Crouzier, T.; Ren, K.; Nicolas, C.; Roy, C.; Picart, C. Layer-by-layer films as a biomimetic reservoir for rhBMP-2 delivery: Controlled differentiation of myoblasts to osteoblasts. *Small* **2009**, *5*, 598–608. [CrossRef] [PubMed]
38. Miller, T.; Goude, M.C.; McDevitt, T.C.; Temenoff, J.S. Molecular engineering of glycosaminoglycan chemistry for biomolecule delivery. *Acta Biomater.* **2014**, *10*, 1705–1719. [CrossRef]
39. Xu, X.; Jha, A.K.; Duncan, R.L.; Jia, X. Heparin-decorated, hyaluronic acid-based hydrogel particles for the controlled release of bone morphogenetic protein 2. *Acta Biomater.* **2011**, *7*, 3050–3059. [CrossRef] [PubMed]
40. Ao, Q.; Wang, S.; He, Q.; Ten, H.; Oyama, K.; Ito, A.; He, J.; Javed, R.; Wang, A.; Matsuno, A. Fibrin Glue/Fibronectin/Heparin-Based Delivery System of BMP2 Induces Osteogenesis in MC3T3-E1 Cells and Bone Formation in Rat Calvarial Critical-Sized Defects. *ACS Appl. Mater. Interfaces* **2020**, *12*, 13400–13410. [CrossRef]
41. Wigmosta, T.B.; Popat, K.C.; Kipper, M.J. Bone morphogenetic protein-2 delivery from polyelectrolyte multilayers enhances osteogenic activity on nanostructured titania. *J. Biomed. Mater. Res. Part A* **2021**, *109*, 1173–1182. [CrossRef] [PubMed]
42. Hannink, G.; Geutjes, P.J.; Daamen, W.F.; Buma, P. Evaluation of collagen/heparin coated TCP/HA granules for long-term delivery of BMP-2. *J. Mater. Sci. Mater. Med.* **2013**, *24*, 325–332. [CrossRef] [PubMed]
43. Hao, W.; Han, J.; Chu, Y.; Huang, L.; Zhuang, Y.; Sun, J.; Li, X.; Zhao, Y.; Chen, Y.; Dai, J. Collagen/Heparin Bi-Affinity Multilayer Modified Collagen Scaffolds for Controlled bFGF Release to Improve Angiogenesis In Vivo. *Macromol. Biosci.* **2018**, *18*, e1800086. [CrossRef] [PubMed]
44. Laub, M.; Chatzinikolaidou, M.; Jennissen, H.P. Aspects of BMP-2 binding to receptors and collagen: Influence of cell senescence on receptor binding and absence of high-affinity stoichiometric binding to collagen. *Mater. Werkst.* **2007**, *38*, 1019–1026. [CrossRef]
45. Meneghetti, M.C.; Hughes, A.J.; Rudd, T.R.; Nader, H.B.; Powell, A.K.; Yates, E.A.; Lima, M.A. Heparan sulfate and heparin interactions with proteins. *J. R. Soc. Interface* **2015**, *12*, 20150589. [CrossRef] [PubMed]
46. Salvi, C.; Lyu, X.; Peterson, A.M. Effect of Assembly pH on Polyelectrolyte Multilayer Surface Properties and BMP-2 Release. *Biomacromolecules* **2016**, *17*, 1949–1958. [CrossRef] [PubMed]
47. Belair, D.G.; Le, N.N.; Murphy, W.L. Design of growth factor sequestering biomaterials. *Chem. Commun.* **2014**, *50*, 15651–15668. [CrossRef] [PubMed]
48. Schonherr, E.; Hausser, H.-J. Extracellular Matrix and Cytokines: A Functional Unit. *Dev. Immunol.* **2000**, *7*, 12. [CrossRef] [PubMed]

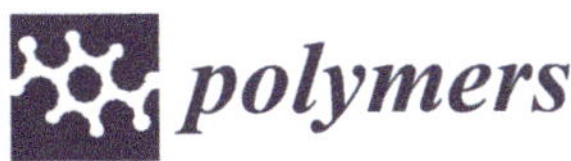 *polymers*

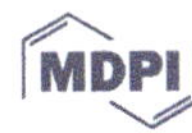

Article

Variation in Hydrogel Formation and Network Structure for Telo-, Atelo- and Methacrylated Collagens

Malachy Kevin Maher [1,2], Jacinta F. White [2], Veronica Glattauer [2], Zhilian Yue [1], Timothy C. Hughes [2], John A. M. Ramshaw [3] and Gordon G. Wallace [1,*]

1   Intelligent Polymer Research Institute, ARC Centre of Excellence for Electromaterials Science, AIIM Facility, Innovation Campus, University of Wollongong, Wollongong, NSW 2519, Australia; mkm290@uowmail.edu.au (M.K.M.); zyue@uow.edu.au (Z.Y.)

2   CSIRO Manufacturing, Clayton, Melbourne, VIC 3168, Australia; jacinta.white@csiro.au (J.F.W.); veronica.glattauer@csiro.au (V.G.); timothy.hughes@csiro.au (T.C.H.)

3   Department of Surgery, St. Vincent's Hospital, University of Melbourne, Melbourne, VIC 3065, Australia; johnamramshaw@gmail.com

*   Correspondence: gwallace@uow.edu.au; Tel.: +61-(0)-2-4221-3127

Abstract: As the most abundant protein in the extracellular matrix, collagen has become widely studied in the fields of tissue engineering and regenerative medicine. Of the various collagen types, collagen type I is the most commonly utilised in laboratory studies. In tissues, collagen type I forms into fibrils that provide an extended fibrillar network. In tissue engineering and regenerative medicine, little emphasis has been placed on the nature of the network that is formed. Various factors could affect the network structure, including the method used to extract collagen from native tissue, since this may remove the telopeptides, and the nature and extent of any chemical modifications and crosslinking moieties. The structure of any fibril network affects cellular proliferation and differentiation, as well as the overall modulus of hydrogels. In this study, the network-forming properties of two distinct forms of collagen (telo- and atelo-collagen) and their methacrylated derivatives were compared. The presence of the telopeptides facilitated fibril formation in the unmodified samples, but this benefit was substantially reduced by subsequent methacrylation, leading to a loss in the native self-assembly potential. Furthermore, the impact of the methacrylation of the collagen, which enables rapid crosslinking and makes it suitable for use in 3D printing, was investigated. The crosslinking of the methacrylated samples (both telo- and atelo-) was seen to improve the fibril-like network compared to the non-crosslinked samples. This contrasted with the samples of methacrylated gelatin, which showed little, if any, fibrillar or ordered network structure, regardless of whether they were crosslinked.

Keywords: collagen; hydrogel; stability; transmission electron microscopy; methacrylation; rheology; gelatin methacrylate

Citation: Maher, M.K.; White, J.F.; Glattauer, V.; Yue, Z.; Hughes, T.C.; Ramshaw, J.A.M.; Wallace, G.G. Variation in Hydrogel Formation and Network Structure for Telo-, Atelo- and Methacrylated Collagens. *Polymers* **2022**, *14*, 1775. https://doi.org/10.3390/polym14091775

Academic Editors: Nunzia Gallo, Marta Madaghiele, Alessandra Quarta and Amilcare Barca

Received: 24 March 2022
Accepted: 23 April 2022
Published: 27 April 2022

Publisher's Note: MDPI stays neutral with regard to jurisdictional claims in published maps and institutional affiliations.

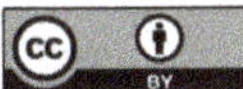

Copyright: © 2022 by the authors. Licensee MDPI, Basel, Switzerland. This article is an open access article distributed under the terms and conditions of the Creative Commons Attribution (CC BY) license (https://creativecommons.org/licenses/by/4.0/).

1. Introduction

Collagen, both in its native form and also in its denatured form, gelatin, is able to form highly hydrated networks, termed hydrogels, which have been widely used in regenerative medicine, through printing or casting [1,2], to create 3D environments for cell proliferation and differentiation [3,4]. Collagen is suitable for use in regenerative medicine because it is abundant in the extracellular matrix (ECM), where it self-assembles and interacts with other collagens and with a wide range of other ECM molecules and cells [5,6].

The collagen family consists of 28 distinct types [7], of which type I collagen, the main component of skin, tendon, ligaments, and bone, is the most abundant. Many collagens are only minor components of the ECM, albeit with specific roles. All collagens share a common structural motif, the triple-helix, in which three individual chains, each in a left-handed polyproline II-like helix, are wound together to form a right-handed, rope-like triple helix [8]. This gives type I collagen a fairly rigid, rod-like structure, approximately 280 nm in length [8]. The amino acid sequence controls the secondary and tertiary molecular structure, with collagens that are characterised by a repeating (Gly-Xaa-Yaa)n sequence; only Gly is small enough to fit within the triple-helical conformation [8]. The Xaa and Yaa positions are most commonly proline and hydroxyproline (Hyp). Furthermore, structural constraints mean that the side chains of the residues in the Xaa position are more accessible, while those in the Yaa are less accessible due to steric hindrance. In denatured collagen, gelatin, the individual chains are flexible and have fewer steric constraints.

A major property of type I collagen is that when heated to 37 °C at neutral pH, purified, soluble type I collagen molecules contain sufficient binding domains to reform into fibrils, which, in turn, entangle to form a hydrogel [9]. During the biosynthesis of collagen, when molecules transit from the cell to the ECM, N- and C-terminal propeptide domains are removed, leaving short, 14- and 26-residue non-triple-helical telopeptide domains at each end of the collagen molecule. The 26-residue C-telopeptide is important in the initiation and rate of fibril formation [10] and, hence, in gelation. Type I collagen lacking the telopeptide domains, due, for example, to enzyme extraction, forms gels much more slowly [11]. Another factor that further limits fibril formation is whether the type I collagen is modified via, for example, succinylation, methylation or deamidation [12].

In order to create 3D collagen templates (scaffolds) that are mechanically stable, stabilisation by chemical or physical crosslinking methods is required. While many stabilisation methods are more suited to the treatment of dry collagen sponges or membranes [5], few are readily applicable to in situ crosslinking, as is required for 3D printing structures, in which rapid gelation is required [13]. One method that has gained importance is the prior methacrylation of gelatin [14] or collagen [15], followed by exposure to UV light with an initiator present, which allows casting or printing. The initial and preferred method of methacrylation for collagen was achieved using methacrylic anhydride [15], although other approaches, involving reactions using carbodiimides [16] and N-hydroxysuccinimide derivatives, are possible [17].

The presence of methacrylate groups, however, has the potential to change or interfere with the native fibril-forming process. This paper, therefore, examines the effects of modifying both telo- and atelo-collagens on the resulting fibril and subsequent network structures in photoinitiated gels, and compares these to the structures found in un-modified, collagen-based hydrogels and with those formed in methacrylated gelatin.

2. Materials and Methods

2.1. Collagen Samples

Rat tail telo-collagen was obtained from tail tendons cut into small sections (~10 mm) and suspended at ~5 mg/mL in 50 mM acetic acid (Chem Supply, Port Adelaide, South Australia, Australia) adjusted to pH 2.5 with HCl (Sigma Aldrich, St. Louis, MO, USA), at 4 °C for 16 h [18]. For preparation of atelo-collagen, pepsin was added at 1 mg/mL. After digestion, samples were clarified by centrifugation at $7500 \times g$ for 120 min at 4 °C. Collagen was precipitated by addition of NaCl (Sigma Aldrich, St. Louis, MO, USA) solution to 0.7 M, and left standing at 4 °C for 16 h. The precipitate was collected by centrifugation, $2500 \times g$ for 30 min, then dialysed exhaustively against 20 mM acetic acid and freeze-dried.

Deamidated collagen was prepared by incubating purified telo-collagen with 5% *w/v* NaOH (Sigma Aldrich, St. Louis, MO, USA) in saturated Na_2SO_4 (Sigma Aldrich, St. Louis, MO, USA) for 4-days [12] and was recovered by neutralising, followed by dialysis and freeze-drying, as previously described [19].

Methacrylated collagen was prepared using telo-and atelo-collagen samples dissolved at 3 mg/mL in 20 mM acetic acid and then adjusted to 200 mM NaCl and taken to pH 7.5 with NaOH, all at 4 °C. A 5-fold molar excess of methacrylic anhydride was added and the pH was maintained at 7.5 using NaOH for 4 h. The reaction was left overnight for completion, and then samples were dialysed exhaustively against 20 mM acetic and freeze-dried. The extent of collagen modification was determined in triplicate using a 2,4,6-

trinitrobenzene sulfonic acid (TNBSA) assay (Thermo Scientific, Waltham, MA, USA) [20], following the manufacturer's instructions.

Methacrylated gelatin (GelMA) was also prepared using a 5-fold molar excess of methacrylic anhydride in 200 mM NaCl at pH 7.5, but at 22 °C, using 300 g Bloom porcine skin gelatin (Sigma Aldrich, St. Louis, MO, USA).

2.2. Circular Dichroism

Collagen and GelMA samples were dissolved in phosphate buffered saline (PBS) at 0.1 mg/mL at 5 °C. Circular dichroism (CD) spectra were collected using samples in 1-mm cuvettes using a JASCO J-815 instrument (Jasco, Easton, MD, USA). Spectra were collected at 400–200-nanometer wavelengths, while temperature scans were performed at 222 nm at 0.3 °C/min from 10–50 °C.

2.3. Rheology

Collagen samples were prepared by dissolving at 30 mg/mL in 20 mM acetic acid at 4 °C. GelMA samples were prepared by dissolving at 10 mg/mL in PBS. Rheology measurements were performed with a Physica MCR 301 Rheometer (Anton Paar, Graz, Austria) fitted with a Peltier temperature controller and connected to an EXFO Acticure 4000 light source. Measurements were obtained using a 15 mm 1° conical plate. Immediately prior to measuring, collagen samples were neutralised to pH of 7.25 ± 0.25 with 1 M NaOH, and the salt concentration was balanced to $1 \times$ PBS using $10 \times$ PBS solution. Samples of 0.1 mL were used and added to the Peltier stage at 4 °C, and set at a gap distance of 500 μm. Samples were then held for a pre-shear period to remove prior memory, using a shear rate of 5 s^{-1} for 2 min at 4 °C. Samples were then taken to 37 °C over 60 s and rheological shear observations were performed for 30 min at a fixed oscillatory frequency of 1 Hz and an amplitude of 1%. Control samples were also held at 4 °C for 30 min to establish that no unwanted rheological changes were occurring. In collagen samples that had been methacrylated, and GelMA samples, lithium phenyl-2,4,6-trimethylbenzoylphosphinate (LAP) (Sigma Aldrich, St. Louis, MO, USA) was dissolved at 0.05%. Samples were then added to the rheometer, and the pre-shear procedure performed, as described above. The samples were exposed to 400 nm light at 20 mW/cm^2 for 60 s, immediately prior to commencing the 30-min rheological testing, again monitoring at a fixed frequency of 1 Hz and amplitude of 1%, at 37 °C.

2.4. Transmission Electron Microscopy

Unmodified collagen samples were gelled after neutralising and heating to 37 °C, as with the rheology measurements, however, the TEM samples were diluted (1 mg/mL) so that a weaker gel that could be pipetted onto an imaging grid. Methacrylated samples had LAP added at 0.05%, followed by exposure to 400 nm light at 20 mW/cm^2 for 30 s prior to taking to 37 °C, following the approach used for the rheology measurements. Gelled samples were examined by transmission electron microscopy (TEM) using a Tecnai 12 transmission electron microscope (FEI, Eindhoven, The Netherlands) at an operating voltage of 120 kV. Samples were prepared on carbon-coated grids (EMSCF200H-CU-TH, ProSciTech, Kirwan, Australia) that were glow-discharged to render them hydrophilic. A 1-microliter drop of sample was applied to an upturned grid held in anti-capillary forceps over moist filter paper, and left for 1 min over moistened filter paper. Excess liquid was then removed with filter paper and the grid was then inverted onto a drop of 2% PTA stain, pH 6.9 on parafilm, for 1 min. The grid was removed from the stain, and excess stain was wicked away with filter paper. Grids were allowed to dry before viewing under the microscope. Images were recorded using a FEI Eagle 4k × 4k CCD camera with AnalySIS v3.2 camera-control software (Olympus, Tokyo, Japan).

3. Results

Samples of both telo- and atelo- rat collagen were readily prepared and methacrylated. The proportion of methacrylation was similar in both the telo- and atelo- collagen samples with 55% (±7%, n = 3) and 52% (±4%, n = 3), respectively, of the Lys residues present in the methacrylated collagens. These values contrasted with the 77% (±3%, n = 3) obtained for the GelMA, which was also modified by the same excess of methacrylic anhydride. These results were consistent with other reports, in which a similar molar excess of reagent was used [21,22].

The chemical modification of collagens can lower the stability of the triple helix [12,23]. This was examined in the present samples through CD spectroscopy (Figure 1), which found that both the methacrylated samples gave similar spectra to the unmodified collagens. The wavelength of the maximum absorption was observed at 222 nm for both.

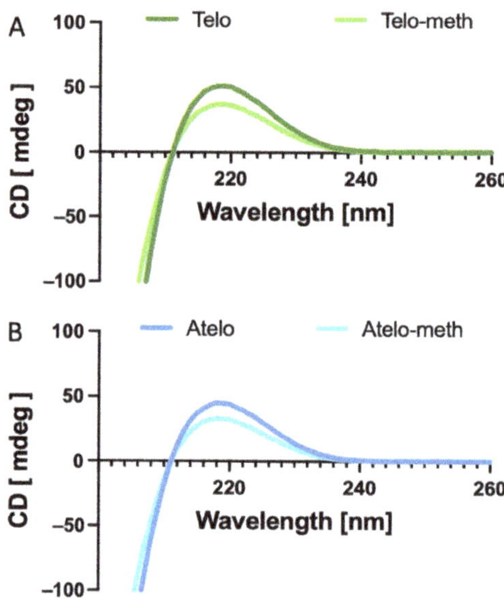

Figure 1. CD spectra of collagens and modified collagens. (**A**) Telo-collagen and methacrylated telo-collagen. (**B**) Atelo-collagen and methacrylated atelo-collagen. In both cases, the modified collagens showed the lower ellipticity.

The thermal response curves, measured at 222 nm (Figure 2), indicated that the methacrylation of both the telo-collagen (Figure 2A) and the atelo-collagen (Figure 2B) led to the destabilisation of the triple helix, with around 2 °C decreases in thermal stability in both cases. The atelo-collagen samples were found to have marginally higher thermal stability compared to those of the telo-collagen, a phenomenon that has been observed previously [24].

Turbidity has frequently been used to study the formation of collagen gels by heating cold, neutral solutions to 37 °C [11,25]. Studies have demonstrated a lag phase (where no change in modulus occurred as molecules heated and began or organise), of around 10 min, depending on the conditions, which suggests that fibril nucleation occurred, followed by an increase in turbidity as fibril formation, thickening and growth continued [26,27]. In the present study, however, photo-rheology was used as it enables quantifiable changes in viscosity and modulus following the irradiation of methacrylated collagen samples for observation. This approach was validated using samples of telo-, atelo- and deamidated telo- rat tail type I collagen (Figure 3A). These rheological data showed that the telo-collagen exhibited rapid gel formation, after a lag period of about 11 min, following the increase in the temperature from 4 to 37 °C, which was consistent with the turbidity data. By contrast, the atelo-collagen showed slower gelation after an extended lag period. The data for the deamidated collagen showed that little, if any, fibril formation or association occurred (Figure 3A). Thus, the absence of the telopeptides significantly decreased both the rate of fibril formation and the modulus that was obtained after 45 min by almost 50%.

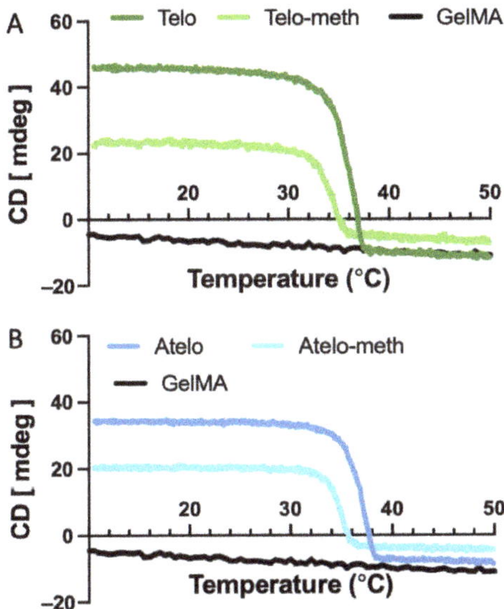

Figure 2. Thermal denaturation of collagens and modified collagens measured using CD spectroscopy at 222 nm. (**A**) Telo-collagen and methacrylated telo-collagen. (**B**) Atelo-collagen and methacrylated atelo-collagen. In both cases, the modified collagens showed the lower stability.

The methacrylation of both collagen samples resulted in a reduced rate of viscosity increase during the thermal gelation process. This was most notable for the methacrylated telo-collagen (Figure 3B), where the reduction in the change in viscosity was about 80%, falling to a level that was much lower than that of the unmodified atelo-collagen. However, the extent of the reduction upon ~50% methacrylation modification was less than for the deamidated collagen where limited, if any, fibril formation occurred. There was also a reduced change in viscosity for the methacrylated atelo-collagen of about 80%, giving a particularly low value as the original unmodified material showed a limited viscosity increase over the 45 min of heating (Figure 3C). In all cases, except for the deamidated collagen, visual inspection found that some form of gel formed, although these forms were typically weak, except for the unmodified telo-collagen, which formed a firm gel. The change in modulus after UV irradiation of the methacrylated collagens was much more rapid (Figure 4), reaching comparable modulus levels around four times more rapidly than any of the thermally gelled materials. A summary of the rheological data indicates that statistically significant differences changes were found when different materials were examined (Figure 5).

The structures of the collagen fibrils, aggregates, and networks in the various hydrogels, with and without UV crosslinking, were examined by TEM (Figure 6). These data showed that the fibrils in the hydrogels formed by thermal treatment of telo-collagen solution were large in diameter, and showed the well-ordered, asymmetrically banded, staggered overlap structure that is observed in native tissues [28,29] (Figure 6A). The asymmetry of these fibrils, a head–tail to head–tail arrangement, was evident from the minor banding seen within the major, 67 nm banding pattern. These large structures overlapped and entangled to provide a network with the stability required for gel formation (Figure 6B).

The diameters of the individual fibrils were typically between 20 and 50 nm, similar to the size seen in immature tissue [30], but not always as well formed. Frequently, larger structures that comprised many small fibrils that had coalesced and entangled to give larger assemblies were seen (Figure 6A,B). By comparison, the fibril-like structures formed by the atelo-collagen were smaller in diameter, and more numerous (Figure 6C), and did not typically show a normal staggered overlap structure (Figure 6C). These fibril-like structures (Figure 6C) could potentially include symmetric, head–tail to tail–head structures, which are found in fibrous-long-spacing (FLS) packing [28]. These would have shown a different staining pattern, but this was also not seen. Rather, the larger fibre bundles of the atelocollagen formed an extended network that was sufficient to stabilise a weak gel, and were augmented by a range of thin structures (Figure 6C), which were possibly only a few molecules thick, which may have been insufficient to show any banded stain pattern [29].

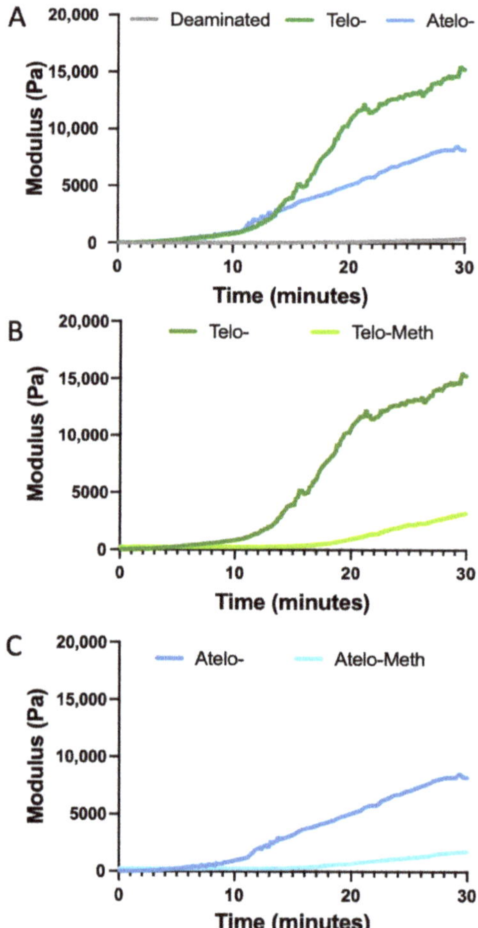

Figure 3. Rheological examination of collagen and modified collagens. (**A**) Telo-collagen, atelo-collagen and deamidated telo-collagen. (**B**) Telo-collagen and methacrylated telo-collagen without UV irradiation. (**C**) Atelo-collagen and methacrylated atelo-collagen without UV irradiation.

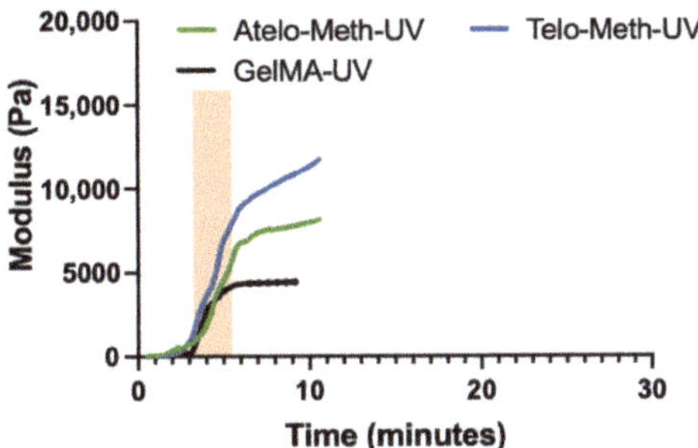

Figure 4. Rheological examination of photo-crosslinking kinetics of methacrylated telo-collagen and methacrylated atelo-collagen, following exposure to UV irradiation. The orange bar represents the UV exposure period.

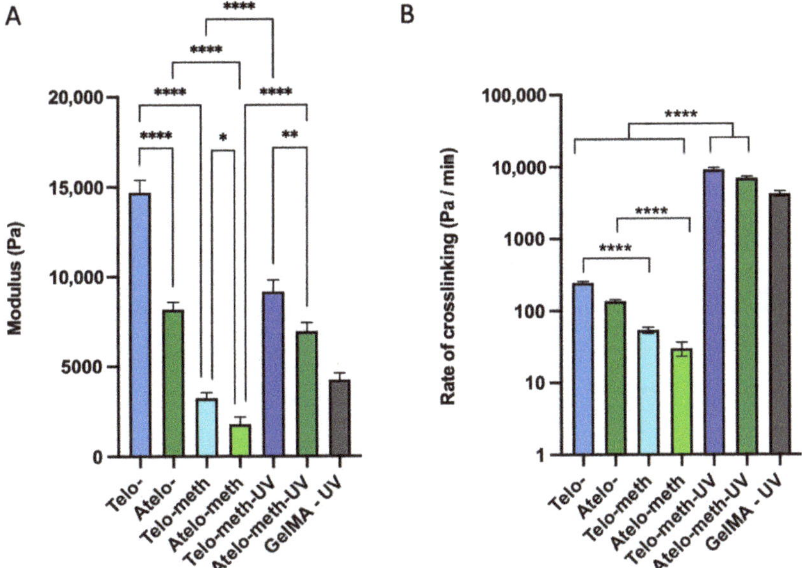

Figure 5. Summary of the rheological crosslinking scans. (**A**) The modulus immediately following the crosslinking period; for fibrillogenesis samples this occurred at 50 min, and for the UV samples this occurred at 5 min (following the 1-min UV exposure). (**B**) The rate of crosslinking during the active phase (50-min window for the fibrillogenesis, and 1-min window for the photo-crosslinked samples). Results of the one way ANOVA show significance between groups with * = $p < 0.05$, ** = $p < 0.01$ and **** = $p < 0.0001$.

The collagen networks of methacrylate-modified collagens after thermal but not UV gelation were distinct from those of unmodified collagens (Figure 6D,E). Long, extensive fibrillar structures were not observed in either the telo- or the atelo-collagen (Figure 6D,E). Some laterally aggregated structures were present, some of which showed apparent non-specific interactions that may have contributed to the increase in viscosity and could have contributed towards a weak gel network. The images obtained revealed no collagen structure, suggesting that most of the collagen was present in the gel as single molecules that were not resolved by the TEM.

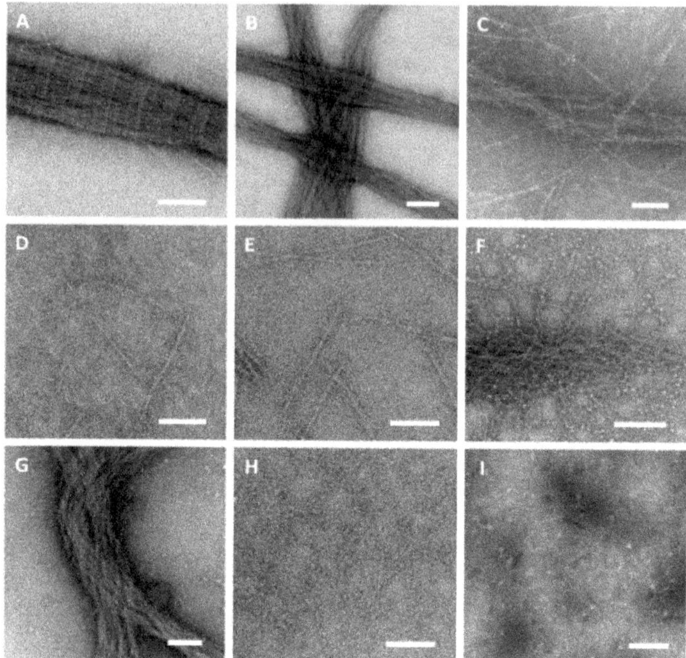

Figure 6. TEM of collagens, methacrylated collagens and GelMA samples after thermal and UV-induced gelation. (**A**) Telo-collagen. (**B**) Telo-collagen. (**C**) Atelo-collagen. (**D**) Methacrylated telo-collagen without UV irradiation. (**E**) Methacrylated atelo-collagen without UV irradiation. (**F**) Methacrylated telo-collagen with UV irradiation. (**G**) Methacrylated atelo-collagen with UV irradiation. (**H**) GelMA without UV irradiation. (**I**) GelMA with UV irradiation. Bars = 100 nm, excepting (**B,F**), where Bar = 200 nm.

The hydrogel structures formed by the methacrylate-modified collagens after UV gelation were distinct from those of the thermally treated samples (Figure 6F,G). The methacrylated telo-collagen showed a mixture of large, poorly formed fibrous bundles, giving a coarse network, which was associated with many small, thin fibrous entities. Small, round structures were also observed, which were interpreted as being due to the LAP catalyst as they were only present in the samples that had LAP added (Figure 6F,G,I) and have been observed previously in resilin samples in which LAP was present [31]. The methacrylated atelo-collagen network (Figure 6G) was similar to that observed with the methacrylated telo-collagen, except that the fibrous bundles were the major component, and the fine network of smaller fibres was not as extensive.

The hydrogel formed by methacrylated gelatin in the absence of UV irradiation (Figure 6H) showed a different, distinct structure. There was no evidence of any re-formed structures of the same length as a collagen molecule. Rather, a range of smaller, indistinct structures of various sizes was present as part of a semi-continuous assembly. The hydrogel formed by the methacrylated gelatin after UV irradiation (Figure 6I) also showed few, if any, apparent structures. Zones of denser, amorphous material were present, along with the structures interpreted as the LAP addition.

4. Discussion

Hydrogels have gained significant interest in tissue engineering and regenerative medicine for the delivery of cells to form new replacement tissues [32,33]. The structure and chemistry of hydrogels can affect the performances of cells [34–36]. For example, the stiffness of hydrogel networks can lead to variations in cellular responses. Various biofabrication and regenerative medicine approaches rely on hydrogels with specific Young's moduli to best facilitate cellular differentiation, diffusion and mechanical robustness [34,35]. The moduli of native soft tissues, such as those of the brain (0.1–1 kPa), muscle (~10 kPa) and pre-mineralised bone (30 kPa), have been established; recreating these environments is essential to directing stem-cell lineage. Stem cells can differentiate towards these lineages via cues such as scaffold stiffness [37,38].

For collagens and gelatines, the structure, organisation, density, and extent of additional crosslinking can all affect and provide control over the Young's modulus to allow the creation of a template with tunable stiffness. The use of these biopolymers in the formation of hydrogel templates can provide the further advantage of providing suitable cellular interactions [5]. Type I collagen contains numerous different cellular interaction sites [39,40]. Some of these binding sites occur on isolated molecules, while others require a larger, properly formed fibrillar site to be present [41]. However, if the collagen is chemically modified, such as through the addition of methacryl functionality, the extent of some interactions, especially those dependent on fibrillar structures, could be reduced or lost [42]. In gelatin, the denaturation of collagen leads to the loss of conformation-dependent sites. However, linear RGD sequences become available, after being hidden by the triple-helical conformation that internalises the Gly residue, so that integrin binding can occur, albeit by a different path to that seen on triple-helical collagen [43].

The formation of collagen hydrogels through warming neutral solutions is well established [9,44], with the variations in the hydrogel structure determined by the source [45], concentration [46], incubation temperature [47], pH [48] and ionic strength [49] of the collagen solution. For laboratory experiments, rat-tail-tendon type I collagen is a preferred source, as this collagen can be acid-extracted so that it retains telopeptides, which enhance fibril formation [11] (Figure 3A). Other collagens that could be acid-extracted in good yield with intact telopeptides include marine collagens [50] and chicken collagen [51]. The presence of telopeptides from xenogeneic species, however, may not be preferable for clinical applications as telopeptides can cause immune responses [52].

The telo-collagen in the thermally produced hydrogels reformed into fibrils analogous to those in native tendons and other tissues, showing an asymmetric banded structure on the TEM (Figure 6A,B). Each fibril was composed of triple-helical collagen molecules arranged in a staggered, overlapped array, resulting in a characteristic 67 nm banding periodicity in which all the molecules were oriented in one direction. Each repeating band consisted of a 30 nm "overlap" zone and a 37 nm "gap" zone, which led to the observed banding through different rates of stain uptake [53]. The collagen in these gels has a native, strong interaction with cells, which leads to the consolidation of the hydrogel into a more tissue-like structure [54].

Atelo-collagen, which is generally obtained through the digestion of tissues by pepsin [55], can also form into hydrogels, but the rate of formation is much slower (Figure 3A). The TEM showed that the structure was less well organised (Figure 6C) but still had a fibrous network that was able to form a hydrogel that could be reorganised and consolidated [56]. However, hydrogels from either telo- or atelo collagen that is subsequently cross-linked retain their size when incubated with cells and do not readily consolidate [57]. The fibrous structure observed in these atelocollagen hydrogels (Figure 6C) was poorly organised and lacked the ordered, asymmetric, staggered overlap structure of native fibrils. A mixture of other centrosymmetric structures may have been present, with at least four fibrous-long-spacing (FLS) packing modes having been observed [58]. In addition, smaller collagen structures were present, also forming a quasi-network structure (Figure 6C). In some cases, the visible material was comparable to the length of a single collagen molecule, but probably comprised in-phase aggregates of collagen molecules, analogous to the segment-long-spacing (SLS) assemblies that can be observed under specific conditions [59]. In other cases, end-to-end assemblies of these structures occurred, leading to smaller fibril-like structures (Figure 6C).

Typically, modified collagens, such as deamidated collagen, do not form into fibrils (Figure 3A), either because of changes to the charge distribution or because of steric hinderance, and probably remain as single molecules. In the present study, neither the telo-nor the atelo-methacrylated collagens showed a major propensity for thermal hydrogel formation, although there was a slight degree of gelation, unlike in the fully deamidated collagen. This reduction was not due to denaturation, as the modified collagens were still triple-helical (Figures 1 and 2), albeit with slightly reduced thermal stability.

Individually, both these modified collagens, although modified using an excess of reagent, were just over 50% modified based on the number of available Lys residues. Similarly, the prepared GelMA was modified to around 80%. The reactivity of Lys residues depends on their pKa values, with those with lower pKa values reacting more readily [60]. In any given protein, the pKa values of the Lys residues vary with the surrounding tertiary structural environment, although often with only small differences [61]. In collagens, Lys residues are found preferentially in the Yaa position [62] and of these, several may be subject to secondary modification to give hydroxylysine, some of which may be additionally glycosylated, potentially further reducing their reactivity. The lower degree of reaction of the collagen compared to the GelMA reflects the changes in the tertiary structure such that the Lys residues of the gelatin were more readily available, while the reactivity of some, potentially those with secondary modifications, was still low, leading to incomplete modification.

The ultrastructure of the methacrylated collagen hydrogels formed by the thermal treatment, as shown by the TEM (Figure 6D,E), were quite distinct from those of the unmodified collagens. Both preparations showed structures that were the length of individual collagen molecules, but were probably wider than single molecules. This suggests that lateral, in-phase assemblies were formed, analogous to SLS aggregates, but not of sufficient width or diameter to enable any fine structure banding to be visible. Additional interactions, however, could lead to a network sufficiently fine to stabilise hydrogels.

By contrast, the networks formed by the UV crosslinking of the methacrylated telo-and atelo-collagens were distinct (Figure 6F,G). The use of UV prior to the thermal treatment allowed little time for any natural associations to occur and the crosslinking led to extensive fibrous material formation that lacked any apparent order. This fibrous material further aggregated to give larger fibrous ropes. For the methacrylated telo-collagen, a significant amount of fine fibre network was also present, but this was less significant for the methacrylated atelo-collagen material (Figure 6F,G).

The TEM also showed that the structure of the methacrylated gelatin hydrogel in the absence of UV irradiation (Figure 6H) was quite distinct from the collagen-based hydrogels. No structures equivalent to full-length collagen molecules were seen, but an array of smaller structures was present. When a normal, unmodified gelatin hydrogel forms, small sections of the individual, denatured chains reassemble to form triple-helical segments, although it is unlikely that these relate to the natural chain organisation [63]. These triple-helical segments allow an initial fine network to form, providing the junctional domains that enable gel formation. With increasing time, the triple-helical domains coalesce to form larger structures, providing what is termed a coarse network [63]. In this non-crosslinked structure, the association of randomly organised chains occurs, while the re-formation of triple-helical segments consolidates the structure. In the samples that were UV-crosslinked, there was no apparent structure associated with the gel, and only regions of amorphous density were seen. However, when a gel is formed, some form of network must be present, with chains possibly only of single molecules. Nevertheless, the high degree of methacrylation, 80%, would have led to the formation of a large number of crosslinks. Gelatin solution is readily digested by proteases, leading to small, non-gelling fragments. When crosslinked methacrylated gelatin is incubated with cells, which typically have a range of cell surface proteases [64], as well as potentially secreting proteases, the extent of crosslinking limits the solubilisation of the gel, either directly, or by limiting the rate of cellular migration until sufficient remodeling has occurred [21].

The methacrylation of a denatured collagen, gelatin, has proven to be a popular method for tissue engineering and for the production of bioinks, where gelation induced by photochemical methods allows the rapid rates of crosslinking and stabilisation that are needed for successful bioprinting. The mechanical properties of methacrylated gelatin and, consequently, its cell and tissue interaction properties, can be tuned by adjusting the nature of the material though variations in the concentration and the extent of crosslinking [21]. Cells bind to gelatin networks, possibly due to the presence of otherwise cryptic RGD sites that are revealed during the denaturation of the collagen. Native collagen has a broader range of highly specific binding sites, including for integrin binding, through a conformationally dependent sequence, while being considerably more stable towards general proteolysis. Native collagen was therefore examined in this study as an alternative material for forming a biologically-based hydrogel network. As with methacrylated gelatin, it was expected that the concentration and extent of crosslinking would influence the characteristics of the hydrogel. For collagen, however, the nature of the networks that are formed can be variable, depending on the conditions under which the collagen extraction is performed. Thus, the hydrogels formed from acid-extracted telo-collagen can be distinct from those of enzyme-extracted atelo-collagen, from which the telopeptides are removed during enzyme solubilisation, giving a further variable for hydrogel formation that is not present in gelatin-based hydrogels.

In conclusion, this study highlights the differences in ultrastructure that were produced in collagen hydrogels that were extracted by varying techniques and as a result of methacrylation. The presence of telopeptides was seen to facilitate fibril formation to a large degree, compared to atelo- forms of collagen. Once methacrylated, the triple helix was seen to be destabilized and to undergo denaturation at lower temperatures compared to the unmodified forms. Methacrylation was also seen to impact fibril formation in both the methacrylated telo- and methacrylated atleo- conditions. Future studies could be targeted to understand how various collagen ultrastructures impact cellular function and the mechanical properties of these hydrogel scaffolds.

Author Contributions: Conceptualization, J.A.M.R. and G.G.W.; methodology, J.A.M.R., M.K.M., V.G., T.C.H., J.F.W. and Z.Y.; formal analysis, J.A.M.R., J.F.W. and M.K.M.; writing—original draft preparation, J.A.M.R. and M.K.M.; writing—review and editing, J.A.M.R., G.G.W., V.G., T.C.H., Z.Y. and M.K.M.; supervision, G.G.W., J.A.M.R., V.G., T.C.H. and Z.Y.; funding acquisition, G.G.W., T.C.H. and V.G. All authors have read and agreed to the published version of the manuscript.

Funding: Financial support was received from the Global Challenges Joint Ph.D. Program between the University of Wollongong and CSIRO. Additional support was received from the Australian National Fabrication Facility (ANFF), Materials Node, the Australian Research Council (ARC) and the Australian Centre for Electromaterials Science (ACES). Gordon Wallace acknowledges the support provided by the ARC through an ARC Laureate Fellowship (FL110100196).

Institutional Review Board Statement: Not applicable.

Informed Consent Statement: Not applicable.

Data Availability Statement: Not applicable.

Conflicts of Interest: The authors declare no conflict of interest.

References

1. Glowacki, J.; Mizuno, S. Collagen scaffolds for tissue engineering. *Biopolymers* **2008**, *89*, 338–344. [CrossRef] [PubMed]
2. Hoque, M.E.; Nuge, T.; Yeow, T.K.; Nordin, N.; Prasad, R. Gelatin based scaffolds for tissue engineering-a review. *Polym. Res. J.* **2015**, *9*, 15.
3. Murphy, C.M.; Haugh, M.G.; O'brien, F.J. The effect of mean pore size on cell attachment, proliferation and migration in collagen–glycosaminoglycan scaffolds for bone tissue engineering. *Biomaterials* **2010**, *31*, 461–466. [CrossRef] [PubMed]
4. Kroehne, V.; Heschel, I.; Schügner, F.; Lasrich, D.; Bartsch, J.; Jockusch, H. Use of a novel collagen matrix with oriented pore structure for muscle cell differentiation in cell culture and in grafts. *J. Cell. Mol. Med.* **2008**, *12*, 1640–1648. [CrossRef] [PubMed]
5. Ramshaw, J.A.; Glattauer, V. *Biophysical and Chemical Properties of Collagen: Biomedical Applications*; IOP Publishing: Bristol, UK, 2019.

6. San Antonio, J.D.; Jacenko, O.; Fertala, A.; Orgel, J.P. Collagen structure-function mapping informs applications for regenerative medicine. *Bioengineering* **2021**, *8*, 3. [CrossRef]

7. Ricard-Blum, S. The collagen family. *Cold Spring Harb. Perspect. Biol.* **2011**, *3*, a004978. [CrossRef] [PubMed]

8. Brodsky, B.; Ramshaw, J.A.M. The collagen triple-helix structure. *Matrix Biol.* **1997**, *15*, 545–554. [CrossRef]

9. Gross, J.; Kirk, D. The heat precipitation of collagen from neutral salt solutions: Some rate-regulating factors. *J. Biol. Chem.* **1958**, *233*, 355–360. [CrossRef]

10. Prockop, D.J.; Fertala, A. Inhibition of the self-assembly of collagen I into fibrils with synthetic peptides: Demonstration that assembly is driven by specific binding sites on the monomers. *J. Biol. Chem.* **1998**, *273*, 15598–15604. [CrossRef]

11. Gelman, R.A.; Poppke, D.C.; Piez, K.A. Collagen fibril formation in vitro. The role of the nonhelical terminal regions. *J. Biol. Chem.* **1979**, *254*, 11741–11745. [CrossRef]

12. Rauterberg, J.; Kühn, K. The renaturation behaviour of modified collagen molecules. *Hoppe Seylers Z. Physiol. Chem.* **1968**, *349*, 611–622. [CrossRef] [PubMed]

13. Bell, A.; Kofron, M.; Nistor, V. Multiphoton crosslinking for biocompatible 3D printing of type I collagen. *Biofabrication* **2015**, *7*, 035007. [CrossRef] [PubMed]

14. van den Bulcke, A.I.; Bogdanov, B.; De Rooze, N.; Schacht, E.H.; Cornelissen, M.; Berghmans, H. Structural and rheological properties of methacrylamide modified gelatin hydrogels. *Biomacromolecules* **2000**, *1*, 31–38. [CrossRef] [PubMed]

15. Brinkman, W.T.; Nagapudi, K.; Thomas, B.S.; Chaikof, E.L. Photo-cross-linking of type I collagen gels in the presence of smooth muscle cells: Mechanical properties, cell viability, and function. *Biomacromolecules* **2003**, *4*, 890–895. [CrossRef]

16. Shreiber, D.; Gaudet, I. Process for the Synthesis of Methacrylate-Derivatized Type-1 Collagen and Derivatives Thereof. U.S. Patent 865,871,1B2, 25 February 2014.

17. Cosgriff-Hernandez, E.; Hahn, M.; Russell, B.; Wilems, T.; Munoz-Pinto, D.; Browning, M.; Rivera, J.; Höök, M. Bioactive hydrogels based on designer collagens. *Acta Biomater.* **2010**, *6*, 3969–3977. [CrossRef] [PubMed]

18. Rajan, N.; Habermehl, J.; Coté, M.-F.; Doillon, C.J.; Mantovani, D. Preparation of ready-to-use, storable and reconstituted type I collagen from rat tail tendon for tissue engineering applications. *Nat. Protoc.* **2006**, *1*, 2753–2758. [CrossRef] [PubMed]

19. Truong, Y.B.; Glattauer, V.; Briggs, K.L.; Zappe, S.; Ramshaw, J.A.M. Collagen-based layer-by-layer coating on electrospun polymer scaffolds. *Biomaterials* **2012**, *33*, 9198–9204. [CrossRef] [PubMed]

20. Habeeb, A.S.A. Determination of free amino groups in proteins by trinitrobenzenesulfonic acid. *Anal. Biochem.* **1966**, *14*, 328–336. [CrossRef]

21. Nichol, J.W.; Koshy, S.T.; Bae, H.; Hwang, C.M.; Yamanlar, S.; Khademhosseini, A. Cell-laden microengineered gelatin methacrylate hydrogels. *Biomaterials* **2010**, *31*, 5536–5544. [CrossRef]

22. Hoch, E.; Schuh, C.; Hirth, T.; Tovar, G.E.; Borchers, K. Stiff gelatin hydrogels can be photo-chemically synthesized from low viscous gelatin solutions using molecularly functionalized gelatin with a high degree of methacrylation. *J. Mater. Sci. Mater. Med.* **2012**, *23*, 2607–2617. [CrossRef] [PubMed]

23. Zhang, Y.; Liu, W.; Li, G.; Shi, B.; Miao, Y.; Wu, X. Isolation and partial characterization of pepsin-soluble collagen from the skin of grass carp (*Ctenopharyngodon idella*). *Food Chem.* **2007**, *103*, 906–912. [CrossRef]

24. Walton, R.S.; Brand, D.D.; Czernuszka, J.T. Influence of telopeptides, fibrils and crosslinking on physicochemical properties of type I collagen films. *J. Mater. Sci. Mater. Med.* **2010**, *21*, 451–461. [CrossRef]

25. Birk, D.E.; Silver, F.H. Collagen fibrillogenesis in vitro: Comparison of types I, II, and III. *Arch. Biochem. Biophys.* **1984**, *235*, 178–185. [CrossRef]

26. Comper, W.; Veis, A. The mechanism of nucleation for in vitro collagen fibril formation. *Biopolym. Orig. Res. Biomol.* **1977**, *16*, 2113–2131. [CrossRef] [PubMed]

27. Zhu, J.; Kaufman, L.J. Collagen I self-assembly: Revealing the developing structures that generate turbidity. *Biophys. J.* **2014**, *106*, 1822–1831. [CrossRef] [PubMed]

28. Doyle, B.; Hulmes, D.J.S.; Miller, A.; Parry, D.A.D.; Piez, K.; Woodhead-Galloway, J. AD-periodic narrow filament in collagen. *Proc. R. Soc. Lond. Ser. B Biol. Sci.* **1974**, *186*, 67–74.

29. White, J.F.; Werkmeister, J.A.; Darby, I.A.; Bisucci, T.; Birk, D.E.; Ramshaw, J.A.M. Collagen fibril formation in a wound healing model. *J. Struct. Biol.* **2002**, *137*, 23–30. [CrossRef] [PubMed]

30. Parry, D.A.; Craig, A. Quantitative electron microscope observations of the collagen fibrils in rat-tail tendon. *Biopolym. Orig. Res. Biomol.* **1977**, *16*, 1015–1031. [CrossRef] [PubMed]

31. Okesola, B.O.; Lau, H.K.; Derkus, B.; Boccorh, D.K.; Wu, Y.; Wark, A.W.; Kiick, K.L.; Mata, A. Covalent co-assembly between resilin-like polypeptide and peptide amphiphile into hydrogels with controlled nanostructure and improved mechanical properties. *Biomater. Sci.* **2020**, *8*, 846–857. [CrossRef] [PubMed]

32. Nguyen, K.T.; West, J.L. Photopolymerizable hydrogels for tissue engineering applications. *Biomaterials* **2002**, *23*, 4307–4314. [CrossRef]

33. Mantha, S.; Pillai, S.; Khayambashi, P.; Upadhyay, A.; Zhang, Y.; Tao, O.; Pham, H.M.; Tran, S.D. Smart hydrogels in tissue engineering and regenerative medicine. *Materials* **2019**, *12*, 3323. [CrossRef] [PubMed]

34. Brandl, F.; Sommer, F.; Goepferich, A. Rational design of hydrogels for tissue engineering: Impact of physical factors on cell behavior. *Biomaterials* **2007**, *28*, 134–146. [CrossRef]

35. Annabi, N.; Tamayol, A.; Uquillas, J.A.; Akbari, M.; Bertassoni, L.E.; Cha, C.; Camci-Unal, G.; Dokmeci, M.R.; Peppas, N.A.; Khademhosseini, A. 25th anniversary article: Rational design and applications of hydrogels in regenerative medicine. *Adv. Mater.* **2014**, *26*, 85–124. [CrossRef] [PubMed]

36. Maher, M.; Castilho, M.; Yue, Z.; Glattauer, V.; Hughes, T.C.; Ramshaw, J.A.M.; Wallace, G.G. Shaping collagen for engineering hard tissues: Towards a printomics approach. *Acta Biomater.* **2021**, *131*, 41–61. [CrossRef] [PubMed]

37. Saha, K.; Keung, A.J.; Irwin, E.F.; Li, Y.; Little, L.; Schaffer, D.V.; Healy, K.E. Substrate modulus directs neural stem cell behavior. *Biophys. J.* **2008**, *95*, 4426–4438. [CrossRef] [PubMed]

38. Engler, A.J.; Griffin, M.A.; Sen, S.; Bonnemann, C.G.; Sweeney, H.L.; Discher, D.E. Myotubes differentiate optimally on substrates with tissue-like stiffness pathological implications for soft or stiff microenvironments. *J. Cell Biol.* **2004**, *166*, 877–887. [CrossRef] [PubMed]

39. Kadler, K.E.; Holmes, D.F.; Trotter, J.A.; Chapman, J.A. Collagen fibril formation. *Biochem. J.* **1996**, *316*, 1–11. [CrossRef] [PubMed]

40. Sweeney, S.M.; Orgel, J.P.; Fertala, A.; McAuliffe, J.D.; Turner, K.R.; Di Lullo, G.A.; Chen, S.; Antipova, O.; Perumal, S.; Ala-Kokko, L.; et al. Candidate cell and matrix interaction domains on the collagen fibril, the predominant protein of vertebrates. *J. Biol. Chem.* **2008**, *283*, 21187–21197. [CrossRef]

41. Orgel, J.; San Antonio, J.; Antipova, O. Molecular and structural mapping of collagen fibril interactions. *Connect. Tissue Res.* **2011**, *52*, 2–17. [CrossRef] [PubMed]

42. Cereceres, S.; Touchet, T.; Browning, M.B.; Smith, C.; Rivera, J.; Höök, M.; Whitfield-Cargile, C.; Russell, B.; Cosgriff-Hernandez, E. Chronic wound dressings based on collagen-mimetic proteins. *Adv. Wound Care* **2015**, *4*, 444–456. [CrossRef] [PubMed]

43. Emsley, J.; Knight, C.G.; Farndale, R.W.; Barnes, M.J.; Liddington, R.C. Structural basis of collagen recognition by integrin α2β1. *Cell* **2000**, *101*, 47–56. [CrossRef]

44. Antoine, E.E.; Vlachos, P.P.; Rylander, M.N. Review of collagen I hydrogels for bioengineered tissue microenvironments: Characterization of mechanics, structure, and transport. *Tissue Eng. Part B Rev.* **2014**, *20*, 683–696. [CrossRef] [PubMed]

45. Kreger, S.; Bell, B.; Bailey, J.; Stites, E.; Kuske, J.; Waisner, B.; Voytik-Harbin, S. Polymerization and matrix physical properties as important design considerations for soluble collagen formulations. *Biopolym. Orig. Res. Biomol.* **2010**, *93*, 690–707. [CrossRef]

46. Miron-Mendoza, M.; Seemann, J.; Grinnell, F. The differential regulation of cell motile activity through matrix stiffness and porosity in three dimensional collagen matrices. *Biomaterials* **2010**, *31*, 6425–6435. [CrossRef] [PubMed]

47. Yang, Y.; Motte, S.; Kaufman, L.J. Pore size variable type I collagen gels and their interaction with glioma cells. *Biomaterials* **2010**, *31*, 5678–5688. [CrossRef] [PubMed]

48. Yamamura, N.; Sudo, R.; Ikeda, M.; Tanishita, K. Effects of the mechanical properties of collagen gel on the in vitro formation of microvessel networks by endothelial cells. *Tissue Eng.* **2007**, *13*, 1443–1453. [CrossRef] [PubMed]

49. Achilli, M.; Mantovani, D. Tailoring mechanical properties of collagen-based scaffolds for vascular tissue engineering: The effects of pH, temperature and ionic strength on gelation. *Polymers* **2010**, *2*, 664–680. [CrossRef]

50. Ramshaw, J.A.M.; Werkmeister, J.A.; Bremner, H.A. Characterization of type I collagen from the skin of blue grenadier (*Macruronus novaezelandiae*). *Arch. Biochem. Biophys.* **1988**, *267*, 497–502. [CrossRef]

51. Cliché, S.; Amiot, J.; Avezard, C.; Gariepy, C. Extraction and characterization of collagen with or without telopeptides from chicken skin. *Poult. Sci.* **2003**, *82*, 503–509. [CrossRef]

52. Werkmeister, J.A.; Ramshaw, J.A.M. Immunology of collagen-based biomaterials. In *Biomaterials and Bioengineering Handbook*; Marcel Dekker: New York, NY, USA, 2000.

53. Chapman, J.A. The staining pattern of collagen fibrils: I. An analysis of electron micrographs. *Connect. Tissue Res.* **1974**, *2*, 137–150. [CrossRef]

54. Bell, E.; Ivarsson, B.; Merrill, C. Production of a tissue-like structure by contraction of collagen lattices by human fibroblasts of different proliferative potential in vitro. *Proc. Natl. Acad. Sci. USA* **1979**, *76*, 1274–1278. [CrossRef]

55. Miller, E.J.; Rhodes, R.K. [2] Preparation and characterization of the different types of collagen. In *Methods in Enzymology*; Elsevier: Amsterdam, The Netherlands, 1982; Volume 82, pp. 33–64.

56. Eckes, B.; Wang, F.; Rittié, L.; Scherr, G.; Zigrino, P. Cell-populated collagen lattice models. In *Fibrosis*; Springer: Berlin, Germany, 2017; pp. 223–233.

57. Redden, R.A.; Doolin, E.J. Collagen crosslinking and cell density have distinct effects on fibroblast-mediated contraction of collagen gels. *Ski. Res. Technol.* **2003**, *9*, 290–293. [CrossRef] [PubMed]

58. Doyle, B.B.; Bendit, E.; Blout, E.R. Infrared spectroscopy of collagen and collagen-like polypeptides. *Biopolym. Orig. Res. Biomol.* **1975**, *14*, 937–957. [CrossRef]

59. Bruns, R.R.; Hulmes, D.J.; Therrien, S.F.; Gross, J. Procollagen segment-long-spacing crystallites: Their role in collagen fibrillogenesis. *Proc. Natl. Acad. Sci. USA* **1979**, *76*, 313–317. [CrossRef] [PubMed]

60. Gaudriault, G.; Vincent, J.-P. Selective labeling of α-or ε-amino groups in peptides by the Bolton-Hunter reagent. *Peptides* **1992**, *13*, 1187–1192. [CrossRef]

61. Ramshaw, J.A.M.; Coyne, J.A.; Lewontin, R.C. The sensitivity of gel electrophoresis as a detector of genetic variation. *Genetics* **1979**, *93*, 1019–1037. [CrossRef]

62. Ramshaw, J.A.M.; Shah, N.K.; Brodsky, B. Gly-XY tripeptide frequencies in collagen: A context for host–guest triple-helical peptides. *J. Struct. Biol.* **1998**, *122*, 86–91. [CrossRef]

Polymers **2022**, *14*, 1775

63. de Wolf, F. Molecular structure of gelatin gels. In *Industrial Proteins in Perspective*; Elsevier: Amsterdam, The Netherlands, 2003; pp. 159–167.
64. Bateman, J.F.; Pillow, J.J.; Mascara, T.; Medvedec, S.; Ramshaw, J.A.M.; Cole, W. Cell-layer-associated proteolytic cleavage of the telopeptides of type I collagen in fibroblast culture. *Biochem. J.* **1987**, *245*, 677–682. [CrossRef] [PubMed]

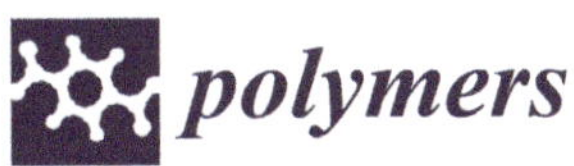 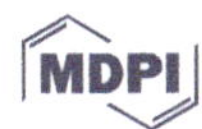

Article

Corneal Stroma Regeneration with Collagen-Based Hydrogel as an Artificial Stroma Equivalent: A Comprehensive In Vivo Study

Egor Olegovich Osidak [1,*], Andrey Yurevich Andreev [1,2,3,4], Sergey Eduardovich Avetisov [2,3], Grigory Victorovich Voronin [2,3], Zoya Vasilievna Surnina [2], Anna Vladimirovna Zhuravleva [5], Timofei Evgenievich Grigoriev [6], Sergey Vladimirovich Krasheninnikov [6], Kirill Konstantinovich Sukhinich [7], Oleg Vadimovich Zayratyants [5] and Sergey Petrovich Domogatsky [1,8]

1   Imtek Ltd., 3rd Cherepkovskaya 15A, 121552 Moscow, Russia
2   Research Institute of Eye Disease, 11A Rossolimo St., 119021 Moscow, Russia
3   I.M. Sechenov First Moscow State Medical University, 8-2 Trubetskaya Str., 119991 Moscow, Russia
4   LEC Ltd., Rozhdestvenskaya, 7, 141006 Mytischi, Russia
5   FSBEI HE A.I. Yevdokimov MSMSU MOH Russia, Rakhmanovsky Lane, 3, 127994 Moscow, Russia
6   National Research Center Kurchatov Institute, Akademika Kurchatova pl.,1, 123182 Moscow, Russia
7   Koltzov Institute of Developmental Biology of the Russian Academy of Sciences, Vavilova 26, 119334 Moscow, Russia
8   FSBI National Medical Research Centre of Cardiology of the Ministry of Health of the Russian Federation, 3 Cherepkovskaya 15A, 121552 Moscow, Russia
*   Correspondence: eosidak@gmail.com

Citation: Osidak, E.O.; Andreev, A.Y.; Avetisov, S.E.; Voronin, G.V.; Surnina, Z.V.; Zhuravleva, A.V.; Grigoriev, T.E.; Krasheninnikov, S.V.; Sukhinich, K.K.; Zayratyants, O.V.; et al. Corneal Stroma Regeneration with Collagen-Based Hydrogel as an Artificial Stroma Equivalent: A Comprehensive In Vivo Study. *Polymers* **2022**, *14*, 4017. https://doi.org/10.3390/polym14194017

Academic Editors: Nunzia Gallo, Marta Madaghiele, Alessandra Quarta and Amilcare Barca

Received: 23 August 2022
Accepted: 22 September 2022
Published: 26 September 2022

Publisher's Note: MDPI stays neutral with regard to jurisdictional claims in published maps and institutional affiliations.

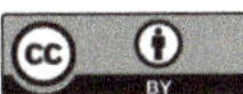

Copyright: © 2022 by the authors. Licensee MDPI, Basel, Switzerland. This article is an open access article distributed under the terms and conditions of the Creative Commons Attribution (CC BY) license (https://creativecommons.org/licenses/by/4.0/).

Abstract: Restoring the anatomical and functional characteristics of the cornea using various biomaterials is especially relevant in the context of a global shortage of donor tissue. Such biomaterials must be biocompatible, strong, and transparent. Here, we report a Viscoll collagen membrane with mechanical and optical properties suitable for replacing damaged stromal tissue. After removing a portion of the stroma, a Viscoll collagen membrane was implanted into the corneas of rabbits. After 6 months, the active migration of host cells into Viscoll collagen membranes was noted, with the preservation of corneal transparency in all experimental animals. Effective integration of the Viscoll collagen membrane with corneal tissue promoted nerve regeneration in vivo, as confirmed by in vivo confocal microscopy. We also demonstrated the safety and efficacy of the Viscoll collagen membrane for corneal stroma regeneration. Thus, in combination with the proposed packaging format that provides long-term storage of up to 10 months, this material has great potential for replacing and regenerating damaged stromal tissues.

Keywords: viscoll collagen membrane; cornea regeneration; stromal replacement; tissue engineering

1. Introduction

Throughout human life, the cornea is constantly in contact with its surrounding environment in a way that is harmful to the delicate tissue. The immediate environment includes high and low temperatures, air pollution and toxic substances, ultraviolet radiation, and other types of radiation. However, owing to its complex structure, which includes the unique nature of trophism, innervation, and a type of cellular regeneration, it remains transparent and is the main refractive lens of the eye [1].

Any damage or disease of the cornea can lead to a complete or partial loss of its properties; in particular, the loss of transparency leads to a significant decrease in visual acuity. The most common diseases include keratoconus, dystrophies of various origins, ulcers, and corneal injury [2].

Donor cornea transplantation is the most common method of surgical treatment for most diseases of the cornea; however, the global shortage of donor tissue significantly complicates its use. Thus, the development of alternative approaches based on tissue engineering and regenerative medicine is necessary to solve this problem [3].

Thus far, advances in the field of tissue engineering have shifted the therapeutic focus to creating an artificial cornea that produces the conditions for restoring specific layers through cellular regeneration [3]. This shift has become possible owing to the development of new, less invasive surgical techniques, including anterior and posterior lamellar keratoplasty, in which only the damaged area of the cornea is replaced, while leaving the surrounding healthy tissue intact [4]. These techniques can improve outcomes in terms of graft survival and the number of postoperative complications compared with penetrating keratoplasty, in which the entire cornea is replaced.

In our previous work, we demonstrated the safety and biocompatibility of a Viscoll collagen membrane based on medical-grade Viscoll collagen [5]. Implantation of this Viscoll collagen membrane resulted in an increased overall thickness of the cornea and its strength characteristics, as well as the maintenance of transparency for up to six months postoperatively. Importantly, the cornea is highly innervated, and nerve regeneration after injury plays a critical role in the restoration of normal function [6,7]. Therefore, it is essential to investigate the regeneration of the replaced corneal tissue and the innervation of the restored area.

The primary aim of this study is to conduct a comprehensive assessment of the suitability of the Viscoll collagen membrane as an artificial analogue of the corneal stroma for the regeneration of its defects. A feature of our manufacturing process of the collagen membrane was increasing the concentration of collagen instead of the standard chemical crosslinking protocols to improve the biomechanical characteristics of the final product. The specific objectives of the current work include the study of the biomechanical characteristics and transparency of the Viscoll collagen membrane in comparison with the stroma from the human cornea; toxicological studies of the Viscoll collagen membrane; and evaluation of the effectiveness of the Viscoll collagen membrane for corneal regeneration during its implantation in the cornea of rabbits, in which a section of the stroma was surgically removed.

2. Materials and Methods

2.1. Animal Experiments

All experiments were carried out in compliance with Directive 2010/63/EU and the Research Institute of Eye Diseases Animal Care and Use Committee guidelines, and the study was approved by the aforementioned institution's review board (№763, date of approval 11 May 2021). The experimental studies involved 10 male Chinchilla rabbits, aged 12–16 weeks and weighing 3.0–3.5 kg. All animals were allowed to adapt to their environment for 2 weeks before surgery. The rabbits received general and local anesthesia before and during surgery. General anesthesia was administered via intramuscular injection of ketamine (50 mg/kg) and xylazine (15 mg/kg). After the surgery, the animals were maintained under controlled conditions: temperature, 22 ± 1 °C; relative humidity, 45%; 10 air changes per hour; and a 12 h light/dark cycle. The rabbits had free access to water and standard compound feed. The surgeries were performed under general anesthesia. The rabbits were euthanized under deep anesthesia (100 mg/kg ketamine and 4 mg/kg xylazine) with 80 mg/kg pentobarbital.

2.2. Collagen Membrane Preparation

The production of Viscoll collagen membrane was certified according to ISO 13485 (Quality System for Medical Devices). Viscoll Collagen Membrane was obtained sterile from initially sterile components as a result of an aseptic manufacturing process (according to ISO 13408) in ISO 5 and ISO 7 class cleanrooms (according to ISO 14644-1) and did not require final sterilization.

The Viscoll collagen membrane was prepared using a previously published method [5] consisting of two stages: gelation and vitrification at constant pressure.

2.2.1. Gelation

Briefly, 0.5 mL of a sterile 30 mg/mL solution of medical grade native porcine collagen type I (Viscoll®; Imtek Ltd., Moscow, Russia) was added to each well of a 24-well plate. To remove air bubbles from the collagen solution, the plates were centrifuged for 30 min using an Avanti J-26XP centrifuge (oscillating bucket rotor JS-5.2; Beckman Coulter, Inc., Brea, CA, USA) at 3200 rpm and 4 °C. To induce collagen gelation, the plates were incubated in an atmosphere of ammonia vapor for 12 h at 20 °C. After incubation, collagen hydrogels were collected, immersed in water for injection (Solopharm, Saint-Petersburg, Russia), and incubated for 24 h at 20 °C.

2.2.2. Plastic Compression and Vitrification

At this stage, collagen hydrogels were placed between two teflon plates, one of which was subjected to a constant load of 3 kg until complete vitrification.

2.2.3. Packaging

For long-term storage, the resulting material was rehydrated in water for injection (Solopharm) for 5 min. Then, the collagen membrane was placed on a square Teflon plate and hermetically packed in sterile primary packaging that met the requirements of ISO 11607-1 (Clinipak®, Klinipak LLC, Moscow, Russia). The material in the primary package was hermetically packed under vacuum into a secondary vacuum package (Figure 1). The obtained material was stored at 4–10 °C for 10 months before use.

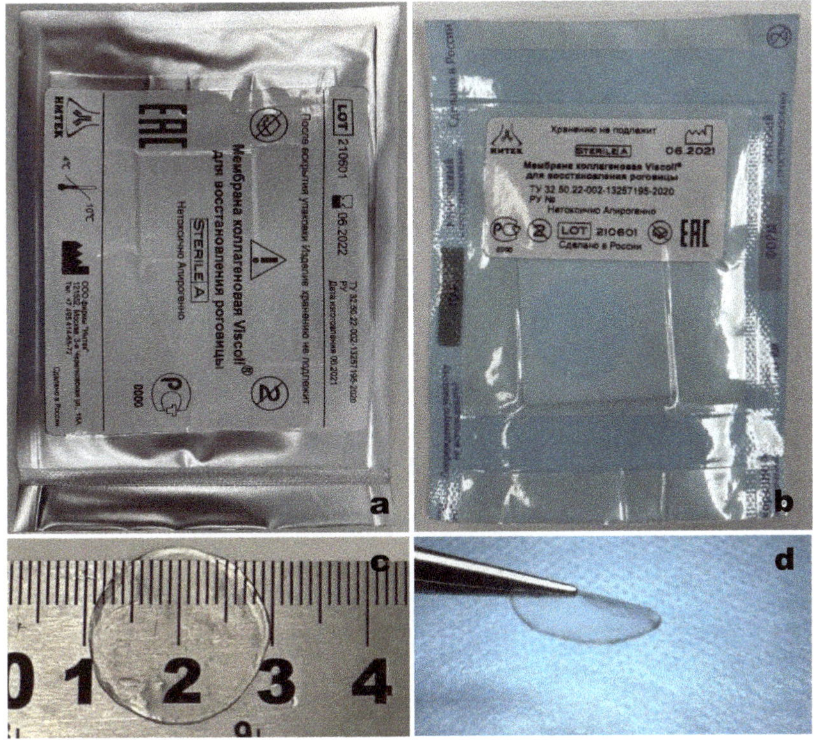

Figure 1. (**a**) Viscoll collagen membrane in vacuum packaging; (**b**) Viscoll collagen membrane in primary packaging; (**c**,**d**) views of the Viscoll collagen membrane ready for use.

2.3. Human Corneal Stroma Samples Preparation

Sections of the human corneal stroma were obtained using a Moria Evolution 3E microkeratome (Moria, Antony, France). The human corneoscleral disc from healthy donors was placed in a chamber with connected irrigation and securely fixed. First, the surface layer of the cornea was removed, including the Bowman's membrane, and then a stromal section of a given thickness was performed directly using a 150 μm microkeratome head. An ultrasonic pachymeter was used to measure the thickness of the central part of the cornea before and after the incision. As a result, stromal samples with an average thickness of 300 ± 20 μm were obtained.

2.4. Optical Properties of Collagen Membranes and Human Cornea

Light transmission through five Viscoll collagen membranes and five human corneal stroma samples were measured in the 380–780 nm wavelength range using a UV-VIS spectrophotometer (PE-5400UV, Ecroskhim, Saint-Petersburg, Russia). All samples were about 300 μm thick. Samples were immersed in 150 mM NaCl before measurement. During the measurement, samples were placed on one side of an empty transparent cuvette. An identical empty cuvette served as a reference.

2.5. Toxicology

Toxicological tests of the Viscoll collagen membrane were performed according to ISO 10993 standards by an independently certified testing laboratory center (IMBIIT, Moscow, Russia). Viscoll collagen membranes were tested according to the following protocols:

- ISO 10993-5: In vitro cytotoxicity. Direct effect of extracts from membranes on L929 mouse fibroblasts.
- ISO 10993-6: Implantation. The study is intended to evaluate the biocompatibility of the test material and tissue within the eye by surgical implantation of the material into the eye of a rabbit for an appropriate period of time. The reverse tolerance of the test material and eye tissues after implantation is evaluated.
- ISO 10993-10: Irritating effect. In vivo. Ocular irritation in rabbits.
- ISO 10993-10: Irritating effect. In vivo. Skin sensitization in guinea pigs.
- ISO 10993-11: Acute systemic toxicity test in rabbits.
- GPM.1.2.4.0005.15: Pyrogenicity. The test is based on the measurement of body temperature in rabbits before and after the injection of membrane extracts.

2.6. Ex Vivo Sewing Test

The cadaveric eye was fixed in a special holder. Non-penetrating trepanation of the cornea was performed at 2/3 of its depth, after which the upper layers of the stroma were removed, and a collagen graft was placed in the formed trepanation bed and fixed with a continuous 10-0 nylon suture. The detailed technique is presented in Supplementary Information (Video S1).

2.7. Surgery

The rabbits received general and local anesthesia before and during surgery. General anesthesia was administered via intramuscular injection of ketamine (50 mg/kg) and xylazine (15 mg/kg). The local anesthesia (2% (*w/v*) lidocaine eye drops) was administered to the right eye of each rabbit. A mark was made on the cornea using an 8 mm-diameter trephine, and an approximately 3 mm-long incision was made along the marking line at 1/3 of the depth, with a disposable blade. An intrastromal pocket was formed through the formed access. To do this, a tunnel was formed along the notch line using a spatula, which was cut with scissors concentrically to the markup. Thus, intraoperative access was expanded by $\frac{1}{2}$ of the circumference, and then, using a stratifier, we formed an intracorneal pocket. Repeated stratification was performed in the formed pocket, thereby highlighting the layer of the underlying stroma that was then removed. In one group of animals, a collagen membrane was implanted into the area where the stroma was excised (first group—

surgery and implantation of membranes). In another group (second group—only surgery), consisting of two rabbits, implantation of the collagen membrane was not performed after the removal of the stroma, and the wound was sutured using 10-0 nylon sutures (MANI Inc., Utsunomiya, Japan). Eye drops containing 0.3% (*w/v*) gentamicin were applied daily for the first 3 days. The detailed technique is presented in Supplementary Information (Video S2).

2.8. Postoperative Observation

Clinical evaluations of the corneas were performed on days 30, 90, and 180 post surgery using slit-lamp microscopy. On days 30, 90, and 180, anterior segment optical coherence tomography (OCT) and in vivo confocal microscopy (IVCM) were performed on the eight rabbits from the first group. The contralateral intact eyes served as the reference.

2.9. Histological and Immunohistological Study

The rabbits were sacrificed on the 180th day after surgery. Corneal samples were excised from four rabbits, fixed in 10% (*v/v*) neutral buffered formalin, dehydrated, and embedded in paraffin wax. Sections of dehydrated, paraffin-embedded samples (5 µm thick) were stained with hematoxylin and eosin using standard techniques and observed under an optical microscope.

For the immunohistochemistry analysis, fixed corneal samples from four rabbits in the first group and two rabbits in the second group and the contralateral intact eyes from both groups were washed in PBS and transferred to 30% (*w/v*) sucrose in PBS. Sections (14 µm thick) were obtained using a cryostat (CM1900, Leica, Weltzar, Germany). The sections were incubated for 1 h at 20–25 °C in blocking solution: 5% (*v/v*) normal goat serum (Sigma-Aldrich, St. Louis, MO, USA), 0.3% (*v/v*) Triton X-100, and 0.01 M PBS (pH 7.4). This was followed by incubation with mouse anti-alpha SMA (1:200; BioLegend, San Diego, CA, USA) in the blocking solution at 4 °C overnight. Thereafter, the sections were washed and incubated for 2 h with goat anti-mouse IgG (AlexaFluor488, 1:600; Abcam, Cambridge, UK) in 0.3% (*v/v*) Triton X-100 and 0.01 M PBS (pH 7.4). Sections were then washed in PBS, and nuclei were stained with DAPI solution (2 µg/mL; Sigma, St. Louis, MI, USA). Histological images were obtained using a BZ-9000E fluorescence microscope (Keyence, Osaka, Japan).

2.10. Mechanical Testing

The tensile strengths of the five collagen membranes were measured using an Instron Universal Testing Instrument (model 5982; Illinois Tool Works, Inc., Glenview, IL, USA) and a 2530-series load cell (model 2530-50N; Illinois Tool Works, Inc.). Mechanical trials were conducted in compliance with the ASTM D5748 standard. This testing method was designed to provide the conditions for biaxial deformation with a constant crosshead speed (1 mm/min). The specimen holder has a diameter of 5 mm. The loading element tip radius was 1.25 mm. During mechanical testing, all the samples were kept in Ringer's solution at 20 °C. During the test, we considered the test samples as conical surfaces of variable height. The obtained experimental dependences in the load-displacement coordinates were recalculated into stress–strain curves using the following formulas.

Sample deformation:

$$\varepsilon = ((S_{tek} - S_0)/S_0) \times 100\%, \tag{1}$$

where S_0 is the initial area of the sample and S_{tek} is the current area of the sample, calculated by the following formula:

$$S_{tek} = \pi R \, (R^2 + \Delta l^2)^{1/2}, \tag{2}$$

where R is the sample radius and Δl is the displacement of the loading element.

The stress was calculated by the following formula:

$$\sigma = P/S_{tek}, \tag{3}$$

where P is the current load on the sample.

Based on the stress–strain curves (Figure 2b), the fracture strain (at the maximum load) and the elastic modulus (in the section of the curve with the maximum slope) were calculated. All calculations were carried out using Instron Bluehill 2 Universal software (Illinois Tool Works, Inc.).

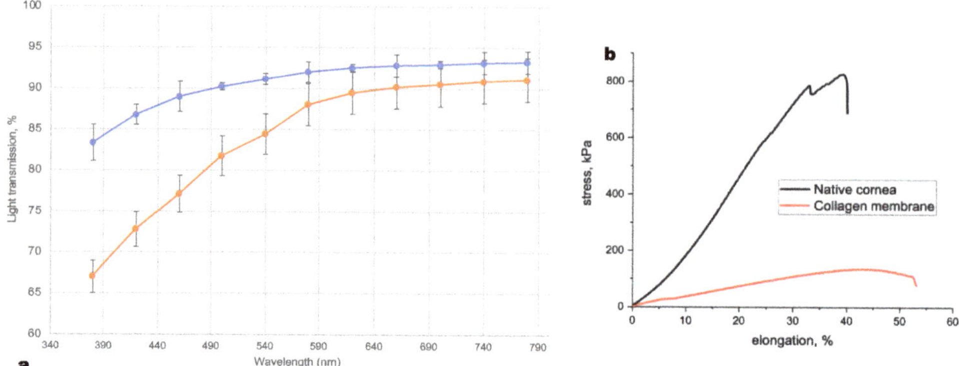

Figure 2. (**a**) Optical properties of the Viscoll collagen membrane (blue line) and stroma of human cornea (orange line). Samples thickness: 300 µm. (**b**) Characteristic stress–tension curves for Viscoll collagen membranes and human cornea samples.

2.11. Statistical Analysis

The basic summary statistics are presented as the mean ± standard deviation. All statistical analyses were performed using Excel 16.4 (Microsoft, Inc., Redmond, DC, USA).

3. Results

3.1. Optical and Physical Properties

Figure 2a shows the mean of light transmission of five samples of membranes and five samples of human cornea stroma as a function of wavelength in the 380–780 nm range. The Viscoll collagen membrane can transmit visible light similar to the human cornea; however, the mechanical properties of the human cornea surpass those of the Viscoll collagen membrane by about six-fold. Still, the mechanical properties of the Viscoll collagen are sufficient for its manipulation and fixation with a surgical suture. This is discussed in more detail below. Table 1 summarizes the optical and mechanical properties of collagen membranes prepared from 3% (w/v) Viscoll collagen solution and stroma of the human cornea.

Table 1. Optical and mechanical properties of Viscoll collagen membrane made from 3% (w/v) collagen solution and stroma of the human cornea.

Sample	Thickness (mm)	Transparency (%)	Young Modulus (kPa)	Stress at Rupture (kPa)	Elongation at Rupture (%)
Viscoll Collagen membrane	0.3	83.3–93.3 (at λ from 380–780 nm)	467 ± 30	137 ± 11	41 ± 5
Stroma of human cornea	0.3	67.0–91.1 (at λ from 380–780 nm)	2859 ± 30	836 ± 6	41 ± 2

3.2. Suturability of the Membranes

To assess the suitability of the membranes for surgical practice, it was necessary to test them under ex vivo conditions during keratoplasty of the cadaveric eye. It was demonstrated that the Viscoll collagen membrane can be fixed with both interrupted and continuous sutures without macroscopic damage to the material (Supplementary Information Video S1). Suture and fixation of the material are possible using standard surgical instruments but require more careful handling; it is not recommended to exert strong pressure on the material when grasping with tweezers, as this can lead to damage.

3.3. Toxicology

Viscoll collagen membranes successfully passed all the necessary toxicological tests. When L929 mouse fibroblasts were cultured with extracts from Viscoll membrane samples, no cytotoxic effects were detected. This sensitizing effect was also studied in sexually mature albino guinea pigs using a method to maximize the sensitizing effect. None of the animals exhibited hypersensitive reactions. When the solution was instilled into the conjunctival sac of rabbits, no irritating effect on the cornea, iris, or conjunctiva was detected. In addition, no chemoses or pathological secretions were observed. Under the conditions of implantation of the collagen membrane samples, no general toxic effects were detected and there were no observable effects on the tissues surrounding the implant compared to those in the controls.

Extracts prepared in a sterile solution of 0.9% sodium chloride for injection did not show pyrogenic reactions when administered intravenously to rabbits. The total temperature increase did not exceed the permissible value ($\sum\Delta t$) of $\leq 1.2\ °C$.

3.4. Clinical Results

Clinical pictures were recorded daily during the first stage of the study. In the early postoperative period, slight corneal oedema was observed in all 10 cases, which was most pronounced in the area of the surgical suture. There were no signs of inflammation, the moisture in the anterior chamber was transparent, and the iris actively reacted to light; 2 weeks after the operation, oedema had largely regressed. The subsequent clinical state was stable; the cornea remained transparent and no signs of inflammation were observed (Figure 3a). However, by the end of the 6th month of observation, against the background of sagging suture material, four rabbits showed signs of corneal neovascularization in the form of superficial "tassels" of newly formed vessels, stretching from the limbus to the operation area and into the suture area. After the removal of the sutures, the vascular reaction stopped and the newly formed vessels quickly became empty (Figure 4). In the second group, the clinical picture was similar, with slight oedema in the postoperative period associated with surgical trauma and subsequent stabilization. In rabbits from the second group, after 6 months of observation, a vascular reaction to the suture material was also noted, but was less pronounced.

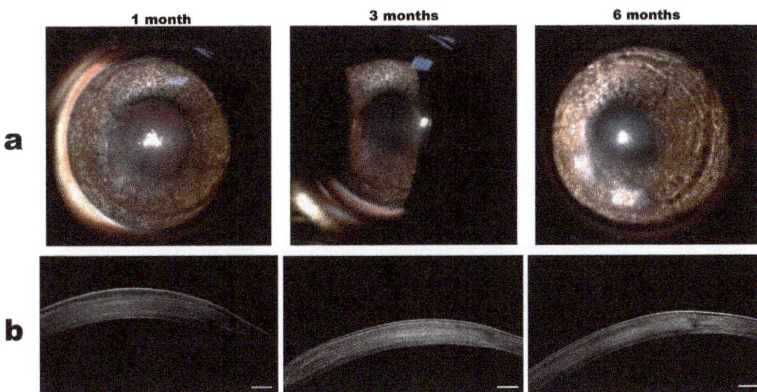

Figure 3. (a) Representative photographs of collagen membranes implanted in the stroma at different follow-up times. (b) Representative OCT images of rabbit corneas at different follow-up times. Scale bar = 250 μm.

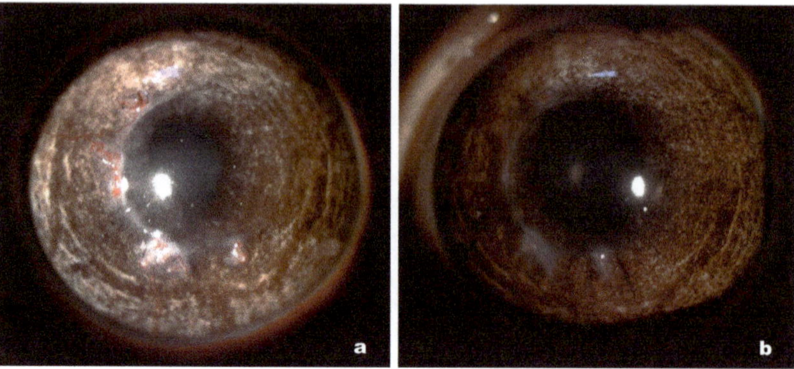

Figure 4. The role of sutures in corneal neovascularization. (**a**) Rabbit cornea with implanted membrane 6 months after surgery (before suture removal); (**b**) same cornea after removal of the sutures (1 week later).

3.5. OCT and In Vivo Confocal Microscopy Results

According to the OCT data, the collagen membrane was in close contact with the corneal stroma throughout the observation period (Figure 3b). One month after the operation, the average thickness of the central region of the cornea in the first group was 365 ± 23 μm, and the boundaries of the implant were visible, making it possible to estimate its thickness, which was 190 ± 15 μm. At 3 and 6 months after surgery, the boundaries of the implant and stroma were indistinct, which indicates good integration of the collagen membrane with the surrounding tissue. Compared to the first month, the average thickness of the central region of the cornea after 3 and 6 months decreased by 316 ± 19 μm and 305 ± 20 μm, respectively. The mean central corneal thickness of the non-operated corneas of the contralateral eye was 230 ± 20 μm.

IVCM was performed to evaluate the anatomical layers of the cornea and the membrane at the cellular level [8]. The surface epithelium and endothelium remained unchanged throughout the experiment and were comparable to those of non-operated corneas (Figure 5). After 6 months, the presence of sub-basal nerves was noted under the epithelium and in the central region of the cornea, indicating regeneration of the sub-basal nerve plexus. Two rabbits were noted to have slightly more macrophages than the other rabbits, with a clear trend towards a decrease by 6 months. The presence of linear structures, which appear due to apoptosis of the stromal cells [9], was observed at 1 and 3 months after the operation; by 6 months, their number had significantly decreased.

3.6. Histological Results

At 6 months after the surgery, the cornea was preserved throughout and was of uniform thickness. The cornea's substantia propria had no visible changes throughout its thickness, and the anterior epithelium and border (Bowman) membranes did not change. The posterior (Descemet's) membrane, as well as the adjacent stromal layer (Dua's layer) were preserved, as was the posterior epithelium (endothelium). The implant was well traced along its entire length; it was not defibrillated and was fully integrated into the corneal stroma. At the border of the cornea with the limbus, there was scant inflammatory infiltration (predominantly perivascular) and slight hyalinosis along this side of the implant. In addition, host cell migration within the material was observed in the samples (Figure 6), which is in agreement with our previous results [5]. The results of immunohistochemical staining of corneal samples 6 months after surgery revealed single stromal cells expressing α-SMA in both groups (Figure 7).

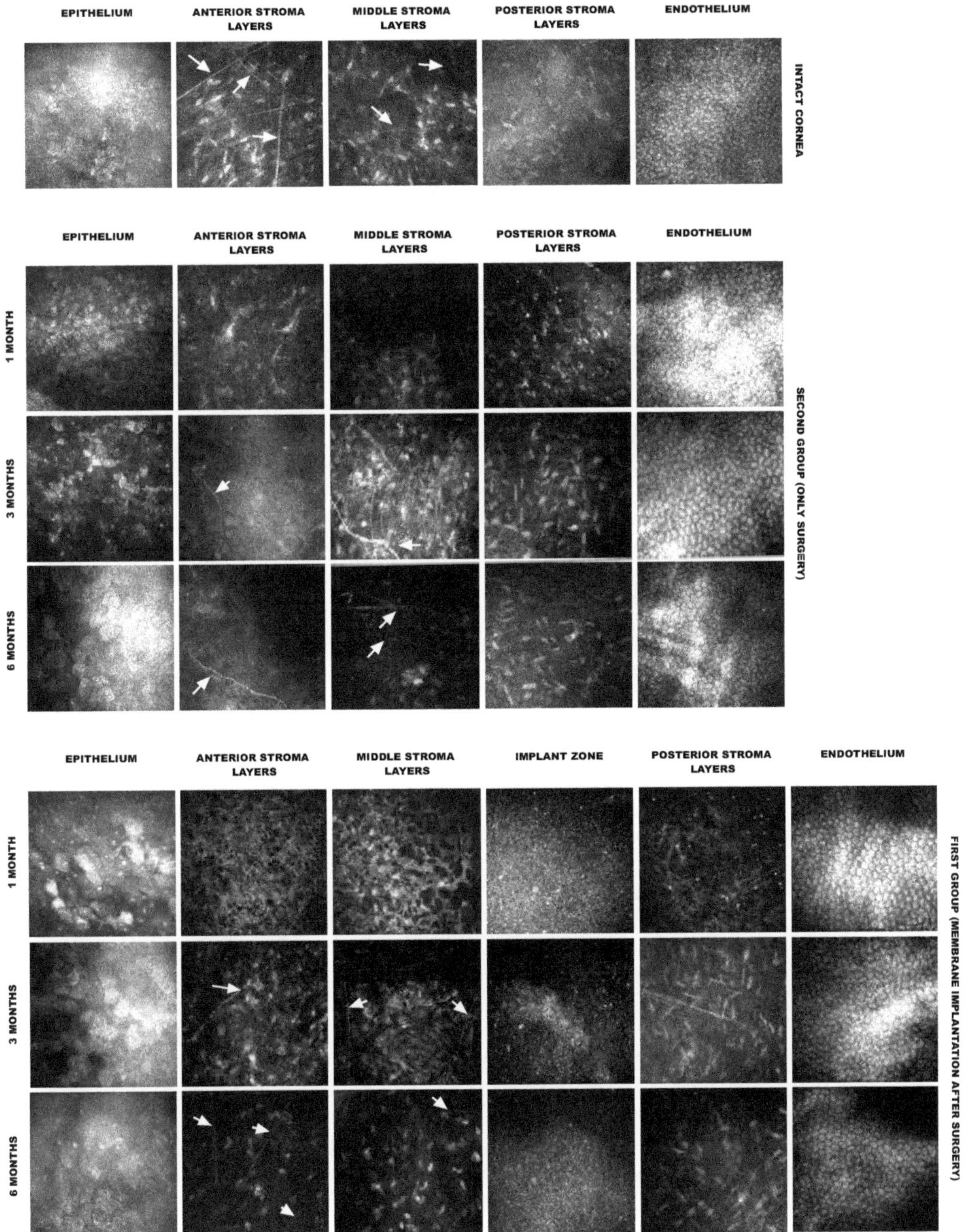

Figure 5. In vivo confocal microscope images of rabbit corneas implanted with the collagen membrane at different observation times. Arrows indicate nerves.

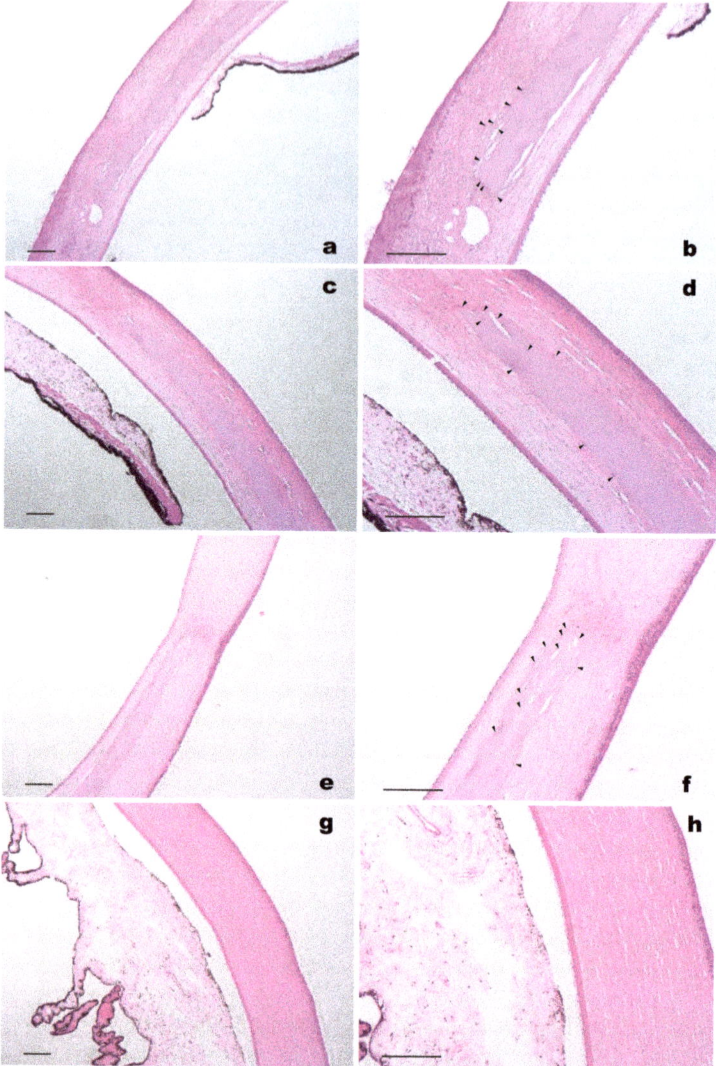

Figure 6. Hematoxylin and eosin staining of a cornea 180 days after the implantation of the collagen membrane: (**a–f**) first group, (**g,h**) intact cornea. Arrows indicate the migration of host cells into the membrane. Scale bar = 100 μm.

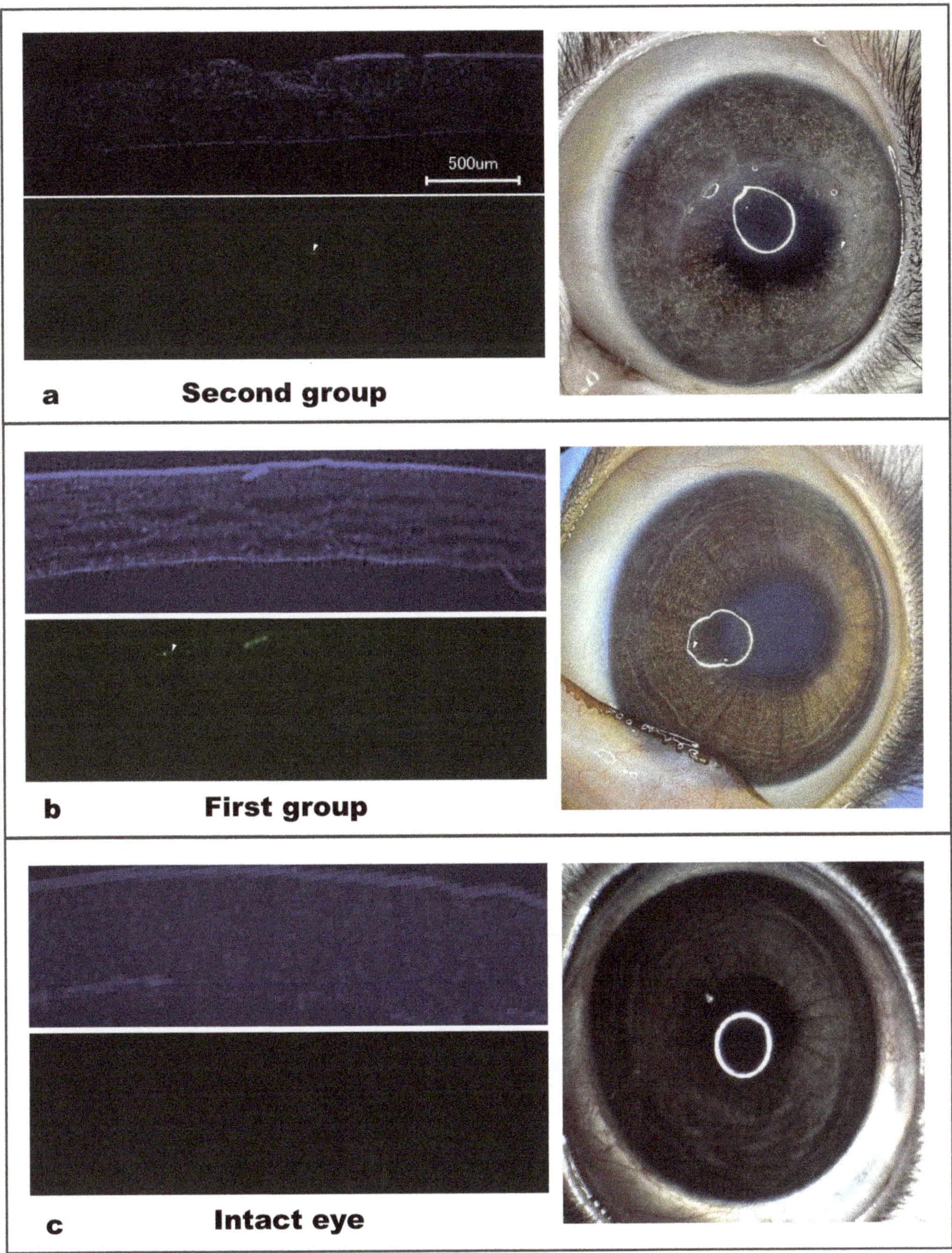

Figure 7. Representative photographs of rabbit eyes and their immunohistochemical analysis 6 months after surgery. (**a**) Second group (only surgery); (**b**) first group (surgery with collagen membrane implantation); (**c**) contralateral control eye. In both groups, the presence of α-SMA-positive fibroblasts was noted. Blue—DAPI staining (nuclei), green—α-SMA staining.

4. Discussion

Given that more than 90% of the human cornea is in the stroma, the solution of creating a fully functional and biocompatible stromal replacement is key to both artificial cornea technology and the ability to restore a healthy stroma in patients with corneal blindness [3]. Therefore, active practical research is being conducted in this direction, among which corneal stroma tissue engineering with cell-free collagen hydrogels [10,11] is a promising approach with potential clinical application. The pioneers in this field are the Griffith et al. group, who were the first to conduct clinical trials of collagen hydrogels, which were prepared from recombinant type III collagen chemically cross-linked with EDC/N-hydroxysuccinimide to impart mechanical strength to the material [12]. Although this work demonstrated the safety of this approach and even the restoration of innervation, in subsequent studies from the same group, the absence of host cell migration into such material was noted four years after surgery in humans [13]; therefore, complete regeneration of the cornea has not been achieved thus far. There may be several reasons for this, but it is most likely that the chemical cross-linking of the collagen material significantly impedes the migration of cells into the implant and, as a result, complete regeneration of the corneal stroma is unattainable.

Many years of experience with collagen experimentation have shown that native highly purified collagen has extremely low antigenic properties and low inflammatory potential [14], leading to the adoption of collagen biomaterials in clinical practice. Therefore, when developing new collagen biomaterials, it is necessary to be guided by the following principle: the fewer structural and property changes to collagen during the process, the more likely it is to obtain an ideal collagen biomaterial. This principle is especially important if the goal of this study is to achieve the clinical application of the biomaterial.

Our approach to the creation of an artificial cornea is to reject the use of any chemical cross-links, as they can impair the biocompatibility of the entire implant [15] and hinder the process of host cell migration into the implant [16], or, in some cases, completely block it [13]. Therefore, to enhance the biomechanical characteristics of the implant, a solution of concentrated medical-grade Viscoll collagen I was used. In contrast to our previous work [5], we used a higher concentration of collagen to manufacture the membrane. This made it possible to increase the mechanical properties of the membrane compared to our previous work [5], but this was not enough to achieve the mechanical properties of the human cornea. It should be noted that this is not a critical disadvantage since the properties of the Viscoll collagen membrane are sufficient for its fixation with a classic surgical suture. At the same time, we had previously shown that its mechanical properties after implantation into the stroma of the cornea will inevitably increase due to the natural process of adaptation of the collagen membrane with the surrounding tissues [5]. Moreover, cells can also enhance the mechanical strength of collagen hydrogels [17]. Thus, the success of the regeneration of the damaged cornea will depend on how effectively the corneal cells will interact with the collagen membrane in vivo.

An important result obtained in this study was that active cell migration was observed in all implanted collagen membranes after 6 months. This is consistent with our previous in vitro results, which demonstrated that collagen hydrogels prepared from a concentrated collagen solution maintained a high survival rate of encapsulated cells, maintained their morphology and functional activity for at least 28 days, and did not interfere with cellular movement [17]. Our cellular migration results were also consistent with earlier in vivo work by our group [5]. These results are in stark contrast with those from the cross-linked recombinant human collagen membrane, where host cell migration into the hydrogel was not observed up to 4 years post operation [13], as well as with the data obtained for cross-linked porcine collagen in a rabbit study, in which only sparse cell migration into the hydrogel was observed at 6 months post surgery [10]. This may be evidence that the chemical cross-linking of collagen hydrogels impairs cell permeability in vivo.

In the study of corneal tissue regeneration, it is extremely important to investigate the issue of innervation of the restored area because nerve regeneration after corneal injury plays a decisive role in restoring normal function.

A study of the micromorphology of the cornea using laser confocal microscopy revealed that the removal of a portion of the stroma during anterior lamellar keratoplasty leads to the initial loss of nerves; however, in all experimental animals, nerve regeneration was confirmed at 6 months after the operation. Similar results were obtained during the implantation of chemically cross-linked collagen membranes into the corneal stroma of animals [10,11,18] and humans [13]. It is worth noting here that the process of reinnervation of implanted donor corneas in humans is very slow, lasting from one to several years [6,19]. The results obtained in this study may indicate that the Viscoll collagen membrane supports, or at least does not interfere with, the process of nerve repair in the cornea after layered keratoplasty.

According to our OCT data, after implantation, there was no migration or displacement of the collagen membrane implant; it took its position and fixed itself within the surrounding tissues. This behavior was also confirmed by histological examination, which showed that the collagen fibers of the stroma were closely intertwined with those of the implant, indicating a good survival rate.

Corneal neovascularization in the peripheral implanted zone was noted in four rabbits in the first group and two rabbits in the second group. Neovascularization is associated with sagging of the suture material due to the gradual integration of collagen with the corneal stroma; this involves natural cross-linking and strengthening of the biomechanics, which significantly weakens the sutures and causes sagging [20]. In such cases, the timely removal of the sutures completely resolves the problem and, according to the results of our study, this should be done 4–5 months after the operation.

Immunohistochemical staining of cryosectioned cornea samples revealed the presence of single α-SMA-positive stromal cells in both groups, whereas none were found in the intact cornea samples. Notably, the presence of these cells did not affect the transparency of the corneas. The presence of α-SMA-positive cells in the corneal stroma was likely induced by the operation itself, during which a part of the stroma was removed. The results provide evidence that the Viscoll collagen membrane does not have an irritating effect on the corneal tissue, which is also consistent with the results of the toxicological tests performed.

Our work has several limitations. (1) The experiments were carried out on a healthy cornea, in which a section of healthy stroma was surgically removed and a collagen membrane was implanted in its place. There is no doubt that the processes of tissue regeneration in various pathologies of the cornea, especially in case of chemical burns, will proceed differently. However, our results strongly suggest that the Viscoll collagen membrane may also be effective in the treatment of pathological conditions of the cornea. It should be noted that in this case, it may be necessary to develop new approaches for the treatment of various corneal pathologies using the Viscoll collagen membrane. (2) Short-term observation: Ideally, for a clear understanding of the reparative processes occurring in the damaged cornea during implantation of the Viscoll collagen membrane, a four-year follow-up is required. At the same time, it is extremely difficult to monitor rabbits that have undergone a full course of anesthesia for more than 6 months. At the same time, the processes of regeneration of the cornea in rabbits proceed faster than in humans. Therefore, to a certain extent, the results could be extrapolated to the regeneration of the human cornea.

Considering the proven safety of the Viscoll collagen membrane and its possible potential for the treatment of various corneal pathologies, especially under the conditions of a global shortage of donor tissue, our results can serve as the basis for future clinical trials.

5. Conclusions

In this study, a Viscoll collagen membrane prepared from a concentrated collagen solution was presented. Viscoll collagen membrane manufacturing technology can be easily scaled up to 5000 units, and the proposed packaging format allows for the maintenance of its key properties for at least 12 months. In addition to its excellent optical and mechanical properties, the Viscoll collagen membrane promotes active cell migration and can be implanted into the corneal stroma using tools and techniques that mimic those used in human corneal keratoplasty. From the aggregate of the presented data, it can be concluded that the Viscoll collagen membrane has the potential to solve the global problem of limited donor tissue for the treatment of corneal blindness. In addition to this study, we have demonstrated good biochemical properties of the Viscoll collagen membrane and the ability of suture fixation; therefore, the next step in our work will be deep anterior lamellar keratoplasty with the Viscoll collagen membrane.

Supplementary Materials: The following supporting information can be downloaded at https://www.mdpi.com/article/10.3390/polym14194017/s1. Video S1: Suturability of the Membranes; Video S2: Surgery.

Author Contributions: Conceptualization, E.O.O. and A.Y.A.; methodology, E.O.O., A.Y.A., S.E.A., G.V.V., Z.V.S., A.V.Z., T.E.G., S.V.K., K.K.S. and O.V.Z.; investigation, E.O.O. and A.Y.A.; validation, S.E.A., T.E.G. and S.P.D.; formal analysis, S.E.A., G.V.V., Z.V.S., A.V.Z., T.E.G., S.V.K., K.K.S. and O.V.Z.; resources, E.O.O.; writing—original draft preparation, E.O.O. and A.Y.A.; writing—review and editing, S.P.D.; visualization, E.O.O. and A.Y.A.; project administration, E.O.O. All authors have read and agreed to the published version of the manuscript.

Funding: This research received no external funding.

Institutional Review Board Statement: All experiments were carried out in compliance with Directive 2010/63/EU and the Research Institute of Eye Diseases Animal Care and Use Committee guidelines, and the study was approved by the aforementioned institution's review board (№763, date of approval: 11 May 2021).

Data Availability Statement: The data presented in this study are available on request from the corresponding author.

Conflicts of Interest: Egor Osidak is a CTO and chief scientist at Imtek Ltd., which produces medical grade collagen Viscoll and Viscoll collagen membrane. Viscoll collagen membrane is undergoing preparation for clinical translation in Russia. The other authors have no competing interests.

References

1. Meek, K.M.; Knupp, C. Corneal Structure and Transparency. *Prog. Retin. Eye Res.* **2015**, *49*, 1–16. [CrossRef] [PubMed]
2. Mahdavi, S.S.; Abdekhodaie, M.J.; Mashayekhan, S.; Baradaran-Rafii, A.; Djalilian, A.R. Bioengineering Approaches for Corneal Regenerative Medicine. *Tissue Eng. Regen. Med.* **2020**, *17*, 567–593. [CrossRef] [PubMed]
3. Matthyssen, S.; Van den Bogerd, B.; Dhubhghaill, S.N.; Koppen, C.; Zakaria, N. Corneal Regeneration: A Review of Stromal Replacements. *Acta Biomater.* **2018**, *69*, 31–41. [CrossRef] [PubMed]
4. Reinhart, W.J.; Musch, D.C.; Jacobs, D.S.; Lee, W.B.; Kaufman, S.C.; Shtein, R.M. Deep Anterior Lamellar Keratoplasty as an Alternative to Penetrating Keratoplasty a Report by the American Academy of Ophthalmology. *Ophthalmology* **2011**, *118*, 209–218. [CrossRef] [PubMed]
5. Andreev, A.Y.; Osidak, E.O.; Grigoriev, T.E.; Krasheninnikov, S.V.; Zaharov, V.D.; Zaraitianc, O.V.; Borzenok, S.A.; Domogatsky, S.P. A New Collagen Scaffold for the Improvement of Corneal Biomechanical Properties in a Rabbit Model. *Exp. Eye Res.* **2021**, *207*, 108580. [CrossRef] [PubMed]
6. Al-Aqaba, M.A.A.; Dhillon, V.K.; Mohammed, I.; Said, D.G.; Dua, H.S. Corneal Nerves in Health and Disease. *Prog. Retin. Eye Res.* **2019**, *73*, 100762. [CrossRef] [PubMed]
7. Shaheen, B.S.; Bakir, M.; Jain, S. Corneal Nerves in Health and Disease. *Surv. Ophthalmol.* **2014**, *59*, 263–285. [CrossRef] [PubMed]
8. Kocaba, V.; Colica, C.; Rabilloud, M.; Burillon, C. Predicting Corneal Graft Rejection by Confocal Microscopy. *Cornea* **2015**, *34* (Suppl. 10), S61–S64. [CrossRef] [PubMed]
9. Lagali, N.; Bourghardt, B.; Germundsson, J.; Eden, U.; Danyali, R.; Rinaldo, M.; Fagerholm, P. *Confocal Laser Microscopy—Principles and Applications in Medicine, Biology, and the Food Sciences*; IntechOpen: London, UK, 2013. [CrossRef]
10. Xeroudaki, M.; Thangavelu, M.; Lennikov, A.; Ratnayake, A.; Bisevac, J.; Petrovski, G.; Fagerholm, P.; Rafat, M.; Lagali, N. A Porous Collagen-Based Hydrogel and Implantation Method for Corneal Stromal Regeneration and Sustained Local Drug Delivery. *Sci. Rep.* **2020**, *10*, 16936. [CrossRef] [PubMed]

11. Haagdorens, M.; Edin, E.; Fagerholm, P.; Groleau, M.; Shtein, Z.; Ulčinas, A.; Yaari, A.; Samanta, A.; Cepla, V.; Liszka, A.; et al. Plant Recombinant Human Collagen Type I Hydrogels for Corneal Regeneration. *Regen. Eng. Transl. Med.* **2021**, *8*, 269–283. [CrossRef]

12. Fagerholm, P.; Lagali, N.S.; Merrett, K.; Jackson, W.B.; Munger, R.; Liu, Y.; Polarek, J.W.; Söderqvist, M.; Griffith, M. A Biosynthetic Alternative to Human Donor Tissue for Inducing Corneal Regeneration: 24-Month Follow-Up of a Phase 1 Clinical Study. *Sci. Transl. Med.* **2010**, *2*, 46ra61. [CrossRef] [PubMed]

13. Fagerholm, P.; Lagali, N.S.; Ong, J.A.; Merrett, K.; Jackson, W.B.; Polarek, J.W.; Suuronen, E.J.; Liu, Y.; Brunette, I.; Griffith, M. Stable Corneal Regeneration Four Years after Implantation of a Cell-Free Recombinant Human Collagen Scaffold. *Biomaterials* **2014**, *35*, 2420–2427. [CrossRef] [PubMed]

14. Lynn, A.K.; Yannas, I.V.; Bonfield, W. Antigenicity and Immunogenicity of Collagen. *J. Biomed. Mater. Res.* **2004**, *71*, 343–354. [CrossRef] [PubMed]

15. Yang, G.; Xiao, Z.; Long, H.; Ma, K.; Zhang, J.; Ren, X.; Zhang, J. Assessment of the Characteristics and Biocompatibility of Gelatin Sponge Scaffolds Prepared by Various Crosslinking Methods. *Sci. Rep.* **2018**, *8*, 1616. [CrossRef] [PubMed]

16. Petsch, C.; Schlötzer-Schrehardt, U.; Meyer-Blazejewska, E.; Frey, M.; Kruse, F.E.; Bachmann, B.O. Novel Collagen Membranes for the Reconstruction of the Corneal Surface. *Tissue Eng. Part A* **2014**, *20*, 2378–2389. [CrossRef] [PubMed]

17. Osidak, E.O.; Kalabusheva, E.P.; Alpeeva, E.V.; Belousov, S.I.; Krasheninnikov, S.V.; Grigoriev, T.E.; Domogatsky, S.P.; Vorotelyak, E.A.; Chermnykh, E.S. Concentrated Collagen Hydrogels: A New Approach for Developing Artificial Tissues. *Materialia* **2021**, *20*, 101217. [CrossRef]

18. Lagali, N.; Griffith, M.; Fagerholm, P.; Merrett, K.; Huynh, M.; Munger, R. Innervation of Tissue-Engineered Recombinant Human Collagen-Based Corneal Substitutes: A Comparative In Vivo Confocal Microscopy Study. *Investig. Ophthalmol. Vis. Sci.* **2008**, *49*, 3895–3902. [CrossRef] [PubMed]

19. Bandeira, F.; Yusoff, N.Z.; Yam, G.H.; Mehta, J.S. Corneal Re-innervation Following Refractive Surgery Treatments. *Neural Regen. Res.* **2019**, *14*, 557–565. [CrossRef] [PubMed]

20. Hsu, C.C.; Chang, H.M.; Lin, T.C.; Hung, K.H.; Chien, K.H.; Chen, S.Y.; Chen, S.N.; Chen, Y.T. Corneal Neovascularization and Contemporary Antiangiogenic Therapeutics. *J. Chin. Med. Assoc.* **2015**, *78*, 323–330. [CrossRef] [PubMed]

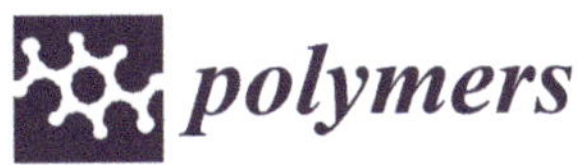 *polymers*

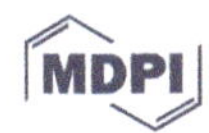

Article

Customizable Collagen Vitrigel Membranes and Preliminary Results in Corneal Engineering

María Dolores Montalvo-Parra [1,2], Wendy Ortega-Lara [1], Denise Loya-García [2], Andrés Bustamante-Arias [2], Guillermo-Isaac Guerrero-Ramírez [2], Cesar E. Calzada-Rodríguez [2], Guiomar Farid Torres-Guerrero [2], Betsabé Hernández-Sedas [2], Italia Tatnaí Cárdenas-Rodríguez [2], Sergio E. Guevara-Quintanilla [2], Marcelo Salán-Gomez [2], Miguel Ángel Hernández-Delgado [2], Salvador Garza-González [2], Mayra G. Gamboa-Quintanilla [2], Luis Guillermo Villagómez-Valdez [2], Judith Zavala [2,*] and Jorge E. Valdez-García [2]

[1] Tecnologico de Monterrey, Escuela de Ingenieria, 2501 Garza Sada Ave., Colonia Tecnologico. C.P., 64849 Monterrey, NL, Mexico
[2] Tecnologico de Monterrey, Escuela de Medicina, 3000 Morones Prieto Ave., Colonia Los Doctores. C.P., 64710 Monterrey, NL, Mexico
* Correspondence: judith.zavala@tec.mx

Citation: Montalvo-Parra, M.D.; Ortega-Lara, W.; Loya-García, D.; Bustamante-Arias, A.; Guerrero-Ramírez, G.-I.; Calzada-Rodríguez, C.E.; Torres-Guerrero, G.F.; Hernández-Sedas, B.; Cárdenas-Rodríguez, I.T.; Guevara-Quintanilla, S.E.; et al. Customizable Collagen Vitrigel Membranes and Preliminary Results in Corneal Engineering. *Polymers* **2022**, *14*, 3556. https://doi.org/10.3390/polym14173556

Academic Editors: Jianxun Ding, Nunzia Gallo, Marta Madaghiele, Alessandra Quarta and Amilcare Barca

Received: 28 May 2022
Accepted: 24 August 2022
Published: 29 August 2022

Publisher's Note: MDPI stays neutral with regard to jurisdictional claims in published maps and institutional affiliations.

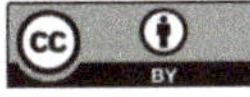

Copyright: © 2022 by the authors. Licensee MDPI, Basel, Switzerland. This article is an open access article distributed under the terms and conditions of the Creative Commons Attribution (CC BY) license (https://creativecommons.org/licenses/by/4.0/).

Abstract: Corneal opacities are a leading cause of visual impairment that affect 4.2 million people annually. The current treatment is corneal transplantation, which is limited by tissue donor shortages. Corneal engineering aims to develop membranes that function as scaffolds in corneal cell transplantation. Here, we describe a method for producing transplantable corneal constructs based on a collagen vitrigel (CVM) membrane and corneal endothelial cells (CECs). The CVMs were produced using increasing volumes of collagen type I: 1X ($2.8\ \mu L/mm^2$), 2X, and 3X. The vitrification process was performed at 40% relative humidity (RH) and 40 °C using a matryoshka-like system consisting of a shaking-oven harboring a desiccator with a saturated K_2CO_3 solution. The CVMs were characterized via SEM microscopy, cell adherence, FTIR, and manipulation in an ex vivo model. A pilot transplantation of the CECs/CVM construct in rabbits was also carried out. The thickness of the CVMs was 3.65–7.2 μm. The transparency was superior to a human cornea (92.6% = 1X; 94% = 2X; 89.21% = 3X). SEM microscopy showed a homogenous surface and laminar organization. The cell concentration seeded over the CVM increased threefold with no significant difference between 1X, 2X, and 3X ($p = 0.323$). The 2X-CVM was suitable for surgical manipulation in the ex vivo model. Constructs using the CECs/2X-CVM promoted corneal transparency restoration.

Keywords: scaffold; collagen vitrigel; tissue engineering; cornea; corneal endothelium

1. Introduction

Tailoring biomaterials for corneal reconstruction via tissue engineering represents an important breakthrough that may alleviate the problem of tissue scarcity. The shortage of corneal graft tissue limits access to a transplant in ~53% of the world's population. Although the cornea is the most frequently transplanted organ worldwide, there is currently only 1 cornea available for every 70 needed [1,2]. Given this situation, alternative solutions are needed to produce tissues for transplantation.

Corneal blindness is one of the four main causes of blindness around the world [3]. It can be caused by diseases, chemical burns, and trauma that affect different corneal layers [4]. The corneal endothelium is the innermost layer of the cornea. It regulates optimal corneal hydration to maintain the clarity needed for proper vision. This tissue does not regenerate and when the cell density decreases to a critical concentration, it produces an irreversible opacity that can only be treated with a corneal transplant [5]. Efforts in cell therapy have demonstrated the ability of corneal endothelial cells (CECs) to proliferate in vitro under the stimulus of supplemented culture media and retain their characteristic polygonal morphology and functional molecular markers, such as tight junctions (ZO-1) and Na-K/ATPase pumps [6–8]. However, given the monolayer nature of the corneal endothelium, CECs injected intracamerally do not always attach effectively to the corneal tissue [9].

Collagen membranes have the potential to serve as scaffolds for CECs in the production of bioengineered corneal tissue, given that type 1 collagen is an abundant protein in the corneal stroma and that it is produced by CECs [10–13]. These membranes are produced via a wide range of methodologies that vary in three main respects: (1) methodology, including desiccation, freeze drying, electrospinning, and 3D printing; (2) conditions, such as the collagen source and concentration, polymerization pH, and temperature; and (3) characterization, including microstructure, transmittance, FTIR, X-ray diffraction, cell adhesion, water uptake, biodegradability, and in vivo biocompatibility [14–16]. This leads to marked variations in parameters that limit the reproducibility of the methodologies and their application in corneal endothelium engineering [17].

Overall, the main challenges in producing collagen membranes for corneal endothelium engineering are the mechanical properties and biocompatibility. Enhancing the cross-linking of collagen fibers in the membranes is a strategy for the improvement of their mechanical properties while maintaining their low immunogenicity. Ultraviolet (UV) light treatment and desiccation in specific conditions are used for this purpose, producing vitrified membranes. Given that these strategies can produce transparent membranes, they have great potential for the restoration of cornea [18–20]. Currently, the protocols for producing collagen–vitrigel membranes (CVM) vary mainly in terms of temperature, time of desiccation, and relative humidity. This modifies the desired characteristics such as thickness, fiber diameter, density, and organization, which affect their application for clinical purposes.

The thickness of membranes is a parameter that is of special interest because it provides two main characteristics that determine their usefulness: surgical manipulation and cell adherence. A thicker collagen membrane is easier to surgically manipulate; however, this increases the distribution of charges, affecting the cell and tissue adherence [21]. A thinner membrane promotes cell and tissue adhesion but can be difficult to manipulate during surgery. For this reason, some collagen membranes reported for corneal engineering are more suitable for the epithelium or stromal layer, in which higher thickness provides the structure and barrier functions that cover different needs.

In this research, we provide a simple and reproducible method to produce CVMs that can be tailored to assemble membranes with different characteristics with potential use in the engineering of different layers of the cornea. We aim to close the gap between the reported methods, leading to the development of standardized protocols that yield reproducible and quantitative characterization, which in turn facilitate comparative research and the development of prototypes for clinical applications [14–20,22–31].

2. Methods

2.1. Matryoshka System Assembly for the Production of Collagen Membranes

For the manufacturing of CVMs, a matryoshka system was assembled (Figure 1).

It consisted of an incubator with a steady temperature (T) bearing a desiccator with a saturated K_2CO_3 solution to control the RH. For this purpose, 50 mL of K_2CO_3 solution were prepared using 1.15 g of K_2CO_3 (Sigma-Aldrich, P5833, St. Louis, MO, USA) per milliliter of bi distilled water. The salt solution was placed in a 200 mL beaker and fixed onto a $330 \times 246 \times 262$ mm desiccator with a clear plastic dome (Thermo Scientific Nalgene, 5310-0250, Cleveland, OH, USA). A closed system was created by placing the sealed desiccator inside a shaking-plate incubator (I5211DS; Labnet International, Edison, NJ, USA). The T and shaking speed of the incubator were set at 40 °C and 30 rpm, respectively. The shaker function was turned on 48 h after the gel was placed inside the matryoshka system to avoid gel tilting. The T and RH were measured with a Monitoring Traceable

Hygrometer (4040CC; Traceable®® Products, Webster, TX, USA) placed inside the desiccator. The T and RH were registered daily until a temperature of 40 °C and RH of 40% were recorded consistently for ~7 days. During this period, no sample was placed inside the system.

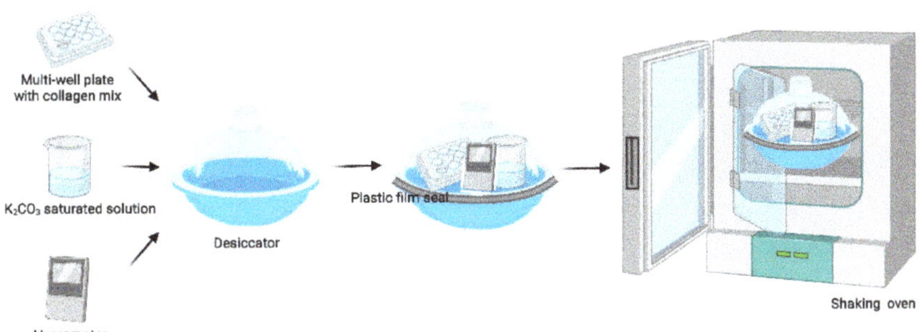

Figure 1. Matryoshka system assembly (created with Biorender.com Available online: https://app.biorender.com (accessed on 21 June 2022).

2.2. Collagen-Based Membrane Production

2.2.1. Collagen Gel Preparation

Collagen type 1 from bovine tail (Gibco) was used. CVM production was based on methods described previously [18,19]. Advanced Dulbecco's Modified Eagle's medium (DMEM) (Gibco–Thermo Fisher Scientific, Grand Island, NY, USA) was prepared with 1% penicillin–streptomycin (Gibco) and 8% qualified fetal bovine serum (Gibco) and kept on ice. Next, 22 mM HEPES (Gibco) was added and mixed with a cold type-I collagen solution (5 mg/mL) at a 1:1 ratio until a uniform yellow mixture was obtained by gentle pipette resuspension. The pipettes were also kept on ice to avoid early gelation. Twelve-well plates were used as casts for 2.2 mL of the collagen mix (2.8 µL/mm^2 of collagen; 1x volume). Gel casts were also prepared at volumes of 2X and 3X collagen. The plates containing the collagen mix were placed in an MCO-18AIC incubator (Sanyo, Osaka, Japan) and kept at 37 °C in 5% CO$_2$ for 2 h until gelation.

2.2.2. Desiccation

The plates containing collagen gels were placed inside the matryoshka system. The temperature and shaking speed of the incubator were set at 40 °C and 30 rpm, respectively. The system remained closed, and T and RH were registered daily. Around day 10–13, the volume of the collagen gels decreased, and membranes were formed. The matryoshka system was then opened and the membranes were rinsed with bi distilled water until the elimination of the phenol red in the medium. The samples were placed back inside the system to complete a period of 37 days of incubation.

2.2.3. Membrane Re Hydration

The plates were removed from the matryoshka system. Bi distilled water was poured into the wells of the plates containing the collagen membranes, left for ~20 min, and then removed. The borders of each membrane were lifted using water pressure. Rounded-tip forceps were used to gently pull out the membranes from the bottom of the well.

2.3. Collagen-Based Membrane Characterization

2.3.1. Optical Microscopy

Membranes were humidified for 20 min and the water excess was removed. The surface of CVM was observed with an Axiovert 40 CFL contrast microscope (Carl Zeiss Microscopy, Jena, Germany) and photographed.

2.3.2. Scanning Electron Microscopy (SEM)

Samples of the membranes were coated with gold using a Quorum QR150 ES sputtering system (Quorum Technologies, Laughton, UK). The surface and transversal ultrastructure were observed and measured with an EVO MA Scanning Electron Microscope (Carl Zeiss Microscopy). The fibers of samples that were desiccated for 7 days (4 samples, 34 fibers per sample) were photographed and measured using NIH ImageJ. Briefly, image calibration to microns was performed, followed by the selection of linear regions of interest and accumulation using the *Analysis>>Measure* route in ImageJ software.

2.3.3. D Confocal Microscopy

Surface regularity and sample thickness were assessed in triplicate using an Axio-CSM 700 50× objective (Carl Zeiss Microscopy). The samples were hydrated for 20 min prior to data collection.

2.3.4. In Vitro Cell Adherence, Viability, and Cytotoxicity

The NIH3T3 cell line was obtained from ATCC (CRL-1658™). The CVMs were cut into circles of 5 mm diameter to fit a 96-well plate. The CVMs were sterilized with Microdacyn (Oculus Innovative Sciences, CA, USA) and rinsed with sterile water. The water was removed and the membranes were left to dry and adhere to the bottom of the wells. NIH3T3 cells were seeded (~10,000) in 100 µL of DMEM F12 (12491-015; Gibco) and incubated overnight at 37 °C in 5% CO_2.

Cytotoxicity and viability tests were performed using Cell Titer Blue (Promega, Madison, WI, USA) according to the manufacturer's instructions. Briefly, 20 µL of Cell Titer Blue was added to each experimental, assay control, and sample control well, followed by gentle resuspension and incubation at 37 °C in 5% CO_2 for 2 h. The same conditions were used to perform a 2–50 × 10^3 cell fluorescence ladder comparison. Fluorescence was recorded on a Synergy HT spectrophotometer (BioTek, Winooski, VT, USA). Triplicates were tested for each membrane concentration in the experimental condition (membrane + cells), the sample control condition (cells alone), the negative control condition (membrane alone), and the assay control condition (medium + Cell Titer Blue).

2.3.5. Fourier-Transformed Infrared Spectra (FTIR)

Functional groups were identified on each membrane sample using an infrared spectrophotometer coupled with a Fourier transform Spectrum 400 apparatus (Perkin Elmer, Waltham, MA, USA) and recorded in the wavenumber range of 4000–400 cm^{-1} at room conditions.

2.3.6. Transmittance Analysis

Samples of 1X, 2X, and 3X membranes were fully hydrated using bi distilled water and placed into clear cuvettes. Absorbance was acquired throughout the UV–VIS spectra (380–700 nm) using a Synergy HT spectrophotometer (BioTek, Winooski, VT, USA) and transformed to transmittance using the Beer–Lambert law equation. Experiments were performed in triplicate.

2.3.7. X-ray Diffraction Analysis (XRD)

XRD was used to assess the crystallinity of the CVM. XRD was recorded in the 2θ range between 10° and 85° with a step size of 0.026 using a PANalytical Empyrean diffractometer (PANalytical, Almelo, The Netherlands) and CuKα radiation (λ = 1.5406 Å). The voltage applied was 45 kV and the current was 40 mA.

2.3.8. Ex Vivo Surgical Manipulation Test

To test the ease of surgically manipulating the CVM before performing transplants in the animal models, an ex vivo test was used. Cow eyes from a local butcher shop were fixated over styrofoam plates. All three CVM types (1X, 2X, and 3X) were stained with Trypan blue by 1 min immersion and transplanted into the anterior chamber, which is similar to a Descemet's stripping endothelial keratoplasty—the surgical procedure for corneal endothelium transplantation. The surgical procedures were performed by two ophthalmic surgeons in order to determine whether the CVM: (1) resisted manipulation with common surgical instruments in this type of surgery to avoiding breakage, (2) was able to introduce them folded through the incision in the periphery of the cornea, and (3) could expand once inside the anterior chamber. Supplementary Video S1 demonstrates the transplantation of a membrane in the ex vivo model.

2.4. Engineered Corneal Endothelium Assembling

We previously reported the ability of CECs to adhere to and proliferate over CVMs [32]. We assembled the CECs/CVM construct for further transplantation to determine its ability to adhere to the corneal stroma and to restore clarity in a corneal opacity model.

This study was approved by the institutional local ethics committee (School of Medicine of Tecnologico de Monterrey), number 2019-003. All the animals were treated according to the Guide for the Care and Use of Laboratory Animals, adhering to the guidelines for the human treatment and ethical use of animals for vision research stated by the National Institutes of Health guide for the care and use of Laboratory animals. White New Zealand rabbits were housed in individual cages and fed ad libitum.

Two 3-month-old male White New Zealand rabbits were used to isolate CECs according to a previous methodology [32,33]. Briefly, White New Zealand rabbits were euthanized with an intravenous pentobarbital lethal dose (90–180 mg/Kg). The endothelium was surgically detached from the corneal stroma. A digestion was made under sterile conditions in a flow hood with 1 mg/mL of collagenase type I (Sigma-Aldrich Co., St. Louis, MO, USA) at 37 °C for 1 h. The CECs were cultured using OptiMEM-I supplemented with 8% FBS, 20 ng/mL of nerve growth factor (NGF; Sigma-Aldrich Co.), 5 ng/mL of epidermal growth factor (EGF; Sigma-Aldrich Co.), 200 mg/L of calcium chloride (Sigma-Aldrich Co.), 20 µg/mL of ascorbic acid (Sigma-Aldrich Co.), 0.08% chondroitin sulfate (Sigma-Aldrich Co.), and 1% antibiotics until confluency. A passage was conducted, and the CECs were cultured using basal media OptiMEM-I supplemented with 8% FBS and 1% antibiotics until confluency. A second passage was carried out, and the CECs were seeded over 2X-CVM (according to the results of the ex vivo model) at a density of 2500 cells/mm^2 overnight. The CECs/CVM construct was analyzed using light microscopy to register the cell polygonal morphology and cell adherence.

2.5. Pilot Study of the Transplantation of Engineered Corneal Endothelium in an Animal Model

In a previous study, we demonstrated the in vivo biocompatibility of CVM in young rabbits [34]. We transplanted the CECs/CVM construct into old rabbits to determine its potential to promote corneal endothelium healing. Five 20-month-old male White New Zealand rabbits were used for the corneal damage model, given that they do not restore corneal clarity after damage according to a previous study [35]. Local and general anesthesia were applied using tetracaine (Ponti Ofteno, Laboratorios Sofía, Jalisco, Mexico) and intramuscular 30 mg/Kg ketamine and 5 mg/Kg xylazine, respectively. A paracenteses was created, and an anterior chamber maintainer was introduced for the injection of 1.2% hyaluronic acid to promote the adhesion of the CECs/CVM construct. The Descemet membrane, along with the corneal endothelium, was surgically removed. After 3 to 5 min, a central corneal opacity was developed and the transplantation of the CECs/CVM constructs was carried out in 4 eyes (experimental group). Supplementary Video S2 demonstrates the transplantation of the construct. Three eyes were transplanted using only the collagen membrane (control group). Post-surgical analgesic and antibiotic schemes were conducted using topical dexamethasone (Soldrin, Pisa, Guadalajara, Jalisco) 1 mg/mL, 1 to 2 drops every 8 h for 48h, subcutaneous flunixin (Sanfer, CDMX, Mexico) 1–2 mg/Kg every 12 h for 3 days, and intravenous enrofloxacin (Bioquin, BioZoo, Jalisco, Mexico) 5–10 mg/Kg every 8 h for 7 days. Clinical follow-up and photodocumentation was conducted daily for

90 days. The rabbits were euthanized with a pentobarbital lethal dose. The corneas were excised and analyzed by light microscopy.

The corneal endothelium was detached and analyzed by immunocytochemistry to analyze the presence of ZO-1 and NA/K-ATPase, molecular markers of CECs. Briefly, the corneal endothelium was fixed with cold 4 °C methanol for 24 h and rinsed 3 times with PBS. Unspecific epitopes were blocked with 5% bovine serum albumin (BSA) (Sigma-Aldrich, Co.) at 37 °C for 30 min. Primary antibodies, rabbit polyclonal for ZO-1 (Invitrogen, Waltham, MA, USA) 1:100, and mouse monoclonal anti-alpha 1 Na-K/ATPase (Abcam, Cambridge, MA, USA) 1:100 were used. The secondary antibody Alexa 488 (2:500) (Abcam) was used for ZO-1 primary antibody, and Alexa 568 (1:500) (Abcam) for Na-K/ATPase primary antibody. DAPI (Sigma-Aldrich Co.) was used as a nuclei counterstain. The images were analyzed using ImageJ software [36].

Statistical Analysis

Statistical comparisons of the experimental groups were carried out using paired Student's *t*-tests or analysis of variance (ANOVA). The significance was set at $p < 0.05$. Microsoft Excel (2013; Redmond, WA, USA) and Systat Sigma Plot (V. 11; San Jose, CA, USA) were used for data processing, statistical analysis, and graph generation.

3. Results

3.1. Matryoshka System Assembling and Stabilization

The temperature inside the system remained constant at 40 °C (SD of ± 0.19 °C at the stabilization phase and SD of ± 0.64 °C in the presence of the samples). The RH at the stabilization phase ranged from 47% to 42% (SD ±1.68%), whereas it ranged from 51% to 33% (SD ± 5.52%) during the sample-desiccation period (Figure 2). A volume of 50 mL of the saturated salt solution lasted for ~100 days when the samples were inside the matryoshka system.

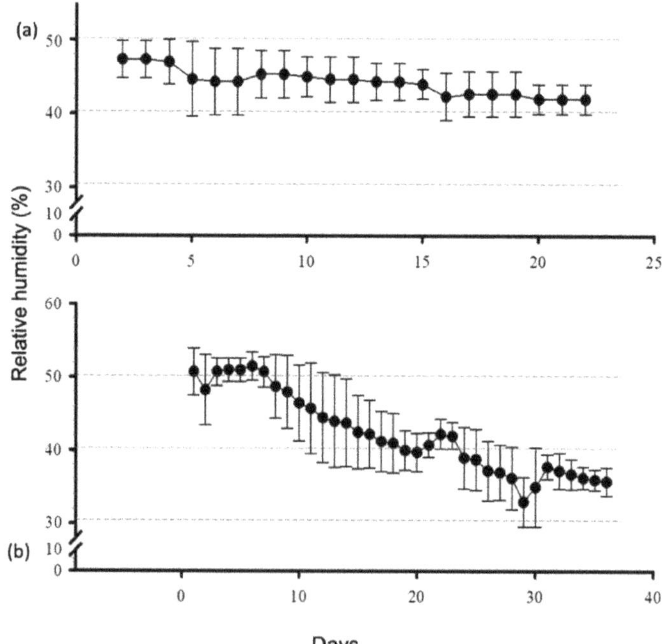

Figure 2. Daily behavior of the relative humidity percentage at the stabilization phase (**a**) and in the presence of 6 mL of collagen gel (**b**).

3.2. Membrane Desiccation and Rehydration

The formation of the membranes occurred when the thickness of the collagen decreased to ~1 mm (Figure 3). Gels at 1X collagen concentration required 10–13 days to reach the membrane state, whereas 2X and 3X required approximately 15 and 20 days, respectively. We also observed that phenol red must be removed during the gel-to-membrane transformation to avoid further interference with transparency. At the end of the 37-day desiccation period, the membranes were completely transparent. Membrane rehydration for ~20 min was necessary to achieve a good retrieval from the cast. A malleable, transparent material was observed in water suspension. The membranes were placed in a water drop on plastic film, the borders were unfolded, and water was removed using a pipette to straighten the membranes, which were left to dry again at room temperature.

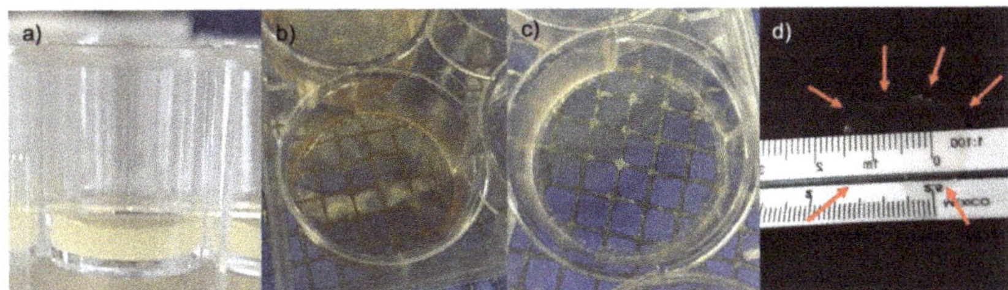

Figure 3. Desiccation process: (**a**) gel before vitrification; (**b**) membrane with phenol red; (**c**) rinsed membrane at day 37; and (**d**) membrane removed from the cast and dried at room temperature.

3.3. Confocal, Optical, and SEM Characterization

A homogeneous surface was observed after 37 days of desiccation in the three membrane types (Figure 4 panel I a). The collagen fibers were observed at day 7 of desiccation with an average diameter of 1.3 µm $\pm$ 0.23 (Figure 4 panel I b). The fibers were not visible at day 37. Confocal microscopy was performed at a thickness of 3.65 µm $\pm$ 0.8 for 1X collagen membranes, 4.8 µm $\pm$ 0.04 for 2X membranes, and 7.2 µm $\pm$ 0.35 for 3X membranes (Figure 4 panel II). the Membrane thickness increased with the collagen concentration and lamina density (Figure 4d–f).

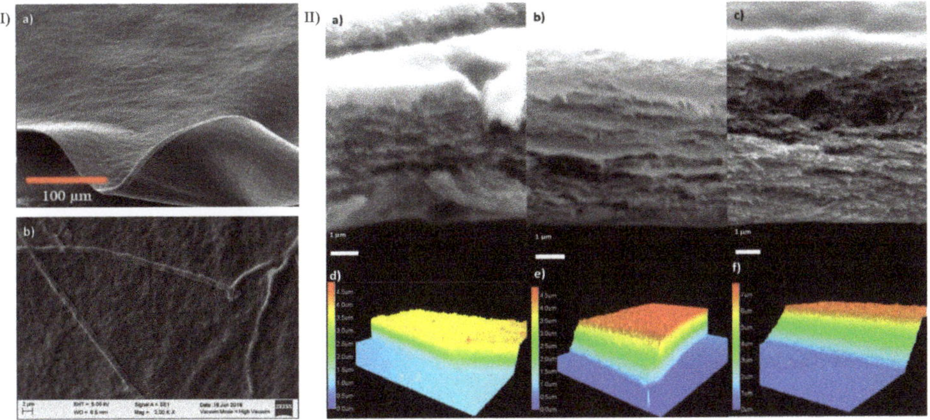

Figure 4. Representative surface and thickness evaluation using material confocal microscopy. Panel (**I**) (**a**) Surface micrograph of a 37-day desiccated 1X membrane. (**b**) Collagen fiber on the surface of a 1X CVM at day 7 of desiccation. Panel (**II**): SEM transversal-view micrograph of a 1X (**a**), 2X (**b**), and 3X (**c**) CVM in wet conditions. (**d**) 1X, (**e**) 2X, and (**f**) 3X CVM showing a thickness of ~3.6, 4.8, and 7.2 µm, respectively.

3.4. Membrane Characterization: Cell Viability, IR Spectra, Transmittance, and X-ray Diffraction

NIH3T3 mouse fibroblasts showed adherence to 1X, 2X, and 3X CVM (Figure 5). A fluorescence analysis indicated that the 10×10^3 cells that were seeded initially proliferated to ~31.7×10^3 cells in wells with no membranes. The populations of cells cultured on 1X, 2X, and 3X CVM increased to ~$35.8 \times 10^3 \pm 5623$, ~$29.6 \times 10^3 \pm 2577$, and $29.5 \times 10^3 \pm 939$ cells, respectively. The cell populations increased threefold within 48 h. One-way ANOVA detected no significant differences between the means of all four samples ($p = 0.323$, n = 3). However, compared with controls, the populations of cells cultured on 1X CVM increased by 12%.

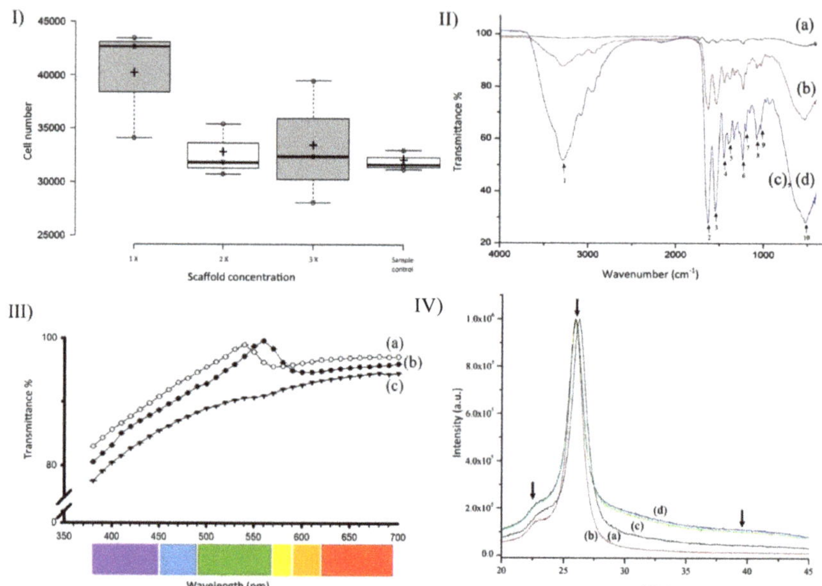

Figure 5. (**I**) **Cell adherence.** NIH3T3 cell count at 48 h when cultured over 1X, 2X, and 3X collagen membranes. Sample control lacks collagen membrane. (**II**) **IR spectra** of pure collagen type 1 (a), 1X collagen membranes (b), 2X collagen membranes (c), and 3X collagen membranes (d). (**III**) **Transmittance.** Percent of transmittance of membranes fabricated using varying collagen volumes: 1X (a), 2X (b), and 3X membranes (c). (**IV**) **X-ray diffraction.** Patterns of pure collagen type 1 (a), 1X (b), 2X (c), and 3X collagen (d) membranes. A 0.6° offset was introduced to detect each pattern clearly. The arrows indicate the 22°, 25.9°, and 39.8° humps for amorphous collagen and the two hydroxyapatite planes.

FTIR studies shows characteristic collagen spectra. The band at 3281 cm^{-1} (Figure 5, II IR spectra, arrow 1), indicating the formation of O–H bonds, is smaller in 3X collagen membranes than in 1X and 2X membranes. Moreover, the fingerprint area corroborated the identity of collagen in the membranes as follows. The Bands at 1660 (Amide I band), 1627, 1635 (β-sheet 2ry structures of Amide I), 1637 (triple helix), and 1679 cm^{-1} (stretching C=O vibrations that are H bonded) were fused into a peak with the least transmittance at 1635 cm^{-1} (Figure 4, IR spectra, arrow 2). The band at 1635 cm^{-1} indicating β-sheet secondary structures was correlated with the laminar structure shown in transversal SEM sections. The band at 1535 cm^{-1} (Figure 4, IR spectra, arrow 3) indicated Amide II, whereas the band at 1240 cm^{-1} (Figure 4, IR spectra, arrow 6) was characteristic of collagen. The contribution of bands at 1446, 1396, and 1202 cm^{-1} is seldom (if at all) reported in the literature (Figure 5, II IR spectra, arrows 4, 5, and 7). The bands at 1084 and 1029 cm^{-1} (Figure 4, IR spectra, arrows 8 and 9) are related to nucleic acids. The band at 1084 cm^{-1}

corresponds to the phosphodiester bonds of the nucleic acid phosphate/sugar backbone. In contrast, the vibration at 1029 cm^{-1} corresponds to collagen and the phosphodiester groups of nucleic acids. Finally, the vibrations at 565 and 527 cm^{-1} (Figure 5, II IR spectra, arrow 10) correspond to phenyl group torsion. All the bands were intensified as the collagen volume increased.

The membranes produced using our method were ~90% transparent in the visible light spectrum (Figure 5, III Transmittance). The average transmittance for 1X membranes was 92.6% $\pm$ 4.91, whereas it was 94% $\pm$ 4.40 for 2X and 89.21% $\pm$ 4.80 for 3X membranes. Lower transmittance values were recorded at violet wavelengths (ranging from 380 to 450 nm): 1X CVM, 80.4%; 2X CVM, 82.98%; and 3X CVM, 77.56%. Moreover, 1X CVM yielded a transmittance peak of 99.6% at 560 nm and 2X CVM had a peak of 99% at 540 nm, both of which are in the green wavelength spectrum. In contrast, 3X CVM exhibited no peak but yielded higher transmittance values (94.7%) at 650 nm. Percent transmittance increased progressively and stabilized at 510 nm (1X) and 590 nm (2X and 3X). Increasing the collagen concentration decreased the transmittance by ~2.5% per added volume, with 1X CVM showing the highest percent transmittance. ANOVA indicated the presence of significant differences ($p \leq 0.001$) between the 3X CVM and the 1X and 2X CVMs.

The XRD patterns of pure collagen type 1 (1X, 2X, and 3X CVM) are shown in Figure 5, IV (X-ray diffraction). All the samples exhibited a typical broad hump around 22°, indicating that the collagen was in an amorphous phase [37,38]. A high-intensity peak was observed at 25.9°, which was related to the hydroxyapatite (HA) 002 plane. A shoulder of the HA 320 plane in the hump was shown at 39.8° compared with datasheet 9-432 from the Joint Committee of Powder Diffraction Standards. All samples showed a similar pattern regardless of the content of collagen.

3.5. Wet Lab with Ex Vivo Model for Surgical Manipulation Test

The 1X CVM did not resist surgical manipulation for folding of introduction through the corneal peripheral incision. It was fragile and fragmented easily. The 2X and 3X CVM resisted surgical manipulation for the folding and introduction into the anterior chamber, and they were also manipulable for unfolding once inside the anterior chamber (Figure 6). Supplementary Video S1 shows the implantation of a 2X membrane into the ex vivo model. Taken together with the cell adherence results, the 2X membranes were selected for further construct assembling and pilot transplantation.

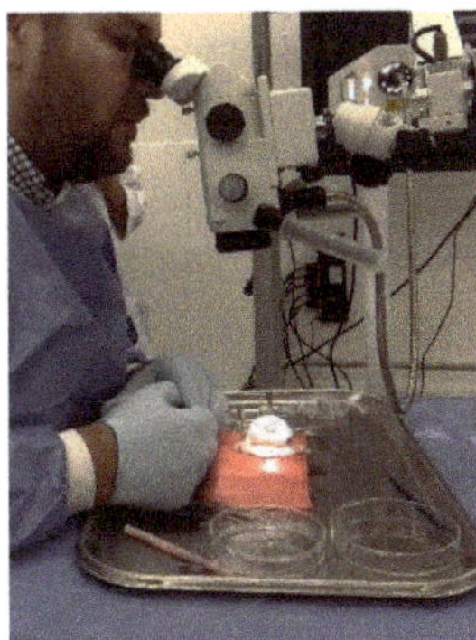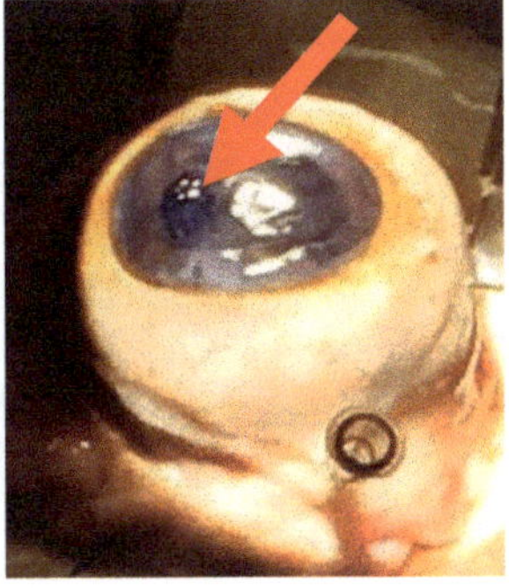

Figure 6. Ex vivo model for surgical manipulation test of collagen membranes. Manipulation of the model under the stereoscope (**left**). Membrane dyed with trypan blue transplanted into the de anterior chamber of the ex vivo model (**right**).

3.6. Engineered Corneal Endothelium

After overnight incubation, there were confluent zones of CEC over the 2X CVM (Figure 7). However, the overall confluence was ~30% in all the membranes. Given that prior analysis demonstrated that the membrane allows cell proliferation, the transplantation of the constructs to the animal model was conducted to evaluate the ability of the CECs to proliferate in vivo over the membrane and to restore corneal clarity.

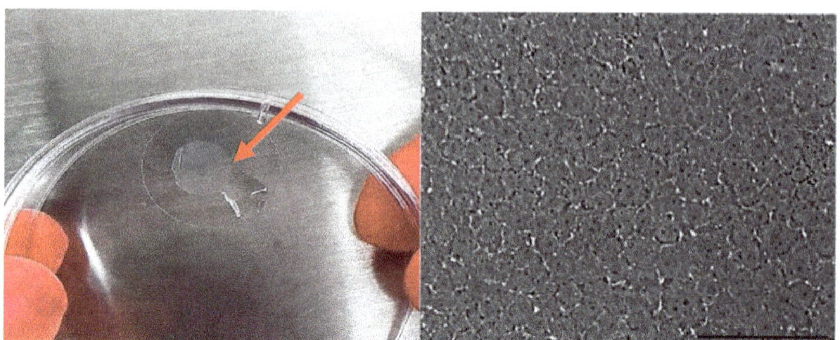

Figure 7. Engineered corneal endothelium (arrow): construct made of CVM and CECs (**left**). Microscopic view of CECs cultured over 2X CVM (**right**). Scale bar = 100 μm.

3.7. Pilot Transplantation

All eyes (7) that underwent surgical removal of the corneal endothelium developed corneal opacity after 5 min. The four eyes transplanted with CECs/CVM constructs (experimental group) showed peripheral corneal clarity and central opacity after 3 weeks, which was maintained consistently for the 90-day follow-up. The three eyes transplanted with CVM (control group) showed full corneal opacity during the 4-week follow-up (Figure 8). No degradation of the CVM was observed.

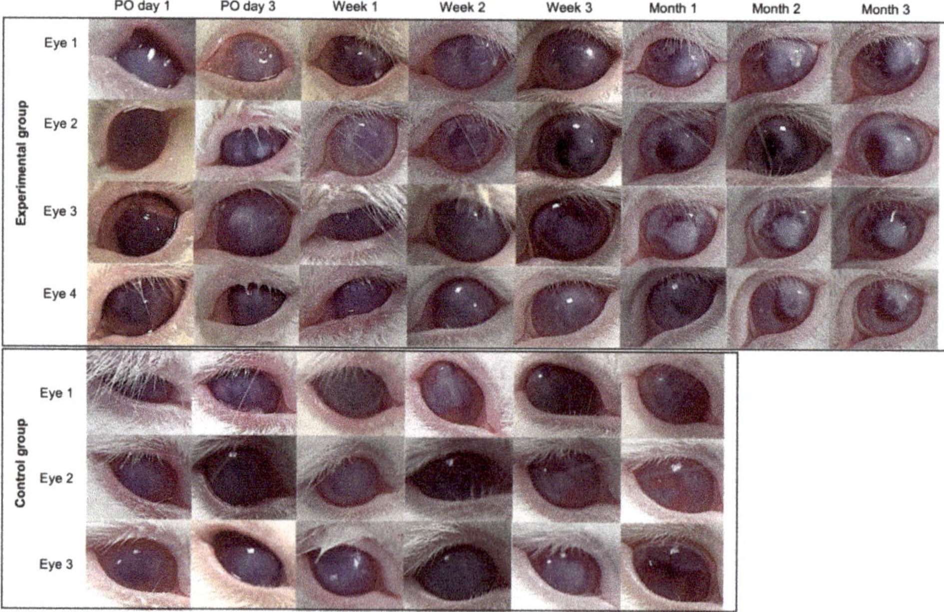

Figure 8. Postoperative follow up of eyes transplanted with CECs/CVM construct and with 2X CVM alone. The eyes with CECs/CVM transplant recovered peripheral transparency, while eyes transplanted with 2X CVM consistently showed edema.

The excised corneas transplanted with construct or CVM showed that the membrane adhered to the stroma. The endothelium of the corneas transplanted with construct showed polygonal cells positive for ZO-1 and Na-K/ATPase by immunocytochemistry analysis throughout the tissue. Light microscopy showed polygonal cells all over the collagen membranes of eyes transplanted with the constructs (Figure 9). No cells were observed in the eyes transplanted with the collagen membranes alone.

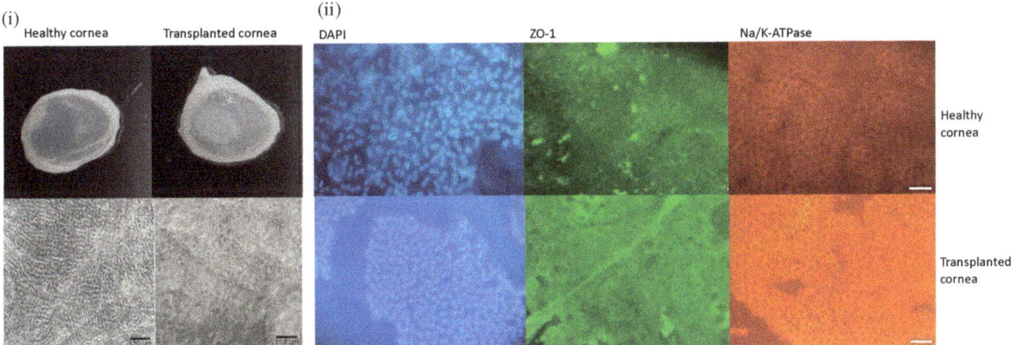

Figure 9. (i) Macroscopic view of representative healthy and transplanted corneas and phase contrast microscopy showing corneal endothelium. Scale bar – 100 μm. (ii) Immunocytochemistry analysis showing the presence of the ZO-1 and Na/k-ATPase markers in the corneal endothelium of a healthy and transplanted cornea. Scale bar = 20 μm.

4. Discussion

Collagen membranes have potential uses in corneal engineering [10,12,19,20,39–42]. The methods reported for producing them include blending and crosslinking, air-drying and freeze drying, and vitrification [18–20,39,40,42–44]. However, multiple fabrication parameters result in a lack of consistency of the resulting material properties, limiting their potential for clinical applications. Here, we present a standardized method to fabricate membranes based on previously reported parameters of collagen type, source, and concentration at 40 °C and 40% RH [18–20]. We increased the desiccation time, as previous reports did not yield functional membranes. We also tested three collagen concentrations, as this has an effect on the mechanical properties and pattern of fiber distribution, which in turn impact cell adhesion and migration [17].

We used a matryoshka desiccation system that provided a stable RH and enabled us to carry out the vitrification process. The RH variation was similar to that reported for commercial humidity chambers. The desiccation time yielded transparent membranes that were easy to remove from the plates.

The thickness of the CVM relied on the time of desiccation more than on the collagen concentration [19]. Overall, our membrane's thickness resembled that of the human corneal endothelium [45] and was 3 to 16 times thinner than that reported previously using collagen [18,20] and other materials such as amniotic membrane, human collagen, silk fibroin, hyaluronic acid, and decellularized extracellular matrix, with a thickness of 20–50 μm [40,46,47]. Our SEM data showed randomly arranged fibrils at the surface of the membranes after short desiccation periods. The fibers observed here were larger by an order of magnitude compared with the sizes of collagen membranes reported previously and resembled the early fibrils reported for collagen gels [19,20,38]. This is attributed to the different order of the neutralization and blending steps used for gel formation [48]. Moreover, the incubation conditions cause an increase in the thickness of fibrils: the lateral fusion of discrete (~4 nm) subunits leads to an increase in fibril diameter, followed by longitudinal growth [40]. Fibril bundling and total unification (greater fibril density and homogeneity) were observed when the drying time was increased and high temperatures were used, leading to the production of the homogeneous and smooth surface observed in 1X, 2X, and 3X CVM. A similar non-fibrillar surface was reported in collagen membranes crosslinked with 1-ethyl-3-(3-dimethyl aminopropyl) carbodiimide (EDC), N-hydroxysuccinimide (NHS), and UV treatment [37,49].

T, RH, and time of desiccation impact CVMs' mechanical strength. Using similar T and RH, Calderon-Colon reported a tensile strength range of 0.69–8.69 MPa. A preliminary analysis of the mechanical behavior of our CVM showed higher strength (9.4 MPa) in the case of the 3X CVM (Supplementary Data) [20,37].

The transmittance of our membranes was higher than that of the human cornea and 10–12% higher than that reported for similar membranes [19,39,41,42,50,51]. The increase in collagen deposition (i.e., membrane thickness) sets a light transmittance threshold and pattern [51]. Therefore, the tailoring of the ultrastructure of these membranes by changing desiccation conditions and collagen concentration allows for the convenient adaptation of their optical transmittance.

FTIR and X-ray diffraction analyses are not often provided in the characterization analysis of this type of membrane. However, they are useful in the demonstration of the crosslinking level, data on the origin of the collagen, and desirable properties regarding biological responses, such as enhancement of mineralization, long-term degradation, and tissue integration [38,48,52].

The three types of CVM allowed for cell adhesion and proliferation [53]. A slightly reduced adhesion ability was observed in the 2X and 3X CVMs, with no significant differences. Contrasting results have been reported in similar membranes: adhesion and proliferation of different corneal cell types (with no data analysis) [18,20,39] and the need for centrifugation and fibrin to enhance cell adhesion [10,40]. Further surgical manipulation in the ex vivo model allowed us to identify the most suitable sample for transplantation purposes. We chose 2X CVMs for transplantation given that they allowed CEC adherence and were easy to surgically manipulate. Previous studies have reported similar results with tests in suturing corneal tissue [39,41]. In addition, this type of wet lab is reported to be a cost-effective technique for the acquisition of surgical abilities in engineered corneal transplantation [54,55].

The transplantation of the CVM/CECs constructs in our pilot study showed that our CVM is suitable for surgical manipulation, adheres to the corneal stroma, and allows CEC proliferation in a model of corneal opacity with high similarities to the human ocular physiology [33]. The transparency was partially restored, even though the cell confluence of the CVM was not full. The effectiveness of corneal endothelium restoration has been proven for collagen membranes fabricated from porcine atelocollagen and bone human collagen [40,54]. Commercially available collagen membranes have shown contrasting results: low adherence to the corneal stroma with low cell viability after transplantation [52] and full recovery of corneal clarity [8]. Similar CVMs have been used only for corneal epithelium healing [37,38].

Although CECs proliferated and covered all of the CVM area, a fibrosis process might take place in the tissue more quickly than the CE can recover [8]. As a pilot study, the transplantation demonstrated for the first time the potential of our CVM for corneal endothelium engineering [55].

5. Conclusions

Here, we present a detailed and reproducible method for producing CVM for corneal engineering. The optimal set of T, RH, and desiccation time conditions in a matryoshka assemblage enabled improvements in transmittance, thickness, fiber size, and promotion of cell adhesion. The CVM produced by this method proved for the first time to have the potential for corneal endothelium healing in a preclinical model. Additionally, we provide a customizable method to produce membranes with potential clinical uses in different ocular sites.

Supplementary Materials: The following supporting information can be downloaded at: https://www.mdpi.com/article/10.3390/polym14173556/s1

Author Contributions: Conceptualization, J.Z. and J.E.V.-G.; data curation, M.D.M.-P., D.L.-G., A.B.-A., G.-I.G.-R., C.E.C.-R., G.F.T.-G., B.H.-S., I.T.C.-R., S.E.G.-Q., M.S.-G., M.Á.H.-D., S.G.-G., M.G.G.-Q. and L.G.V.-V.; formal analysis, M.D.M.-P., W.O.-L., D.L.-G., A.B.-A., G.-I.G.-R., C.E.C.-R., G.F.T.-G., B.H.-S., I.T.C.-R., S.E.G.-Q., M.S.-G., M.Á.H.-D., S.G.-G., M.G.G.-Q. and L.G.V.-V.; funding acquisition, J.E.V.-G.; investigation, M.D.M.-P., J.Z. and J.E.V.-G.; methodology, M.D.M.-P., D.L.-G., A.B.-A., G.-I.G.-R., C.E.C.-R., G.F.T.-G., B.H.-S., I.T.C.-R., S.E.G.-Q., M.S.-G., M.Á.H.-D., S.G.-G., M.G.G.-Q. and L.G.V.-V.; project administration, J.Z.; resources, W.O.-L., J.Z. and J.E.V.-G.; supervision, J.Z. and J.E.V.-G.; validation, M.D.M.-P., W.O.-L., D.L.-G., A.B.-A., G.-I.G.-R., C.E.C.-R., G.F.T.-G., B.H.-S., I.T.C.-R., S.E.G.-Q., M.S.-G., M.Á.H.-D., S.G.-G., M.G.G.-Q. and L.G.V.-V.; visualization, M.D.M.-P.; Writing—original draft, M.D.M.-P. and C.E.C.-R.; writing—review and editing, J.Z. All authors have read and agreed to the published version of the manuscript.

Funding: This research was funded by CONACyT Grant PN6558.

Institutional Review Board Statement: This study was conducted in accordance with the International Guide for the Use and Care of Laboratory Animals and approved by the Institutional Review Board of Instituto Tecnologico y de Estudios Superiores de Monterrey (Protocol code 2019-003, date of approval 20 May 2022 for the Isolation of Corneal Cells; and Protocol code 2019-021, date of approval 06 November 2019 for the Transplantation to animal models).

Informed Consent Statement: Not applicable.

Conflicts of Interest: The authors declare no conflict of interest.

References

1. Gain, P.; Jullienne, R.; He, Z.; Aldossary, M.; Acquart, S.; Cognasse, F.; Thuret, G. Global Survey of Corneal Transplantation and Eye Banking. *JAMA Ophthalmol.* **2016**, *134*, 167–173. [CrossRef] [PubMed]
2. Liu, S.; Wong, Y.L.; Walkden, A. Current Perspectives on Corneal Transplantation. *Clin. Ophthalmol.* **2022**, *16*, 631–646. [CrossRef] [PubMed]
3. Bourne, R.R.A.; Steinmetz, J.D.; Saylan, M.; Mersha, A.M.; Weldemariam, A.H.; Wondmeneh, T.G.; Sreeramareddy, C.T.; Pinheiro, M.; Yaseri, M.; Yu, C.; et al. Causes of Blindness and Vision Impairment in 2020 and Trends over 30 Years, and Prevalence of Avoidable Blindness in Relation to VISION 2020: The Right to Sight: An Analysis for the Global Burden of Disease Study. *Lancet. Glob. Health* **2021**, *9*, e144–e160. [CrossRef]
4. Wang, H.; Zhang, Y.; Li, Z.; Wang, T.; Liu, P. Prevalence and Causes of Corneal Blindness. *Clin. Exp. Ophthalmol.* **2014**, *42*, 249–253. [CrossRef] [PubMed]
5. Zavala, J.; López Jaime, G.R.; Rodríguez Barrientos, C.A.; Valdez-Garcia, J. Corneal Endothelium: Developmental Strategies for Regeneration. *Eye* **2013**, *27*, 579–588. [CrossRef]
6. Ong, H.S.; Ang, M.; Mehta, J. Evolution of Therapies for the Corneal Endothelium: Past, Present and Future Approaches. *Br. J. Ophthalmol.* **2021**, *105*, 454. [CrossRef]
7. Kinoshita, S.; Koizumi, N.; Ueno, M.; Okumura, N.; Imai, K.; Tanaka, H.; Yamamoto, Y.; Nakamura, T.; Inatomi, T.; Bush, J.; et al. Injection of Cultured Cells with a ROCK Inhibitor for Bullous Keratopathy. *N. Engl. J. Med.* **2018**, *378*, 995–1003. [CrossRef]
8. Mimura, T.; Yamagami, S.; Yokoo, S.; Usui, T.; Tanaka, K.; Hattori, S.; Irie, S.; Miyata, K.; Araie, M.; Amano, S. Cultured Human Corneal Endothelial Cell Transplantation with a Collagen Sheet in a Rabbit Model. *Investig. Ophthalmol. Vis. Sci.* **2004**, *45*, 2992–2997. [CrossRef]
9. Levis, H.J.; Peh, G.S.L.; Toh, K.P.; Poh, R.; Shortt, A.J.; Drake, R.A.L.; Mehta, J.S.; Daniels, J.T. Plastic Compressed Collagen as a Novel Carrier for Expanded Human Corneal Endothelial Cells for Transplantation. *PLoS ONE* **2012**, *7*, 11. [CrossRef]
10. Duncan, T.J.; Tanaka, Y.; Shi, D.; Kubota, A.; Quantock, A.J.; Nishida, K. Flow-Manipulated, Crosslinked Collagen Gels for Use as Corneal Equivalents. *Biomaterials* **2010**, *31*, 8996–9005. [CrossRef]
11. Walckling, M.; Waterstradt, R.; Baltrusch, S. Collagen Remodeling Plays a Pivotal Role in Endothelial Corneal Dystrophies. *Investig. Ophthalmol. Vis. Sci.* **2020**, *61*, 1. [CrossRef] [PubMed]
12. Nocera, A.D.; Comín, R.; Salvatierra, N.A.; Cid, M.P. Development of 3D Printed Fibrillar Collagen Scaffold for Tissue Engineering. *Biomed. Microdevices* **2018**, *20*, 26. [CrossRef] [PubMed]
13. Marin, M.M.; Ianchis, R.; Alexa, R.L.; Gifu, I.C.; Kaya, M.G.A.; Savu, D.I.; Popescu, R.C.; Alexandrescu, E.; Ninciuleanu, C.M.; Preda, S.; et al. Development of New Collagen/Clay Composite Biomaterials. *Int. J. Mol. Sci.* **2022**, *23*, 401. [CrossRef]
14. Dems, D.; Rodrigues Da Silva, J.; Hélary, C.; Wien, F.; Marchand, M.; Debons, N.; Muller, L.; Chen, Y.; Schanne-Klein, M.C.; Laberty-Robert, C.; et al. Native Collagen: Electrospinning of Pure, Cross-Linker-Free, Self-Supported Membrane. *ACS Appl. Bio Mater.* **2020**, *3*, 2948–2957. [CrossRef]

15. Antoine, E.E.; Vlachos, P.P.; Rylander, M.N. Tunable Collagen I Hydrogels for Engineered Physiological Tissue Micro-Environments. *PLoS ONE* **2015**, *10*, e0122500. [CrossRef]

16. Takezawa, T.; Ozaki, K.; Nitani, A.; Takabayashi, C.; Shimo-Oka, T. Collagen Vitrigel: A Novel Scaffold That Can Facilitate a Three-Dimensional Culture for Reconstructing Organoids. *Cell Transpl.* **2004**, *13*, 463–473. [CrossRef] [PubMed]

17. Calderón-Colón, X.; Xia, Z.; Breidenich, J.L.; Mulreany, D.G.; Guo, Q.; Uy, O.M.; Tiffany, J.E.; Freund, D.E.; McCally, R.L.; Schein, O.D.; et al. Structure and Properties of Collagen Vitrigel Membranes for Ocular Repair and Regeneration Applications. *Biomaterials* **2012**, *33*, 8286–8295. [CrossRef]

18. Ambrose, W.M.I.; Salahuddin, A.; So, S.; Ng, S.; Márquez, S.P.; Takezawa, T.; Schein, O.; Elisseeff, J. Collagen Vitrigel Membranes for the In Vitro Reconstruction of Separate Corneal Epithelial, Stromal, and Endothelial Cell Layers. *J. Biomed. Mater. Res. B Appl. Biomater.* **2009**, *90*, 818–831. [CrossRef]

19. Ni, M.; Tong, W.H.; Choudhury, D.; Rahim, N.A.A.; Iliescu, C.; Yu, H. Cell Culture on MEMS Platforms: A Review. *Int. J. Mol. Sci.* **2009**, *10*, 5411. [CrossRef]

20. Antoine, E.E.; Vlachos, P.P.; Rylander, M.N. Review of Collagen I Hydrogels for Bioengineered Tissue Microenvironments: Characterization of Mechanics, Structure, and Transport. *Tissue Eng. Part B Rev.* **2014**, *20*, 683. [CrossRef]

21. Hollister, S.J. Scaffold Engineering: A Bridge to Where? *Biofabrication* **2009**, *1*, 012001. [CrossRef] [PubMed]

22. Girlanda, R. Deceased Organ Donation for Transplantation: Challenges and Opportunities. *World J. Transplant.* **2016**, *6*, 451. [CrossRef] [PubMed]

23. PAHO/WHO | Pan American Health Organization. Organ Donation and Transplants. Available online: https://www.paho.org/en/topics/organ-donation-and-transplants (accessed on 25 May 2022).

24. Dong, C.; Lv, Y. Application of Collagen Scaffold in Tissue Engineering: Recent Advances and New Perspectives. *Polymers* **2016**, *8*, 42. [CrossRef]

25. Chen, X.; Zhao, Y.; Li, X.; Xiao, Z.; Yao, Y.; Chu, Y.; Farkas, B.; Romano, I.; Brandi, F.; Dai, J. Functional Multichannel Poly(Propylene Fumarate)-Collagen Scaffold with Collagen-Binding Neurotrophic Factor 3 Promotes Neural Regeneration After Transected Spinal Cord Injury. *Adv. Healthc. Mater.* **2018**, *7*, 14. [CrossRef] [PubMed]

26. Inzana, J.A.; Olvera, D.; Fuller, S.M.; Kelly, J.P.; Graeve, O.A.; Schwarz, E.M.; Kates, S.L.; Awad, H.A. 3D Printing of Composite Calcium Phosphate and Collagen Scaffolds for Bone Regeneration. *Biomaterials* **2014**, *35*, 4026–4034. [CrossRef] [PubMed]

27. Sensini, A.; Gualandi, C.; Zucchelli, A.; Boyle, L.A.; Kao, A.P.; Reilly, G.C.; Tozzi, G.; Cristofolini, L.; Focarete, M.L. Tendon Fascicle-Inspired Nanofibrous Scaffold of Polylactic Acid/Collagen with Enhanced 3D-Structure and Biomechanical Properties. *Sci. Rep.* **2018**, *8*, 17167. [CrossRef]

28. Bertram, U.; Steiner, D.; Poppitz, B.; Dippold, D.; Köhn, K.; Beier, J.P.; Detsch, R.; Boccaccini, A.R.; Schubert, D.W.; Horch, R.E.; et al. Vascular Tissue Engineering: Effects of Integrating Collagen into a PCL Based Nanofiber Material. *Biomed. Res. Int.* **2017**, *2017*, 9616939. [CrossRef]

29. Do Amaral, R.J.F.C.; Zayed, N.M.A.; Pascu, E.I.; Cavanagh, B.; Hobbs, C.; Santarella, F.; Simpson, C.R.; Murphy, C.M.; Sridharan, R.; González-Vázquez, A.; et al. Functionalising Collagen-Based Scaffolds With Platelet-Rich Plasma for Enhanced Skin Wound Healing Potential. *Front. Bioeng. Biotechnol.* **2019**, *7*, 371. [CrossRef]

30. Montalvo-Parra, M.D.; Vidal-Paredes, I.A.; Calzada-Rodríguez, C.E.; Cárdenas-Rodríguez, I.T.; Torres-Guerrero, G.F.; Gómez-Elizondo, D.; López-Martínez, M.; Zavala, J.; Valdez-García, J.E. Experimental Design of a Culture Approach for Corneal Endothelial Cells of New Zealand White Rabbit. *Heliyon* **2020**, *6*, 10. [CrossRef]

31. Rodríguez-Barrientos, C.-A.; Trevino, V.; Zavala, J.; Montalvo-Parra, M.-D.; Guerrero-Ramírez, G.-I.; Aguirre-Gamboa, R.; Valdez-García, J.-E. Arresting Proliferation Improves the Cell Identity of Corneal Endothelial Cells in the New Zealand Rabbit. *Mol. Vis.* **2019**, *25*, 745–755.

32. Valdez-García, J.E.; Mendoza, G.; Zavala, J.; Zavala-Pompa, A.; Brito, G.; Cortés-Ramírez, J.A.; Elisseeff, J. In Vivo Biocompatibility of Chitosan and Collagen–vitrigel Membranes for Corneal Scaffolding: A Comparative Analysis. *Curr. Tissue Eng.* **2015**, *5*, 123–129. [CrossRef]

33. Valdez-Garcia, J.E.; Lozano-Ramirez, J.F.; Zavala, J. Adult White New Zealand Rabbit as Suitable Model for Corneal Endothelial Engineering. *BMC Res. Notes* **2015**, *8*, 28. [CrossRef]

34. Schneider, C.A.; Rasband, W.S.; Eliceiri, K.W. NIH Image to ImageJ: 25 Years of Image Analysis. *Nat. Methods* **2012**, *9*, 671–675. [CrossRef] [PubMed]

35. Tanaka, Y.; Baba, K.; Duncan, T.J.; Kubota, A.; Asahi, T.; Quantock, A.J.; Yamato, M.; Okano, T.; Nishida, K. Transparent, Tough Collagen Laminates Prepared by Oriented Flow Casting, Multi-Cyclic Vitrification and Chemical Cross-Linking. *Biomaterials* **2011**, *32*, 3358–3366. [CrossRef]

36. Kadler, K.E.; Holmes, D.F.; Trotter, J.A.; Chapman, J.A. Collagen Fibril Formation. *Biochem. J.* **1996**, *316 Pt 1*, 1–11. [CrossRef] [PubMed]

37. Long, K.; Liu, Y.; Li, W.; Wang, L.; Liu, S.; Wang, Y.; Wang, Z.; Ren, L. Improving the Mechanical Properties of Collagen-Based Membranes Using Silk Fibroin for Corneal Tissue Engineering. *J. Biomed. Mater. Res. A* **2015**, *103*, 1159–1168. [CrossRef]

38. Chae, J.J.; McIntosh Ambrose, W.; Espinoza, F.A.; Mulreany, D.G.; Ng, S.; Takezawa, T.; Trexler, M.M.; Schein, O.D.; Chuck, R.S.; Elisseeff, J.H. Regeneration of Corneal Epithelium Utilizing a Collagen Vitrigel Membrane in Rabbit Models for Corneal Stromal Wound and Limbal Stem Cell Deficiency. *Acta Ophthalmol.* **2015**, *93*, e57–e66. [CrossRef]

39. Huibertus van Essen, T.; Lin, C.C.; Hussain, A.K.; Maas, S.; Lai, H.J.; Linnartz, H.; van den Berg, T.J.T.P.; Salvatori, D.C.F.; Luyten, G.P.M.; Jager, M.J. A Fish Scale-Derived Collagen Matrix as Artificial Cornea in Rats: Properties and Potential. *Investig. Ophthalmol. Vis. Sci.* **2013**, *54*, 3224–3233. [CrossRef]

40. Vázquez, N.; Chacón, M.; Rodríguez-Barrientos, C.A.; Merayo-Lloves, J.; Naveiras, M.; Baamonde, B.; Alfonso, J.F.; Zambrano-Andazol, I.; Riestra, A.C.; Meana, Á. Human Bone Derived Collagen for the Development of an Artificial Corneal Endothelial Graft. In Vivo Results in a Rabbit Model. *PLoS ONE* **2016**, *11*, e0167578. [CrossRef]

41. Achilli, M.; Mantovani, D. Tailoring Mechanical Properties of Collagen-Based Scaffolds for Vascular Tissue Engineering: The Effects of PH, Temperature and Ionic Strength on Gelation. *Polymers* **2010**, *2*, 664–680. [CrossRef]

42. Offeddu, G.S.; Ashworth, J.C.; Cameron, R.E.; Oyen, M.L. Multi-Scale Mechanical Response of Freeze-Dried Collagen Scaffolds for Tissue Engineering Applications. *J. Mech. Behav. Biomed. Mater.* **2015**, *42*, 19–25. [CrossRef] [PubMed]

43. Zhu, B.; Li, W.; Lewis, R.V.; Segre, C.U.; Wang, R. E-Spun Composite Fibers of Collagen and Dragline Silk Protein: Fiber Mechanics, Biocompatibility, and Application in Stem Cell Differentiation. *Biomacromolecules* **2015**, *16*, 202–213. [CrossRef] [PubMed]

44. Eghrari, A.O.; Riazuddin, S.A.; Gottsch, J.D. Overview of the Cornea: Structure, Function, and Development. *Prog. Mol. Biol. Transl. Sci.* **2015**, *134*, 7–23. [CrossRef]

45. Liu, Y.; Ren, L.; Wang, Y. Crosslinked Collagen-Gelatin-Hyaluronic Acid Biomimetic Film for Cornea Tissue Engineering Applications. *Mater. Sci. Eng. C Mater. Biol. Appl.* **2013**, *33*, 196–201. [CrossRef] [PubMed]

46. Holmes, D.F.; Capaldi, M.J.; Chapman, J.A. Reconstitution of Collagen Fibrils in Vitro; the Assembly Process Depends on the Initiating Procedure. *Int. J. Biol. Macromol.* **1986**, *8*, 161–166. [CrossRef]

47. Christiansen, D.L.; Huang, E.K.; Silver, F.H. Assembly of Type I Collagen: Fusion of Fibril Subunits and the Influence of Fibril Diameter on Mechanical Properties. *Matrix Biol.* **2000**, *19*, 409–420. [CrossRef]

48. Nair, M.; Calahorra, Y.; Kar-Narayan, S.; Best, S.M.; Cameron, R.E. Self-Assembly of Collagen Bundles and Enhanced Piezoelectricity Induced by Chemical Crosslinking†. *Nanoscale* **2019**, *11*, 15120. [CrossRef]

49. Beems, E.M.; van Best, J.A. Light Transmission of the Cornea in Whole Human Eyes. *Exp. Eye Res.* **1990**, *50*, 393–395. [CrossRef]

50. Park, S.N.; Park, J.C.; Kim, H.O.; Song, M.J.; Suh, H. Characterization of Porous Collagen/Hyaluronic Acid Scaffold Modified by 1-Ethyl-3-(3-Dimethylaminopropyl)Carbodiimide Cross-Linking. *Biomaterials* **2002**, *23*, 1205–1212. [CrossRef]

51. Choi, J.S.; Kim, E.Y.; Kim, M.J.; Giegengack, M.; Khan, F.A.; Khang, G.; Soker, S. In Vitro Evaluation of the Interactions between Human Corneal Endothelial Cells and Extracellular Matrix Proteins. *Biomed. Mater.* **2013**, *8*, 014108. [CrossRef]

52. Spinozzi, D.; Miron, A.; Lie, J.T.; Rafat, M.; Lagali, N.; Melles, G.R.J.; Dhubhghaill, S.N.; Dapena, I.; Oellerich, S. In Vitro Evaluation and Transplantation of Human Corneal Endothelial Cells Cultured on Biocompatible Carriers. *Cell Transpl.* **2020**, *29*, 963689720923577. [CrossRef]

53. Srirampur, A.; Mansoori, T. A Simplified Ex Vivo Model to Learn the Correct Orientation of Descemet Membrane Endothelial Graft. *Indian J. Ophthalmol.* **2021**, *69*, 151–152. [CrossRef]

54. Yoshida, J.; Yokoo, S.; Oshikata-Miyazaki, A.; Amano, S.; Takezawa, T.; Yamagami, S. Transplantation of Human Corneal Endothelial Cells Cultured on Bio-Engineered Collagen Vitrigel in a Rabbit Model of Corneal Endothelial Dysfunction. *Curr. Eye Res.* **2017**, *42*, 1420–1425. [CrossRef] [PubMed]

55. Ahearne, M.; Fernández-Pérez, J.; Masterton, S.; Madden, P.W.; Bhattacharjee, P. Designing Scaffolds for Corneal Regeneration. *Adv. Funct. Mater.* **2020**, *30*, 1908996. [CrossRef]

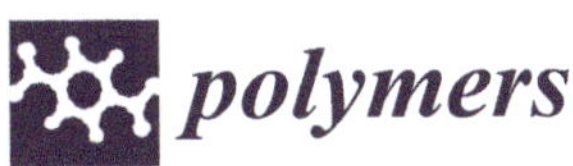 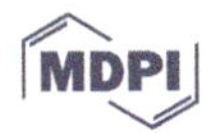

Communication

pH-Dependent Release of Vancomycin from Modularly Assembled Collagen Laminates

Michelle Fiona Kilb [1], **Ulrike Ritz [2]**, **Daniela Nickel [3]** and **Katja Schmitz [1,***]

1   Clemens-Schöpf-Institute of Organic Chemistry and Biochemistry, Technical University of Darmstadt, Alarich-Weiss-Straße 8, 64287 Darmstadt, Germany
2   Department of Orthopaedics and Traumatology, BiomaTiCS, University Medical Center, Johannes Gutenberg University, Langenbeckstraße 1, 55131 Mainz, Germany
3   Berufsakademie Sachsen–Staatliche Studienakademie Glauchau, University of Cooperative Education, Kopernikusstraße 51, 08371 Glauchau, Germany
*   Correspondence: katja.schmitz@tu-darmstadt.de; Tel.: +49-6151-16-21015

Citation: Kilb, M.F.; Ritz, U.; Nickel, D.; Schmitz, K. pH-Dependent Release of Vancomycin from Modularly Assembled Collagen Laminates. *Polymers* **2022**, 14, 5227. https://doi.org/10.3390/polym14235227

Academic Editors: Nunzia Gallo, Marta Madaghiele, Alessandra Quarta and Amilcare Barca

Received: 28 October 2022
Accepted: 29 November 2022
Published: 1 December 2022

Publisher's Note: MDPI stays neutral with regard to jurisdictional claims in published maps and institutional affiliations.

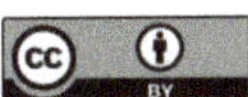

Copyright: © 2022 by the authors. Licensee MDPI, Basel, Switzerland. This article is an open access article distributed under the terms and conditions of the Creative Commons Attribution (CC BY) license (https://creativecommons.org/licenses/by/4.0/).

Abstract: To prevent surgical site infections, antibiotics can be released from carriers made of biomaterials, such as collagen, that support the healing process and are slowly degraded in the body. In our labs we have developed collagen laminates that can be easily assembled and bonded on-site, according to medical needs. As shown previously, the asymmetric assembly leads to different release rates at the major faces of the laminate. Since the pH changes during the wound healing and infection, we further examined the effect of an acidic and alkaline pH, in comparison to pH 7.4 on the release of vancomycin from different collagen samples. For this purpose, we used an additively manufactured sample holder and quantified the release by HPLC. Our results show that the pH value does not have any influence on the total amount of released vancomycin (atelocollagen sponge pH 5.5: 71 ± 2%, pH 7.4: 68 ± 8%, pH 8.5: 74 ± 3%, bilayer laminate pH 5.5: 61 ± 6%, pH 7.4: 69 ± 4% and pH 8.5: 67 ± 3%) but on the time for half-maximal release. At an acidic pH of 5.5, the swelling of the atelocollagen sponge is largely increased, leading to a 2–3 h retarded release, compared to the physiological pH. No changes in swelling were observed at the basic pH and the compound release was 1–2 h delayed. These effects need to be considered when choosing the materials for the laminate assembly.

Keywords: collagen; composite material; controlled release; vancomycin; swelling; pH dependence; rose bengal; crosslinking

1. Introduction

Surgical site infections (SSIs) are a common complication in trauma medicine that prolong recovery times and deteriorate the clinical outcome [1,2]. To prevent such infections, antibiotics can be administered systemically or locally. A local application avoids some side effects resulting from the systemic application. However, high local concentrations of antibiotics can interfere with the healing processes [3], so that a temporally and spatially controlled release is desirable. In particular, the controlled release from biomaterials that can remain inside the body are of interest, as the carrier does not have to be removed [4] and the appropriate drug amount can be directly applied [5].

Biocompatible materials that release drugs with an initial burst, followed by a slow release of smaller amounts to sustain the local concentrations are convenient. Different delivery systems with tunable properties for wound healing drugs have been developed, ranging from microspheres and nanoparticles to injectable hydrogels [4]. Zirak et al. developed porous ceramic microspheres coated with poly(lactic-co glycolic acid) (PLGA) that allow a controlled release of vancomycin and are cell compatible [6]. Microspheres without coating showed an in vitro burst release that can be explained by dominating the bioresorption while coating with the PLGA lead to a dominating effect of diffusion [6]. Somu et al. used self-assembled lysozyme nanoparticles conjugated with curcumin as a drug delivery system, in which the carrier itself is antimicrobially active [7]. Nutan et al. demonstrated that the release of the model drug 5-fluorouracil from the amphiphilic co-network gels and hydrogels, as well as their degradation, can be controlled by gel composition [8] and Singh Chandel et al. developed hydrogels, based on alkylated dextran copolymers that are suitable for the release of the hydrophobic antimycotic griseofulvin and the hydrophilic antibiotic ornidazole alike [9]. Some of these materials even exhibit regenerative properties that can be used for wound healing. Singh Chandel et al. developed water-based injectable hydrogels, based on poly[(2-dimethylamino)ethylmethacrylate]-b-poly(N-isopropyl acrylamide) and poly(ethylene glycol) that enable the proliferation of cells, the platelet adhesion and the adsorption of fibrinogen to support wound healing [10].

Among the biocompatible materials, the biodegradable polymers that lead to the non-toxic degradation products are particularly attractive. Poly(lactic acid) (PLA) and poly(glycolic acid) (PGA) and copolymers thereof (PLGA) belong to the most frequently used polymers in the compound delivery since they are degraded to metabolites that can be further processed in the body [11]. Commonly used biodegradable biomaterials are the polysaccharides hyaluronic acid and chitosan, as well as the protein collagen [12]. Collagen has been used for the sustained release for decades as it is inexpensive, easy to handle and its degradation products are non-toxic and non-immunogenic [12]. Furthermore, it can stimulate bone recovery by promoting the proliferation and differentiation of mesenchymal stem cells [13,14]. In previous studies, we assembled commercially available collagen sheets to collagen laminates by the photochemical crosslinking with rose bengal (RB) and green light (RGX) [15–17]. This convenient and inexpensive method has already been used for different clinical applications [18,19]. Using an additively manufactured sample holder we could show that the direction and time course of the antibiotic release at pH 7.4 can be controlled by the way such laminates are loaded and assembled [16]. The release studies were carried out with the model antibiotic vancomycin which is a frequently used antibiotic to prevent SSIs [1].

Healing wounds are characterized by the dynamic changes of the physiological environment [5]. The pH values observed during healing and infection can differ significantly from the physiological pH. The stages of the physiological cutaneous wound healing are characterized by the pH values ranging from pH 9.0 to 5.5 within 14 days post operation [20]. A decrease of the pH value has been reported for the cultivation of *Staphylococcus aureus* on rat jaw bones [21] and in osteotomy hematoma within 4 h after bone injury, where a pH value of 6.62 $\pm$ 0.33 was measured [22]. As the pH changes during wound healing and infection, we were interested in the effect of the pH on the direction and duration of the vancomycin release from the collagen laminates. For this purpose, we analyzed the release of vancomycin from commercially available sponge-like "Atelocollagen" and a two-layer laminate composed of Atelocollagen and a thin film of "Collagen Solutions" (AC-laminate) under acidic conditions and alkaline conditions. To adhere to the physiologically relevant pH range, a pH of 5.5 was chosen as a commonly used pH value to simulate the acidic conditions at sites of bacterial infection [23,24] and a basic pH of 8.5 was used, which is representative for the initial mean value of wounds after second degree burns [25].

2. Materials and Methods

2.1. Fabrication of the Collagen Samples

Collagen laminates were composed of two different commercially available collagen sheets that had already been characterized before [17]. "Atelocollagen" refers to the first type of collagen, which is an atelocollagen sponge (CLS-01) fabricated from bovine dermal type I collagen from Koken Co., Ltd. (Tokyo, Japan). "Collagen Solutions" describes a non-perforated film of bovine type I collagen from the tendon purchased from Collagen Solutions (London, UK). All buffer components were purchased from Carl Roth GmbH + Co. KG (Karlsruhe, Germany).

The fabrication of the collagen laminates using RGX was performed as described by Kilb et al. [16]. In detail, the collagen sheets with a size of 1 cm $\times$ 1 cm were loaded with

0.01% (*w/v*) RB (Alfa Aesar, Haverhill, MA, USA) in a phosphate buffered saline (PBS, 137 mM sodium chloride, 2.7 mM potassium chloride, 1.5 mM potassium dihydrogen phosphate, 8.1 mM disodium hydrogen phosphate, pH 7.4) in the dark at room temperature (RT). The loading was carried out by swelling the sheets for 2 h in a Petri dish (SARSTEDT, Nümbrecht, Germany) in a total volume that fits the loading capacity. The latter was determined as the weight difference of a dry collagen sample and of the sample after swelling with PBS [17]. For the fabrication of AC-laminates, the loaded Atelocollagen and Collagen Solutions sheets were placed onto each other with 20 µL of 0.01% (*w/v*) RB solution in PBS in-between. The stacked sheets were crosslinked to each other by exposure to green light (λ = 565 nm, M565L3, Thorlabs GmbH, Bergkirchen, Germany) for 10 min.

Single RGX-modified collagen sheets were similarly prepared and directly exposed to green light after loading with 0.01% (*w/v*) RB in PBS.

2.2. Release of Vancomycin

The release of vancomycin was determined, as described by Kilb et al. [16]. All buffer components were purchased from Carl Roth GmbH + Co. KG (Karlsruhe, Germany).

For the release of vancomycin from the crosslinked Atelocollagen and AC-laminates, the collagen samples were prepared, as described in Section 2.1 with the modification that the 0.01% (*w/v*) RB solution in PBS used for the loading of Atelocollagen was supplemented with vancomycin hydrochloride (Carl Roth GmbH + Co. KG, Karlsruhe, Germany), corresponding to an uptake of 1 mg vancomycin. The preparation of the Collagen Solutions sheet for the laminate was performed as described in Section 2.1. The respective collagen sample was placed between both parts of the sample holder that was fabricated from a standard white resin V4 (Formlabs, Somerville, MA, USA) [16]. The sample holder was placed into a cavity of a non-treated 24-well tissue culture plate (VWR International, Radnor, PA, USA) that was filled with 1 mL of PBS, MES buffer (140 mM sodium chloride, 9.6 mM MES, pH 5.5) or Tris buffer (140 mM sodium chloride, 9.6 mM Tris base, pH 8.5). In the upper part of the sample holder, 1 mL of PBS, MES buffer or Tris buffer was added as well. The incubation was performed at 37 °C and the liquid from the upper and lower parts of the sample holder was completely withdrawn at different time points. In the next step, 1 mL of fresh buffer was added to both cavities of the sample holder. The vancomycin content was analyzed by the reversed-phase HPLC, as described by Eckes et al. [17] and Kilb et al. [16]. A detailed description can be found in the Supplementary Materials.

2.3. Determination of the Swelling Degree of Collagen Samples

The swelling degree of the collagen laminates and the single RGX-modified collagen sheets was determined by a method reported previously by Eckes et al. and Braun et al. [15,17]. In brief, the collagen samples were prepared, as described in Section 2.1. The samples were freeze-dried overnight and the dry weight (m_{dry}) of each sample was determined in triplicates. Each collagen sample was transferred to a well of a non-treated, flat bottom 24-well microplate (VWR, Radnor, PA, USA) and incubated for 2 h in 2 mL of the appropriate buffer (PBS pH 7.4, MES pH 5.5 or Tris pH 8.5) at 37 °C. The non-absorbed liquid was removed from the samples by carefully blotting the samples on green paper towels and the wet weight (m_{wet}) of the samples was determined in triplicates. The swelling degree was calculated from the triplicates, according to equation 1. The significance levels of the differences between the experimentally determined mean swelling degrees were analyzed by a Kruskal–Wallis–ANOVA at p = 0.05 with OriginPro 2021b (OriginLab Corporation, Northampton, MA, USA).

$$\text{Swelling degree [\%]} = ((m_{wet} - m_{dry})/m_{dry}) \times 100\% \qquad (1)$$

3. Results

3.1. Release of Vancomycin from the RGX-Modified Atelocollagen

As the pH value changes during the physiological cutaneous wound healing from pH 9.0 to pH 5.5 and the microbial contamination also leads to a moderately acidic environment at the sites of infection [20,23,24], the release of vancomycin from a single RGX-modified sheet of Atelocollagen was examined at pH 5.5 and pH 8.5. The release was compared to the release data at pH 7.4, that has been published previously [16]. As shown in Figure 1a–c, the total amount of released vancomycin after 24 h of incubation did not differ between pH 5.5, pH 7.4 and pH 8.5 (pH 5.5: 71 ± 2%, pH 7.4: 68 ± 8% [16] and pH 8.5: 74 ± 3%). For pH 5.5, the time for the half-maximal release was reached three hours later than at pH 7.4 and for pH 8.5, the time for the half-maximal release was reached one hour later than under the physiological pH (pH 5.5: 41 ± 1% (4 h), pH 7.4: 32 ± 6% (1 h) [16] and pH 8.5: 39 ± 3% (2 h)). At pH 5.5, equal amounts of vancomycin were released into the upper and the lower cavity, similar to the release results at the physiological pH [16]. At pH 8.5, only slightly more vancomycin was detected in the upper cavity after 8 h.

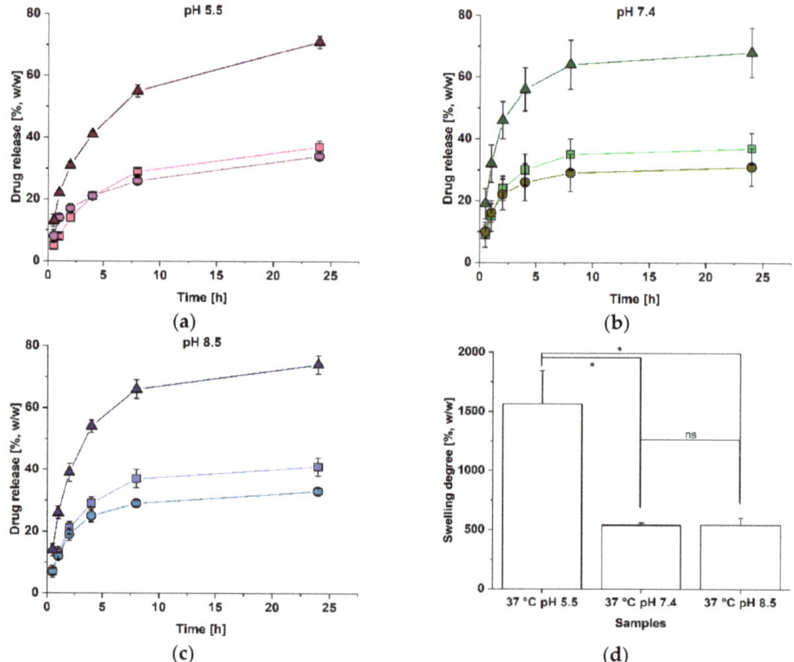

Figure 1. Vancomycin release and swelling properties of the RGX-modified Atelocollagen at different pH values. The release of vancomycin was determined over 24 h in the upper chamber (squares), lower chamber (dots) and in total (triangles). The amount of released vancomycin was calculated according to the amount (1 mg) loaded into the Atelocollagen layer. Error bars represent the standard deviation (n = 3); (**a**) Release at pH 5.5; (**b**) Release at pH 7.4 (data obtained from Kilb et al. [16]); (**c**) Release at pH 8.5; (**d**) Swelling degree after 2 h of incubation at 37 °C at different pH values. A Kruskal–Wallis–ANOVA was used to determine the significance of the difference of the mean swelling degrees at $p \leq 0.05$, indicated by an asterisk. Non-significant differences are indicated by ns.

To analyze whether the elongated times for the half-maximal release at pH 5.5 and pH 8.5 can be explained by the pH-dependent swelling, the swelling degrees of the RGX-modified Atelocollagen at pH 5.5, pH 7.4 and pH 8.5 were examined and compared. The result in Figure 1d shows that the mean swelling degrees differed significantly between pH 7.4 and pH 5.5, as a 65% lower swelling degree was reached at pH 7.4. No significant difference was found between pH 7.4 and pH 8.5 (pH 5.5: 1562 ± 283%, pH 7.4: 539 ± 20% and pH 8.5: 541 ± 64%).

3.2. Release of Vancomycin from the Two-Layer Heterogenous Laminates (AC-Laminates)

To study the release from the asymmetric bilayer-laminates, the AC-laminates were examined that had already shown a collagen-sheet-dependent release of vancomycin at pH 7.4. [16] As higher amounts of vancomycin were released, if antibiotics had been loaded into the Atelocollagen layer, [16] this setup was also chosen to study the release at other pH values. The laminate was positioned in the sample holder with Atelocollagen facing the upper chamber, as previous experiments had shown that this setup facilitated the handling and that an unequal release is independent from the orientation of the laminate in the sample holder [16]. Release studies were performed at pH 5.5 and pH 8.5 and compared to the published release data at pH 7.4 [16]. As shown in Figure 2a–c, the amounts of the totally released vancomycin reached similar amounts after 24 h under all conditions (pH 5.5: 61 ± 6%, pH 7.4: 69 ± 4% [16] and pH 8.5: 67 ± 3%). Compared to the physiological pH, the time for the half-maximal release was reached two hours later at pH 5.5 and pH 8.5 (pH 5.5: 33 ± 3% (4 h), pH 7.4: 38 ± 5% (2 h) [16] and pH 8.5: 45 ± 2% (4 h)). Similar to the findings at pH 7.4 [16], more vancomycin was released at the surface of Collagen Solutions at pH 5.5 and pH 8.5, even though vancomycin was loaded into Atelocollagen.

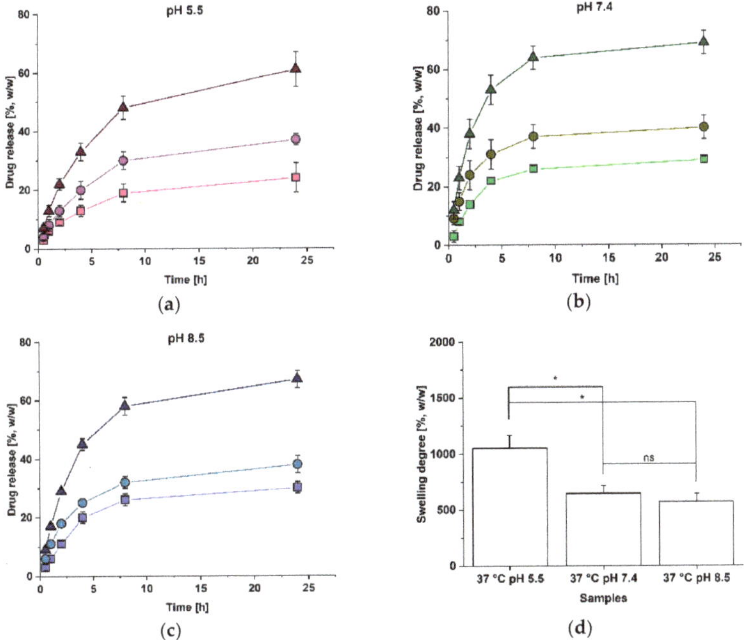

Figure 2. Vancomycin release and the swelling properties of the AC-laminates at different pH values. The release of vancomycin was determined over 24 h in the upper chamber (squares), the lower chamber (dots) and in total (triangles). The amount of the released vancomycin was calculated according to the amount (1 mg) loaded into the Atelocollagen layer. This layer of the AC-laminate was facing the upper chamber of the sample holder. Error bars represent the standard deviation (n = 3); (**a**) Release at pH 5.5; (**b**) Release at pH 7.4 (data obtained from Kilb et al. [16]); (**c**) Release at pH 8.5; (**d**) Swelling degree after 2 h of incubation at 37 °C at different pH values. A Kruskal–Wallis–ANOVA was used to determine the significance of the difference of the mean swelling degrees at $p \leq 0.05$, indicated by an asterisk. Non-significant differences are indicated by ns.

The swelling analysis was performed to analyze whether the elongated times for the half-maximal release at pH 5.5 and pH 8.5 might be explained by the pH-dependent differences in the swelling. As for the single Atelocollagen sheets, the swelling degrees at pH 5.5 and pH 7.4 differed significantly, since the swelling at pH 7.4 was about 39% lower than at pH 5.5. At pH 8.5, the AC-laminate reached a similar swelling degree as at pH 7.4 and the swelling degree significantly differed from pH 5.5 (pH 5.5: 1053 ± 114%, pH 7.4: 643 ± 69% and pH 8.5: 568 ± 73%). As the swelling degree of a single RGX-modified sheet of Atelocollagen was significantly higher than a single sheet of the RGX-modified Collagen Solutions (see Figure S2), the swelling effect of the Collagen Solutions layer in the AC-laminate can be neglected.

4. Discussion

As the pH value changes during the wound healing [20] and might have an influence on the release of antibiotics and other drugs from the collagen materials, the release of vancomycin from the RGX-modified Atelocollagen and a modularly assembled collagen laminate composed of Atelocollagen and Collagen Solutions was examined under acidic and alkaline conditions. The results are summarized in Table 1.

Table 1. Overview of the results. The data indicated by the asterisk refers to a previous publication by Kilb et al. and was added to the table for comparison [16].

Laminate or Single Sheet		Released Vancomycin		Swelling Degree	Release Direction
Name	Property	After 24 h	Half-Max. Release		
A (RGX)	pH 5.5	71 ± 2%	41 ± 1% (4 h)	1562 ± 283%	Equal
A (RGX)	pH 7.4	68 ± 8% *	32 ± 6% (1 h) *	539 ± 20%	Equal *
A (RGX)	pH 8.5	74 ± 3%	39 ± 3% (2 h)	541 ± 64%	Unequal after 8 h and 24 h (upper > lower cavity)
AC	pH 5.5	61 ± 6%	33 ± 3% (4 h)	1053 ± 114%	Unequal (C > A)
AC	pH 7.4	69 ± 4% *	38 ± 5% (2 h) *	643 ± 69%	Unequal (C > A) *
AC	pH 8.5	67 ± 3%	45 ± 2% (4 h)	568 ± 73%	Unequal (C > A)

The total maximum releases were similar under all tested conditions, indicating that the total amounts of released vancomycin from both samples are not influenced by the pH value.

Noticeably, the swelling at pH 5.5 was significantly enhanced, compared to pH 7.4 and pH 8.5. During the swelling, an osmotic pressure gradient across the solvent-polymer interface leads to the uptake of fluid [26]. The resulting swelling is limited by the polymeric network structure [27] and at an equilibrium state, the osmotic force equals the elastic force of the network contracting in the opposite direction and thereby limiting the swelling [28]. The minimum swelling takes place at the isoelectric point [26]. For collagen, the pH-dependent swelling has already been reported in the literature [29]. As the isoelectric point of Atelocollagen lies close to pH 8 [30], the polymer bears a positive net charge at a pH of 5.5, resulting in a repulsion of the electric charges, which permits the biopolymer fibers to stretch out longer so that the swelling degree increases, in contrast to pH 7.4 and pH 8.5 [29]. Since pH 7.4 and pH 8.5 lie near the isoelectric point of Atelocollagen, the net charge is low and the swelling behavior does not differ between pH 7.4 and pH 8.5, as the data confirm.

At a pH of 5.5, the times for the half-maximal release were two to four times longer, compared to pH 7.4. As the swelling degrees for both samples at pH 5.5 were significantly larger than at pH 7.4, the elongated times for the half-maximal release might be explained by the different swelling properties of the samples at an acidic pH value. We have previously assumed that the influx of the buffer during the swelling retards the release of vancomycin [16] so that an increased swelling degree and therefore increased fluid influx leads to elongated times for the half-maximal release. The same effect also accounts for the retarded release at the Atelocollagen side of an AC-laminate that has been observed at pH 7.4 [16]. As expected, at pH 5.5, with increased swelling of Atelocollagen, this effect is more pronounced. For the AC-laminate, the swelling effect of Atelocollagen dominates, compared to the swelling of Collagen Solutions (see Figure S2). The release of equal amounts of vancomycin into both directions for Atelocollagen at pH 5.5 meets the expectations as both release areas can be considered as equal to each other [16].

At a pH of 8.5, the samples of RGX-modified Atelocollagen and the AC-laminate showed an elongated time for the half-maximal release, compared to pH 7.4. These findings cannot be explained by swelling, since the swelling degrees did not differ between pH 8.5 and pH 7.4 for either sample. Compared to pH 5.5, the times for the half-maximal release were either equal or shorter. This might be explained by electrostatic interactions between vancomycin and collagen, since vancomycin is negatively charged under alkaline conditions [31] and might interact with the remaining positively charged areas of the collagen chains. In the literature, strong electrostatic interactions between negatively charged rose bengal and positively charged amino groups of a collagen-like peptide have already been reported [32]. At pH 5.5, vancomycin is positively charged and should be repelled by the positive net charge of the biopolymer. However, this may be counteracted by the stronger effect of swelling.

In light of these findings, Atelocollagen should rather be omitted for antibiotic delivery if signs of an infection are already eminent as this would slow down the antibiotic release. A (collagen) material with a pH between 5 and 6 and a more rigid structure with less swelling propensity would be preferable. Moreover, the retarded release of drugs to support wound or bone healing, while infection lasts and pH is lower, could be desirable, e.g., for the therapeutically used growth factors.

5. Conclusions and Outlook

As the pH value changes during the wound healing as well as infection [20], the release of vancomycin from the RGX-modified atelocollagen sponge and a modularly assembled laminate composed of Atelocollagen and Collagen Solutions were analyzed. The total amount of vancomycin released over 24 h was independent of pH (atelocollagen sponge pH 5.5: 71 ± 2%, pH 7.4: 68 ± 8%, pH 8.5: 74 ± 3%, bilayer laminate pH 5.5: 61 ± 6%, pH 7.4: 69 ± 4% and pH 8.5: 67 ± 3%). At pH 5.5, the swelling of the atelocollagen sponge was increased, leading to an elongated time for half-maximal release, compared to the physiological pH. At pH 8.5, where the swelling was comparable to pH 7.4, the time for half-maximal release was also elongated, compared to pH 7.4, which may be explained by the electrostatic interactions between vancomycin and collagen. The latter might be counteracted by the strong swelling at pH 5.5. Thus, when choosing collagen materials to improve wound healing, the interplay between the swelling of collagen and the electrostatic interactions between collagen and the antibiotic that both depend on their isoelectric point, need to be considered. These effects could be used to withhold the bioactive compounds while infections—that lead to lower pH values—last. In future studies, further commercially available collagen materials should be tested, in terms of the antibiotic release at different pH values. Furthermore, the release of other biomolecules from collagen laminates, e.g., antimicrobial peptides or bone morphogenetic proteins, should be characterized. In order to understand the mechanism of the drug release from collagen laminates and to enable the customized design of collagen laminates for drug delivery, the release of vancomycin from different collagen laminates at different conditions will be modelled mathematically, in future studies.

6. Patents

Schmitz, K.; Ritz, U.; Nickel, D.; Oechsner, M.; Beyrich, T.; Rommens, P.M. "Antimikrobielle, gewebsregenerierende Laminate für die regenerative Medizin" (DE102017126149_A1).

Supplementary Materials: The following supporting information can be downloaded at: https://www.mdpi.com/article/10.3390/polym14235227/s1, Figure S1: Calibration curve of vancomycin from 0 to 1 mg/mL, Figure S2: Comparison of the swelling properties of the RGX-modified Collagen Solutions (grey) and Atelocollagen (white).

Author Contributions: Conceptualization, M.F.K. and K.S.; methodology, M.F.K.; validation, M.F.K.; formal analysis, M.F.K.; investigation, M.F.K.; data curation, M.F.K.; writing—original draft preparation, M.F.K.; writing—review and editing, M.F.K., U.R., D.N. and K.S.; visualization, M.F.K.; supervision, K.S.; project administration, M.F.K. and K.S.; funding acquisition, U.R., D.N. and K.S. All authors have read and agreed to the published version of the manuscript.

Funding: This research was funded by Deutsche Forschungsgemeinschaft, project number 400569699. We acknowledge the support from the Deutsche Forschungsgemeinschaft (DFG-German Research Foundation) and the Open Access Publishing Fund of Technical University of Darmstadt.

Institutional Review Board Statement: Not applicable.

Informed Consent Statement: Not applicable.

Data Availability Statement: The data presented in this study are available upon request from the corresponding author.

Acknowledgments: The published data is part of the doctoral thesis of Michelle Fiona Kilb.

Conflicts of Interest: The authors declare no conflict of interest. The funders had no role in the design of the study; in the collection, analyses, or interpretation of the data; in the writing of the manuscript; or in the decision to publish the results.

References

1. Chiang, H.-Y.; Herwaldt, L.A.; Blevins, A.E.; Cho, E.; Schweizer, M.L. Effectiveness of local vancomycin powder to decrease surgical site infections: A meta-analysis. *Spine J.* **2014**, *14*, 397–407. [CrossRef] [PubMed]
2. Horan, T.C.; Gaynes, R.P.; Martone, W.J.; Jarvis, W.R.; Emori, T.G. CDC definitions of nosocomial surgical site infections, 1992: A modification of CDC definitions of surgical wound infections. *Infect. Control Hosp. Epidemiol.* **1992**, *13*, 606–608. [CrossRef] [PubMed]
3. Braun, J.; Eckes, S.; Rommens, P.M.; Schmitz, K.; Nickel, D.; Ritz, U. Toxic Effect of Vancomycin on Viability and Functionality of Different Cells Involved in Tissue Regeneration. *Antibiotics* **2020**, *9*, 238. [CrossRef] [PubMed]
4. Pachuau, L. Recent developments in novel drug delivery systems for wound healing. *Expert Opin. Drug Deliv.* **2015**, *12*, 1895–1909. [CrossRef]
5. Derakhshandeh, H.; Kashaf, S.S.; Aghabaglou, F.; Ghanavati, I.O.; Tamayol, A. Smart Bandages: The Future of Wound Care. *Trends Biotechnol.* **2018**, *36*, 1259–1274. [CrossRef]
6. Zirak, N.; Maadani, A.M.; Salahinejad, E.; Abbasnezhad, N.; Shirinbayan, M. Fabrication, drug delivery kinetics and cell viability assay of PLGA-coated vancomycin-loaded silicate porous microspheres. *Ceram. Int.* **2022**, *48*, 48–54. [CrossRef]
7. Somu, P.; Paul, S. Surface conjugation of curcumin with self-assembled lysozyme nanoparticle enhanced its bioavailability and therapeutic efficacy in multiple cancer cells. *J. Mol. Liq.* **2021**, *338*, 116623. [CrossRef]
8. Nutan, B.; Chandel, A.K.S.; Bhalani, D.V.; Jewrajka, S.K. Synthesis and tailoring the degradation of multi-responsive amphiphilic conetwork gels and hydrogels of poly(β-amino ester) and poly(amido amine). *Polymer* **2017**, *111*, 265–274. [CrossRef]
9. Chandel, A.K.S.; Nutan, B.; Raval, I.H.; Jewrajka, S.K. Self-Assembly of Partially Alkylated Dextran-graft-poly(2-dimethylamino) ethyl methacrylate Copolymer Facilitating Hydrophobic/Hydrophilic Drug Delivery and Improving Conetwork Hydrogel Properties. *Biomacromolecules* **2018**, *19*, 1142–1153. [CrossRef]
10. Chandel, A.K.S.; Kannan, D.; Nutan, B.; Singh, S.; Jewrajka, S.K. Dually crosslinked injectable hydrogels of poly(ethylene glycol) and poly(2-dimethylamino)ethyl methacrylate-b-poly(N-isopropyl acrylamide) as a wound healing promoter. *J. Mater. Chem. B* **2017**, *5*, 4955–4965. [CrossRef]
11. Hofmann, G.O.; Kluger, P.; Fische, R. Biomechanical evaluation of a bioresorbable PLA dowel for arthroscopic surgery of the shoulder. *Biomaterials* **1997**, *18*, 1441–1445. [CrossRef] [PubMed]
12. Gibbs, D.M.R.; Black, C.R.M.; Dawson, J.I.; Oreffo, R.O.C. A review of hydrogel use in fracture healing and bone regeneration. *J. Tissue Eng. Regen. Med.* **2016**, *10*, 187–198. [CrossRef] [PubMed]
13. Akhir, H.M.; Teoh, P.L. Collagen type I promotes osteogenic differentiation of amniotic membrane-derived mesenchymal stromal cells in basal and induction media. *Biosci. Rep.* **2020**, *40*, BSR20201325. [CrossRef]
14. Somaiah, C.; Kumar, A.; Mawrie, D.; Sharma, A.; Patil, S.D.; Bhattacharyya, J.; Swaminathan, R.; Jaganathan, B.G. Collagen Promotes Higher Adhesion, Survival and Proliferation of Mesenchymal Stem Cells. *PLoS ONE* **2015**, *10*, e0145068. [CrossRef] [PubMed]

15. Braun, J.; Eckes, S.; Kilb, M.F.; Fischer, D.; Eßbach, C.; Rommens, P.M.; Drees, P.; Schmitz, K.; Nickel, D.; Ritz, U. Mechanical characterization of rose bengal and green light crosslinked collagen scaffolds for regenerative medicine. *Regen. Biomater.* **2021**, *8*, rbab059. [CrossRef] [PubMed]
16. Kilb, M.F.; Moos, Y.; Eckes, S.; Braun, J.; Ritz, U.; Nickel, D.; Schmitz, K. An Additively Manufactured Sample Holder to Measure the Controlled Release of Vancomycin from Collagen Laminates. *Biomedicines* **2021**, *9*, 1668. [CrossRef]
17. Eckes, S.; Braun, J.; Wack, J.S.; Ritz, U.; Nickel, D.; Schmitz, K. Rose Bengal Crosslinking to Stabilize Collagen Sheets and Generate Modulated Collagen Laminates. *Int. J. Mol. Sci.* **2020**, *21*, 7408. [CrossRef]
18. Alexander, W. American society of clinical oncology, 2010 annual meeting and rose bengal: From a wool dye to a cancer therapy. *Pharm. Ther.* **2010**, *35*, 469–478.
19. Redmond, R.W.; Kochevar, I.E. Medical Applications of Rose Bengal- and Riboflavin-Photosensitized Protein Crosslinking. *Photochem. Photobiol.* **2019**, *95*, 1097–1115. [CrossRef]
20. Schreml, S.; Meier, R.J.; Wolfbeis, O.S.; Landthaler, M.; Szeimies, R.-M.; Babilas, P. 2D luminescence imaging of pH in vivo. *Proc. Natl. Acad. Sci. USA* **2011**, *108*, 2432–2437. [CrossRef]
21. Junka, A.; Szymczyk, P.; Ziółkowski, G.; Karuga-Kuzniewska, E.; Smutnicka, D.; Bil-Lula, I.; Bartoszewicz, M.; Mahabady, S.; Sedghizadeh, P.P. Bad to the Bone: On In Vitro and Ex Vivo Microbial Biofilm Ability to Directly Destroy Colonized Bone Surfaces without Participation of Host Immunity or Osteoclastogenesis. *PLoS ONE* **2017**, *12*, e0169565. [CrossRef] [PubMed]
22. Berkmann, J.C.; Martin, A.X.H.; Ellinghaus, A.; Schlundt, C.; Schell, H.; Lippens, E.; Duda, G.N.; Tsitsilonis, S.; Schmidt-Bleek, K. Early pH Changes in Musculoskeletal Tissues upon Injury-Aerobic Catabolic Pathway Activity Linked to Inter-Individual Differences in Local pH. *Int. J. Mol. Sci.* **2020**, *21*, 2513. [CrossRef] [PubMed]
23. Cicuéndez, M.; Doadrio, J.C.; Hernández, A.; Portolés, M.T.; Izquierdo-Barba, I.; Vallet-Regí, M. Multifunctional pH sensitive 3D scaffolds for treatment and prevention of bone infection. *Acta Biomater.* **2018**, *65*, 450–461. [CrossRef] [PubMed]
24. Onat, B.; Bütün, V.; Banerjee, S.; Erel-Goktepe, I. Bacterial anti-adhesive and pH-induced antibacterial agent releasing ultra-thin films of zwitterionic copolymer micelles. *Acta Biomater.* **2016**, *40*, 293–309. [CrossRef]
25. Ono, S.; Imai, R.; Ida, Y.; Shibata, D.; Komiya, T.; Matsumura, H. Increased wound pH as an indicator of local wound infection in second degree burns. *Burns* **2015**, *41*, 820–824. [CrossRef]
26. ELDEN, H.R. Rate of swelling of collagen. *Science* **1958**, *128*, 1624–1625. [CrossRef]
27. Flory, P.J.; Rehner, J. Statistical Mechanics of Cross—Linked Polymer Networks II. Swelling. *J. Chem. Phys.* **1943**, *11*, 521–526. [CrossRef]
28. Ganji, F.; Vasheghani-Farahani, S.; Vasheghani-Farahani, E. Theoretical Description of Hydrogel Swelling: A Review. *Iran. Polym. J.* **2010**, 375–398.
29. Zhang, Q.; Liu, L.; Zhou, H.; Wu, X.; Yao, K.D. pH-responsive swelling behavior of collagen complex materials. *Artif. Cells Blood Substit. Immobil. Biotechnol.* **2000**, *28*, 255–262. [CrossRef]
30. Lefter, C.-M.; Maier, S.S.; Maier, V.; Popa, M.; Desbrieres, J. Engineering preliminaries to obtain reproducible mixtures of atelocollagen and polysaccharides. *Mater. Sci. Eng. C Mater. Biol. Appl.* **2013**, *33*, 2323–2331. [CrossRef]
31. Pfeiffer, R.R. Structural features of vancomycin. *Rev. Infect. Dis.* **1981**, *3*, S205–S209. [CrossRef] [PubMed]
32. Alarcon, E.I.; Poblete, H.; Roh, H.; Couture, J.-F.; Comer, J.; Kochevar, I.E. Rose Bengal Binding to Collagen and Tissue Photobonding. *ACS Omega* **2017**, *2*, 6646–6657. [CrossRef] [PubMed]

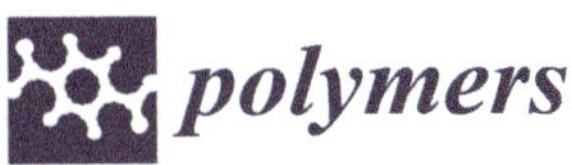

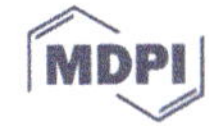

Article

Electrospun Collagen Scaffold Bio-Functionalized with Recombinant ICOS-Fc: An Advanced Approach to Promote Bone Remodelling

Priscila Melo [1,2], Giorgia Montalbano [1], Elena Boggio [3,4], Casimiro Luca Gigliotti [3,4], Chiara Dianzani [5], Umberto Dianzani [4], Chiara Vitale-Brovarone [1] and Sonia Fiorilli [1,*]

[1] Department of Applied Sciences and Technologies, Politecnico di Torino, Corso Duca Degli Abruzzi 24, 10129 Torino, Italy
[2] School of Engineering, Newcastle University, Newcastle Upon Tyne NE1 7RU, UK
[3] NOVAICOS s.r.l.s, Via Amico Canobio 4/6, 28100 Novara, Italy
[4] Department of Health Sciences, Università del Piemonte Orientale, Via Solaroli 17, 28100 Novara, Italy
[5] Department of Drug Science and Technology, Università degli Studi di Torino, Via Pietro Giuria 9, 10125 Torino, Italy
* Correspondence: sonia.fiorilli@polito.it

Citation: Melo, P.; Montalbano, G.; Boggio, E.; Gigliotti, C.L.; Dianzani, C.; Dianzani, U.; Vitale-Brovarone, C.; Fiorilli, S. Electrospun Collagen Scaffold Bio-Functionalized with Recombinant ICOS-Fc: An Advanced Approach to Promote Bone Remodelling. *Polymers* **2022**, *14*, 3780. https://doi.org/10.3390/polym14183780

Academic Editors: Nunzia Gallo, Marta Madaghiele, Alessandra Quarta and Amilcare Barca

Received: 29 July 2022
Accepted: 6 September 2022
Published: 9 September 2022

Publisher's Note: MDPI stays neutral with regard to jurisdictional claims in published maps and institutional affiliations.

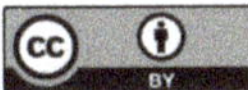

Copyright: © 2022 by the authors. Licensee MDPI, Basel, Switzerland. This article is an open access article distributed under the terms and conditions of the Creative Commons Attribution (CC BY) license (https://creativecommons.org/licenses/by/4.0/).

Abstract: The treatment of osteoporotic fractures is a severe clinical issue, especially in cases where low support is provided, e.g., pelvis. New treatments aim to stimulate bone formation in compromised scenarios by using multifunctional biomaterials combined with biofabrication techniques to produce 3D structures (scaffolds) that can support bone formation. Bone's extracellular matrix (ECM) is mainly composed of type I collagen, making this material highly desirable in bone tissue engineering applications, and its bioactivity can be improved by incorporating specific biomolecules. In this work, type I collagen membranes were produced by electrospinning showing a fibre diameter below 200 nm. An optimized one-step strategy allowed to simultaneously crosslink the electrospun membranes and bind ICOS-Fc, a biomolecule able to reversibly inhibit osteoclast activity. The post-treatment did not alter the ECM-like nanostructure of the meshes and the physicochemical properties of collagen. UV-Vis and TGA analyses confirmed both crosslinking and grafting of ICOS-Fc onto the collagen fibres. The preservation of the biological activity of grafted ICOS-Fc was evidenced by the ability to affect the migratory activity of ICOSL-positive cells. The combination of ICOS-Fc with electrospun collagen represents a promising strategy to design multifunctional devices able to boost bone regeneration in osteoporotic fractures.

Keywords: type I collagen; electrospinning; ICOS-Fc; cell migration; bone remodelling; osteoporosis

1. Introduction

Bone injuries and unsuccessful fracture healing represent one of the most critical clinical burdens nowadays, often caused by pathological conditions, such as osteoporosis (OP), where the dynamic balance between the activity of bone-forming cells, osteoblasts (Ob), and resorptive ones, osteoclasts (Oc), is severely compromised [1,2]. Due to the increase in the ageing population, and the limitations associated with the currently available pharmacological treatments, the total number of people affected by impaired bone healing is predicted to sensibly grow in the coming future [3]. This unmet clinical need results in the urgency of ad hoc medical devices and personalized treatments, not only capable of stimulating bone tissue regeneration in elderly people, but also specifically adapted for the fracture type, the anatomical location, and the specific clinical requirements [4]. To face this challenge, in the field of bone tissue engineering (BTE), the combination of smart biomaterials, biofabrication technologies, and specific biological cues is under investigation to develop multifunctional 3D scaffolds capable of supporting cell proliferation, cell guidance, and to promote the restoration of the tissue's innate natural balance [5]. In this frame, the processing of biopolymers able to induce osteogenesis, such as silk fibroin [6] and collagen [7], is widely reported for manufacturing fibrous scaffolds mimicking both the composition and the architecture of bone extracellular matrix (ECM). To this purpose, electrospinning (ESP) technologies represent one of the most exploited tools to produce biomimetic nanofibrous constructs, with fibre diameters ranging from a few microns to less than 100 nm. Moreover, the resulting electrospun matrices are normally characterized by high flexibility and large exposed surface area which makes them particularly suitable for functionalization with bioactive molecules [8].

Since collagen type I is the main component of bone ECM, its use alone, or in combination with other natural or synthetic polymers, has been widely reported for ESP of scaffolds able to promote cell adhesion and proliferation [6,9–11]. Despite the excellent biocompatibility and bioactivity of collagen, its processing with electrospinning technologies has frequently been associated with partial denaturation of the protein, mainly caused by the solvents and process parameters used. In addition, the poor stability in aqueous media and the fast degradation kinetics of collagen require an adequate chemical crosslinking of the scaffolds often compromises the original nanofibrous structure obtained by electrospinning, as well as the final biocompatibility [12–14].

Although the inclusion of osteoconductive inorganic phases, such as nanohydroxyapatite [15], or mesoporous bioactive glasses (MBGs) [16] has often been chosen as an effective strategy to improve both stability and multifunctionality of collagen-based constructs, an alternative, or complementary method, is represented by the functionalization of the fibrous meshes with specific biological cues. This can be achieved through the encapsulation or the direct covalent binding of bioactive molecules to obtain specific cell stimulation [17]. Thanks to their large exposed and accessible surface area the electrospun matrices, made of either natural or synthetic polymers, have been functionalized with growth factors and stimulatory chemicals (bone morphogenic proteins [18] and osteogenic factors [19]), to induce cell differentiation and stimulate regeneration [20], when the physiological bone remodelling is compromised or delayed (i.e., osteoporosis/osteopenia, autoimmune diseases, and bone tumours).

With this perspective, the recombinant biomolecule ICOS-Fc, patented by the authors (WO/2016/189428), successfully proved to be active on bone resorption by reversibly inhibit osteoclast activity and has consequently emerged as a powerful therapeutic approach to treat osteolytic diseases. Indeed, this recombinant biomolecule is able to bind the surface receptor (ICOSL) expressed by several cell types, including osteoclasts, and, consequently, to substantially affect their activity [17,21,22]. Accordingly, in vitro and in vivo findings have demonstrated that ICOS-Fc prevents differentiation and bone erosive activity of osteoclasts and the development of osteoporosis (OP) in mice [21].

In this work, inspired by the breakthrough of these results, the authors aimed at the design of a bioactive collagen-based device biofunctionalized with ICOS-Fc molecule, potentially intended for the stimulation of physiological bone regeneration in compromised clinical situations. In addition, the peculiar flexibility provided by the electrospun membrane makes the designed device particularly suitable for the treatment of injuries not surgically mendable due to their anatomical location (e.g., pelvic fractures) and the common frailty context of the patient.

In that light, in this study the authors proved the successful development of a *one-step* strategy to simultaneously crosslink and functionalize the electrospun collagen membrane, with the preservation of the biomimetic nanostructure imparted by the electrospinning process and ICOS-Fc biological functionality.

At first, the retention of the collagen structural integrity upon ESP process was assessed, since the protein degradation is a commonly reported issue when organic solvents are involved [13]. Secondly, an EDC/NHS crosslinking strategy has been optimized to promote the simultaneous crosslinking of collagen molecules and the covalent attachment of ICOS-Fc (through the carboxylic groups exposed on Fc residue) to free amine moieties exposed by the protein chains. The following scheme (Figure 1) outlines the multistep procedure applied to obtain crosslinked biofunctionalized collagen membranes.

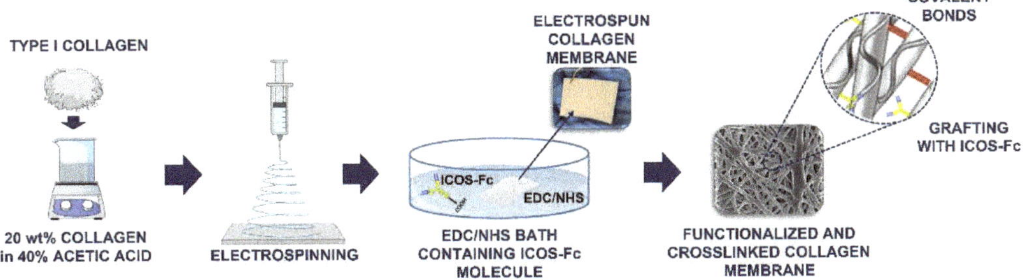

Figure 1. Schematic outline of the electrospun crosslinked collagen membranes functionalized with ICOS-Fc molecules.

Finally, in vitro biological assays aimed at proving the effective binding of ICOS-Fc onto the electrospun membrane and the overall biocompatibility of the final device. Moreover, as proof of retained functionality for the anchored ICOS-Fc, the ability to inhibit the motility of human osteosarcoma cells expressing ICOSL (ICOS-Fc surface receptor) has been investigated, in analogy to the studies performed using the free form of the functional molecule [21].

To the best of the authors' knowledge, this strategy is not yet reported in the literature and, therefore, represents a valuable contribution to the field of BTE.

2. Materials and Methods

2.1. Materials

Type I collagen was extracted from rat tail (N-COL) by NOVAICOS. ICOS-Fc, ICOSL (Sino-Biological, Inc., Beijing, China) and anti-ICOS-Fc antibody (C398.4A) were produced and provided by NOVAICOS. The following materials were purchased from Sigma Aldrich: glacial acetic acid (AA), N-(3-Dimethylaminopropyl)-N'-ethylcarbodiimide hydrochloride (EDC), 1-Hydroxy-2,5-pyrrolidinedione (NHS), pure ethanol (EtOH), and double distilled water (ddH$_2$O).

2.1.1. Collagen Extraction and Preparation of ESP Solution

Type I collagen was extracted from rat tail tendons (N-COL), using a protocol developed in-house, in line with the one reported by Rajan et al. [23]. Briefly, the collagen fibres were dissected into small portions and dried under a biological hood. The dried fibres were weighted and transferred in 0.2% acetic acid (0.2%AA) creating a stock solution. The collagen was stirred at 4 °C for 3 days, and then triturated using a standard hand blender, in an ice bath to prevent overheating. The obtained homogenized mixture was centrifuged at 3500 rpm, at 4 °C for 45 min, then filtered and stored at 4 °C. Prior to use, the collagen was aliquoted in 50 mL tubes, and frozen at −20 °C for 24 h. The samples were then lyophilized with a Lyovapor L-200 freeze-dryer (Büchi, Switzerland) under vacuum (<0.1 mbar) for 72 h. 1 g of N-COL was added to 5 mL of a solution of acetic acid (40% v/v) in ddH$_2$O (40%AA), to achieve a final concentration of N-COL 20% w/w (named hereafter 20N-COL). The solution was left to stir overnight, at room temperature, to ensure full dissolution of the collagen.

2.1.2. Production of ICOS-Fc Recombinant Molecule

Based on the work of Di Niro et al. [24], the extracellular portion of human ICOS was cloned as a fusion protein to the human IgG1 Fc region, generating the ICOS-Fc recombinant protein. After stable transfection, cells were able to express and secrete ICOS-Fc in the culture supernatant as a soluble protein. The human ICOS-Fc was harvested and purified from the supernatant via protein G affinity chromatography.

2.2. Assessment of the Structural Integrity of Extracted Collagen before and after ESP

2.2.1. Circular Dichroism Analysis (CD)

The CD analysis was performed on N-COL as provided and after being dissolved in 40%AA (20N-COL). The 20N-COL sample was prepared as in Section 2.1.1, transferred into a 5 mL Eppendorf, frozen at $-20\ ^{\circ}$C overnight and then lyophilized under vacuum ($<$0.1 mbar) for 24 h. Then, 5 mg of each sample (N-COL and 20N-COL) was added to 5 mL of ddH$_2$O under stirring at room temperature, attaining a concentration of 1 mg/mL. To avoid the signal saturation (absorbance higher than 1.0), a calibration step was performed for each sample where collagen was diluted up to a concentration of 0.1 mg/mL. The CD analysis was performed on diluted samples (0.1 mg/mL), using a JASCO J-815 Circular Dichroism Spectropolarimeter, equipped with a Xe arc lamp, to record data in the far-UV spectral range. A total number of 3 scans were recorded for each sample at 50 nm/sec scanning rate and at 20 $^{\circ}$C to obtain the final averaged CD spectra, and the data analysed with the Spectra Analysis software, purchased by JASCO. All the tests were performed using a quartz circular cuvette with a path length of 0.1 mm in the 180–260 nm wavelength range. Correction of spectra were performed considering the correspondent solvent medium as baseline (ddH$_2$O).

2.2.2. Sodium Dodecyl Sulphate–Polyacrylamide Gel Electrophoresis (SDS-PAGE)

The SDS-PAGE analysis was performed on lyophilized samples of N-COL and 20N-COL (prepared as in Section 2.1.1). The solutions for SDS-PAGE were prepared through the in-house standard procedure for this assay. Briefly, the control samples, N-COL as extracted (2 mg/mL) and type I collagen from rat tail, Roche (the commercial reference sample, 3 mg/mL), were dissolved in 0.2%AA to ensure preservation of N-COL whilst attaining full dissolution. Solutions reached a final concentration of 2 mg/mL, deemed ideal to obtain a reliable result from the SDS-PAGE analysis. The dissolution of 20N-COL samples proved to be difficult, meaning the aforementioned procedure had to be adapted and optimized. In details, 100 mg of lyophilized 20N-COL were added to 50 mL of 0.2%AA and the solution left stirring overnight, at 4 $^{\circ}$C. The resultant solution was homogenized with a hand blender and left stirring for 2 additional days, at 4 $^{\circ}$C. To ensure the final solution possessed the amount of protein needed for the analysis, a Bicinchoninic Acid Protein Assay (BCA) was performed. Since the BCA assay demands a fully homogeneous solution, free of undissolved material and possible agglomerates, the solution was re-blended and filtered through a 100 μm strainer. At this stage, the resulting sample was quantified using BCA, revealing a final concentration of 1.7 mg/mL.

For the SDS-PAGE analysis, 2 and 4 μg of each preparation (N-COL, 20N-COL, and Roche collagen) were resuspended into a loading buffer, heated for 5 min at 95 $^{\circ}$C, and then loaded into the gel wells to perform the run. To visualize the bands, a Coomassie gel staining solution was prepared by mixing 0.1 Coomassie brilliant blue R-250 (Sigma-Aldrich, Burlington, MA, USA) in a solution of 45% methanol and 10%AA. This solution was added to the protein bands for 30 min, and then replaced by a Coomassie gel de-staining solution consisting in 10%AA and 10% methanol. The de-staining solution was left to develop overnight, until the bands were clearly detectable. Pre-stained protein size markers (Thermo-Fisher, Waltham, MA, USA) were used to estimate the apparent size of the collagen subunits.

2.3. Processing and Functionalization of the Electrospun Collagen Membranes

2.3.1. ESP of 20N-COL

The 20N-COL solution was prepared using the method described previously in Section 2.1.1, then transferred to a 10 mL syringe and electrospun for 3 h onto a plate collector covered by aluminium foil, at flow rate of 300 μL/h, a voltage of 22 kV and a working distance of 12 cm. The obtained membranes (20N-COL/ESP) were left to air dry overnight, at room temperature.

2.3.2. Crosslinking and Functionalization of the Electrospun Membranes

The electrospun collagen-based scaffolds were cut into 1×1 cm squares (n = 3), placed in 12-well plates, and incubated at 4 °C overnight. Then, 10 mM of EDC and 5 mM of NHS were added to pure EtOH (previously incubated at 4 °C) and stirred for 5 min. Then, 2 mL of the resultant crosslinking solution was added to each well, followed by the addition of ICOS-Fc at different concentrations: 50, 75, and 100 µg/mL. Samples were incubated for 8 h, at 4 °C then quickly washed 3 times with EtOH and frozen at −20 °C, overnight. Finally, the meshes were lyophilized under vacuum (<0.1 mbar) for 24 h. Crosslinked and functionalized samples will be referred as 20N-COL/ICOS-Fc. Unfunctionalized crosslinked samples were also prepared as reference and will be addressed as 20N-COL/ESP+CL.

2.4. Assessment of ICOS-Fc Binding and Functionality

ELISA-like assays were performed to measure the amount of residual functional ICOS-Fc in the supernatants recovered after the crosslinking/biofunctionalization reaction (i.e., the unbound ICOS-Fc), allowing to assess indirectly the successful grafting of the biomolecule and the retention of its functionality (as the ability to bind ICOSL). The molecule was added in triplicate at different concentrations, 50, 75, and 100 µg/mL, and samples incubated for 8 h, at 4 °C. The electrospun membranes were then removed and the related supernatant was collected and centrifuged at 13 000 rpm for 15 min to allow the precipitation of residual ICOS-Fc (i.e., the unbound ICOS-Fc). The EtOH was substituted with ddH$_2$O for performing the ELISA-like assays.

2.4.1. ELISA-like Assay with ICOSL as Capture

ELISA plates were coated by overnight incubation at 4 °C with 1 µg/mL of human ICOSL-His (Sino-Biological, Beijing, China) in Phosphate Buffer Solution (PBS) 1X, pH 7.4. After washing 5 times with 0.05% Tween-20 in PBS 1X (pH 7.4), non-specific binding was blocked by incubating in the same solution at room temperature for 1 h. Subsequently, samples were added in duplicate and incubated at 37 °C for 2 h and then washed 5 times with horseradish peroxidase (HRP)-conjugated SV5 (Thermo-Fisher) and incubated for 1 h, at room temperature. TMB (tetra-methyl-benzidine) (Merck Life Science, Darmstadt, Germany) (5 times) was added to each well and the reaction stopped by adding H$_2$SO$_4$ 2N (Merck Life Science). A plate reader spectrophotometer at 450 nm (Packard SpectraCount, Meriden, CT, USA) was used to analyse all the samples and the results were recorded as optical density (OD).

2.4.2. ELISA-like Assay with Anti-ICOS (Clone C398.A) as Capture

The ELISA assay was also performed with anti-ICOS (clone C398.4A) as capture, which can bind and detect ICOS-Fc also if non-functional, allowing to evidence any potential denaturation occurred during the binding step. To this purpose, ELISA plates were coated with 1 µg/mL of mAb anti-ICOS clone C398.4A, by overnight incubation in PBS 1X, pH 7.4, at 4 °C. The washing and reading steps used were described in the previous Section 2.4.1.

2.5. Physicochemical Characterization of Electrospun Membranes

The morphology of the 20N-COL/ESP and 20NCOL/ESP+CL was analysed with Field Emission Scanning Electron Microscopy (FESEM) using a ZEISS MERLIN instrument (Carl Zeiss AG, Oberkochen, Germany). The analysis was performed on 3 samples, each one mounted onto an aluminium stub and coated with a 7 nm-thin platinum layer. The fibre and pore diameter were estimated by collecting 5 measurements from each image. Since pores were irregularly shaped, the largest distance between pore edges was considered. The final value was obtained using OriginPro2016 and presented as mean ± standard deviation (SD).

The Attenuated Total Reflection-Fourier Transform Infra-Red spectroscopy (ATR-FTIR) analysis was performed on 5 different of samples, corresponding to different phases of the process: (1) collagen as supplied (N-COL); (2) 20N-COL solution lyophilized (20N-COL); (3) electrospun membranes (20N-COL/ESP); (4) crosslinked without ICOS-Fc

(20N-COL/ESP+CL); and (5) crosslinked membranes functionalized with ICOS-Fc (20N-COL/ICOS-Fc). FTIR spectra were obtained in the 4000–650 cm^{-1} range, and collected with a Bruker Equinox 55 spectrometer, equipped with MCT cryodetector, at a spectral resolution of 4 cm^{-1} and accumulation of 32 scans, by using the attenuated total reflection (ATR) mode.

The Thermogravimetric Analysis (TGA) analysis was performed with a TGA/SDTA851 (Mettler Toledo, USA) using a heating rate of 10 °C/min, within the temperature range of 23–700 °C, in air. The data were collected with STARe software and treated on OriginPro2016. The measurement of residual free amines was conducted for 20N-COL/ESP, 20N-COL/ESP+CL and 20N-COL/ICOS-Fc (50 µg/mL).

2.6. Measurement of Free Amine Residues with 2,4,6-Trinitrobenzene Sulfonic Acid Assay (TNBS)

Since both ICOS-Fc binding and crosslinking involves the reaction of collagen amine groups, TNBS—a UV-absorbing chromophore—was used to show the changes in the free primary amino groups of collagen, before and after crosslinking and functionalization [25]. The measurement of residual free amines was conducted for 20N-COL/ESP, 20N-COL/ESP+CL and 20N-COL/ICOS-Fc (50 µg/mL). For the analysis, 1 mL of 4% (w/v) sodium bicarbonate (NaHCO$_3$, pH 8.5) was added to each sample (11 mg), followed by 1 mL of 0.5% (w/v) TNBS. The samples were placed in a dynamic shaker at 40 °C and incubated for 3 h under mild agitation. Subsequently, 3 mL of 6 M HCl were added to each sample, followed by 1 h incubation in the dynamic shaker, under mild agitation at 90 °C. Prior to the analysis, the dissolved samples were diluted in ddH$_2$O (1:20), then transferred into a 5 mL cuvette for the spectrophotometry analysis. Samples were measured in triplicate and a buffer made of TNBS-only solution was used as control. The absorbance was measured in double mode with a UV-Vis-NIR spectrophotometer (Carry 5000 1.12, Agilent, Santa Clara, CA, USA) and the data obtained through the instrument's software (Scan 3.0). The peak of interest was identified as 346 nm [26,27] on the data that was later processed in OriginPro2016.

2.7. Biological Assessment of ICOS-Fc Functionalized Collagen Scaffolds

The electrospun membranes for the following biological assays were prepared by ESP the 20N-COL solution onto round cover slips (15 mm diameter) for 15 min, using the process parameters described in Section 2.3.1. After ESP, samples were frozen at −20 °C and lyophilized. Subsequently, they were placed in a 24-well plate, immersed in 1 mL of crosslinking solution containing ICOS-Fc at a concentration of 50 µg/mL, then incubated for 1 h at 4 °C. The incubation time was established according to the indications provided by Ribeiro et al. which suggest it should match the amount of collagen present in each membrane [15]. Prior to cell seeding, samples were gradually rehydrated in EtOH/ddH$_2$O at the following concentration (v/v): 100% EtOH, 90%, 70%, 60%, 50%, 40%, 30%, 15%, 10%, and 100% ddH$_2$O.

2.7.1. Cells for Biocompatibility and Migration Assays

Human osteosarcoma cell line U2OS (ICOSL positive) was obtained from the American Type Culture Collection (Manassas, VA, USA) and grown as a monolayer in DMEM (Gibco, Life Technologies, Carlsbad, CA, USA) while human osteosarcoma cell line HOS (ICOSL negative) was obtained from Sigma-Aldrich and cultured in MEM (Gibco) + 1% non-essential amino acids (Sigma-Aldrich). All media were supplemented with 10% Fetal Bovine Serum (FBS), 100 U/mL penicillin, and 100 µg/mL streptomycin (Gibco), and cells maintained at 37 °C in a 5% CO$_2$ humidified atmosphere.

2.7.2. Cytocompatibility of 20N-COL and 20N-COL/ICOS-Fc Membranes

Sterilisation of 20N-COL/ESP+CL and 20N-COL/ICOS-Fc samples were performed under UV-light for 30 min. Before seeding, samples were incubated in DMEM for 30 min. U2OS cells were then seeded onto the samples, plating 30×10^3, 7.5×10^3, and 1.5×10^3 cells in 1 mL/well for 3–5–7 days, respectively, in complete DMEM medium (Gibco) and the samples incubated at 37 °C, in a 5% CO_2 humidified atmosphere. At each time point, viable cells were evaluated by adding XTT [2,3-Bis(2-methoxy-4-nitro-5-sulfophenyl)-2H-tetrazolium-5-carbox-anilide)] reagent (Trevigen, Helgerman CT, Gaithersburg, MD, USA) for 3 h at 37 °C. A plate reader spectrophotometer at 490 nm (Packard SpectraCount) was used to read all samples and cell viability was calculated according to the following formula:

$$\text{cell viability} = ((\text{absorbance of sample})/(\text{absorbance of control (cells alone)})) \times 100$$

2.7.3. Assessment of Cell Motility

Prior to cell seeding, samples were gradually rehydrated in EtOH/ddH$_2$O using protocol described in Section 2.6. The cells were seeded on the collagen membranes for 30 min at 37 ° C, then, detached, counted, and used for the migration assay (2×10^3 cells in 50 µL/well). To perform the Boyden chamber migration assay (BD Biosciences, Milan, Italy) cells were plated onto the apical side of 50 µg/mL Matrigel-coated filters (8.2 mm diameter and 0.5 µm pore size; Neuro Probe, Inc.; BIOMAP snc, Milan, Italy) with the addition of serum-free medium. In parallel, medium containing 20% FBS was placed in the basolateral chamber as a chemoattractant and after 6 h, cells on the apical side were wiped off with Q-tips. Methanol and crystal-violet were subsequently used to stain the cells present at the bottom of the filter and cell count was carried out with an inverted microscope. The data have been expressed as percentages and reported as mean $\pm$ SEM (n = 5) of the percentage of migration versus control migration. Five independent experiments were performed.

3. Results

3.1. Physicochemical Characterization of Collagen and Electrospun Membranes

In order to promote the successful creation of nanofibrous electrospun membranes, a highly concentrated collagen-containing solution (20% *w/v*) was prepared by dissolving lyophilized type I rat tail collagen (N-COL), in an aqueous solution of 40% acetic acid (40%AA). The first essential goal of this study was the assessment of the supramolecular structure of collagen to confirm its preservation upon extraction and dissolution in the acidic medium. This was investigated by performing SDS-PAGE analysis and CD on the collagen, before and after its dissolution.

The results from SDS-PAGE analysis performed on all collagen samples (N-COL, 20N-COL, and type I rat tail collagen from Roche) showed the presence of both α bands, as well as β and γ bands, meaning the chains were not degraded (Figure 2A) [28,29]. This confirms the identity and purity of extracted collagen in the case of N-COL, and its preservation after contact with an acidic solution (20N-COL). Moreover, the N-COL and 20N-COL samples presented the same bands of collagen produced by Roche (chosen as commercial benchmark), confirming their high quality. Both collagen samples, as extracted (N-COL) and after dissolution in acidic medium (20-NCOL), revealed very similar CD patterns (Figure 2B), characteristic of the collagen triple-helix conformation, with a weak positive band at 220 nm, and strong negative band at 198 nm [30]. Overall, this preliminary assessment demonstrated that the dissolution in 40%AA did not significantly alter the structural integrity of N-COL.

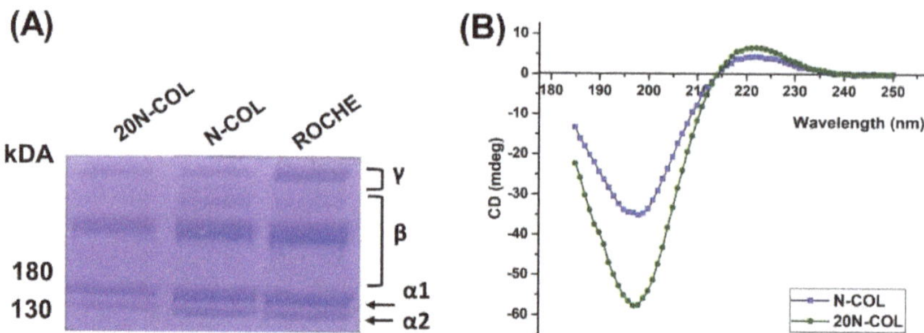

Figure 2. Structural integrity analysis of collagen using (**A**) SDS−PAGE and (**B**) CD.

The obtained acidic solution of 20N-COL was subsequently used to produce nanofibrous scaffolds. To this aim, the solution was electrospun setting the applied voltage and the material flow at 22 kV and 300 µL/h, respectively, using a plate collector and keeping constant conditions of temperature and humidity. The size and morphology of the electrospun collagen fibres was assessed with FESEM (Figure 3A) revealing a homogeneous diameter, approximately 120 nm, and a cylindrical shape. The electrospun collagen membranes were subsequently chemically crosslinked using EDC/NHS in order to avoid premature dissolution in aqueous-based media and improve their mechanical strength. As visible in Figure 3B, the fibre morphology did not change significantly after crosslinking. However, the diameter increased to approximately 140 nm as a result of fibre merging, similarly to what is reported after crosslinking of collagen and other natural polymer-based electrospun structures [31,32]. The average pore diameter, after crosslinking, was reported as 1 µm $\pm$ 0.31, thus obtaining a porosity capable of promoting nutrient exchange and cell migration [33].

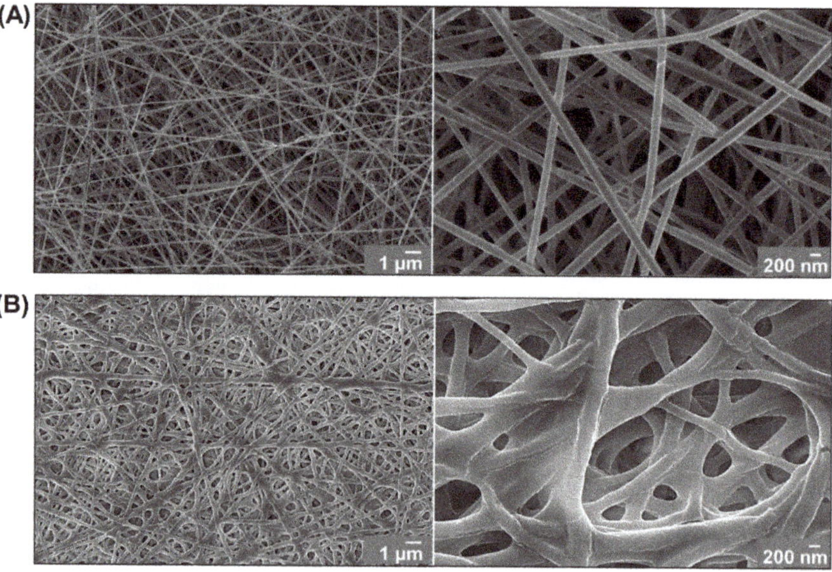

Figure 3. FESEM micrographs of electrospun collagen membranes before (**A**) and after crosslinking with EDC/NHS (**B**).

3.2. Efficiency of the Crosslinking-Biofunctionalization Strategy

To assess the ICOS-Fc grafting onto collagen fibres, ELISA-like assays were performed on the EDC/NHS solution recovered after incubation with the electrospun membranes. The assays aimed to indirectly prove ICOS-Fc grating onto collagen fibres by analysing the presence of the molecule in the supernatant (unbound ICOS-Fc), which was expected to significantly decrease due to its binding to collagen amines. A subtractive calculation method allowed an estimation of the grafted amount based on the obtained concentrations.

ELISA-like assays have been conducted by using recombinant ICOSL or anti-ICOS mAb C398.4A to capture ICOS-Fc, since the first can detect ICOS-Fc only in its functional form. At variance, anti-ICOS mAb C398.4A can detect the presence of ICOS-Fc in the supernatant regardless of the potential alterations to its functionality, which could possibly be caused by the reagents used in the crosslinking reaction. The tests performed on samples incubated for 8 h, containing different concentrations of ICOS-Fc for the functionalization step (Figure 4), revealed concentrations of ICOS-Fc between 3 and 0.002 µg/mL, using both capture tests, implying successful binding of ICOS-Fc to the collagen fibres and no significant damage of the molecule due to the crosslinking medium.

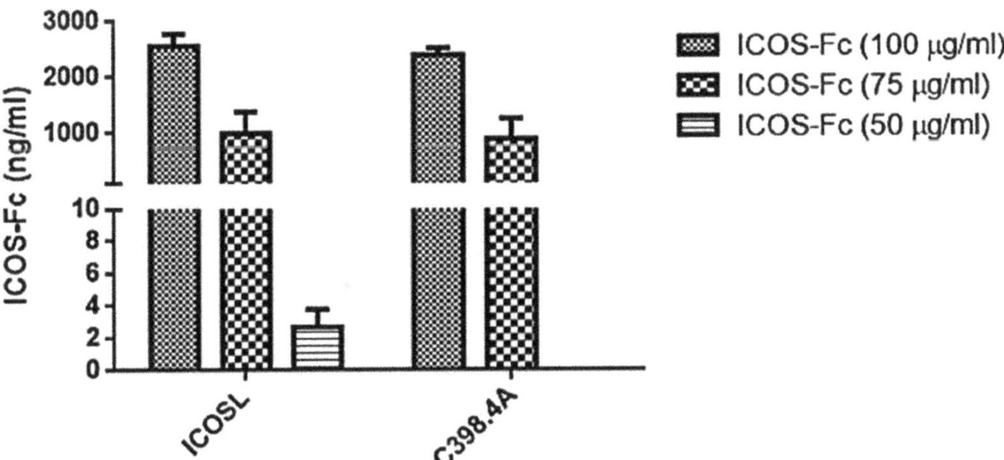

Figure 4. Values of ICOS-Fc obtained from ELISA assay using ICOS-L and C398.4A as capture molecules. Analysis of supernatants obtained from 20N-COL membranes incubated for 8 h in the presence of different concentrations of ICOS-Fc (100–75–50 µg/mL). The graph shows the concentration (ng/mL) as mean and standard error obtained from three independent experiments.

The obtained results show that the three investigated ICOS-Fc concentrations, added during the crosslinking step, allowed for the functionalization of the collagen membranes. The highest concentration of functional ICOS-Fc detected in the supernatant was ca 2.5 µg/mL, measured when the membranes were soaked into a 100 µg/mL solution, meaning that ca 97.5% of the molecules attached to the membrane. Attachment of the molecule was successfully achieved even for lower concentrations like 50 µg/mL where the amount of ICOS-Fc in the supernatant was neglectable for both capture methods, meaning almost 100% binding. This was the concentration used for the remaining tests presented in this section.

Overall, the ELISA assays suggest that ICOS-Fc molecules were effectively bound to the collagen structures with a full retention of the functionality upon the incubation.

As a confirmation of the effective protein crosslinking, and demonstration of the functionalization with ICOS-Fc, an assay to quantify free amines was performed on electrospun collagen prior to crosslinking (20N-COL/ESP), after crosslinking without ICOS-Fc (20N-COL/ESP+CL) and with ICOS-Fc (20N-COL/ICOS-Fc) (Figure 5).

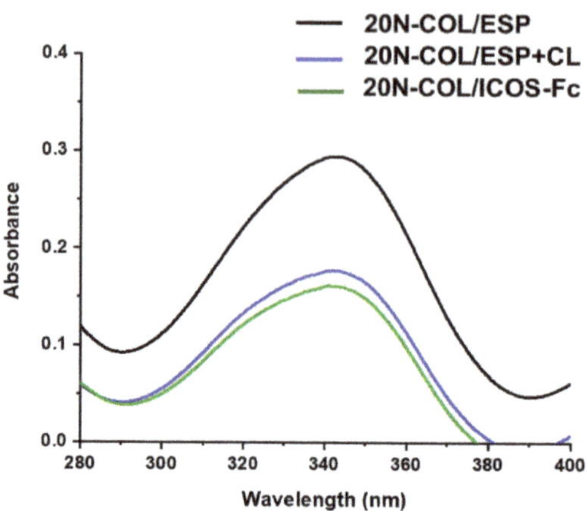

Figure 5. UV-Vis spectra obtained from the free amine analysis of electrospun collagen membranes, as produced (20N-COL/ESP), crosslinked without functionalization (20N-COL/ESP+CL), and crosslinked with addition of ICOS-Fc (20N-COL/ICOS).

The graph obtained from the UV-Vis analysis shows a significant reduction in the free amines in collagen once the sample is crosslinked (20-N-COL/ESP+CL), demonstrating that the covalent bonding between collagen chains has occurred. Moreover, a further small reduction is revealed upon ICOS-Fc functionalization (20N-COL/ICOS-Fc), suggesting the concurrent binding ICOS-Fc to the free amines, without impairing the crosslinking reaction.

The ATR-FTIR analysis (Figure 6) allowed to study the tertiary structure of collagen before (N-COL) and after processing.

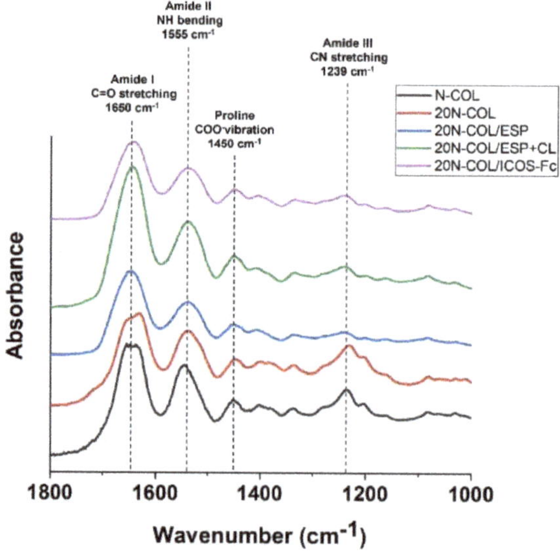

Figure 6. ATR-FTIR spectroscopy of samples produced with N−COL: as supplied (N−COL), after dissolution in acidic medium (20N−COL), after ESP (20N−COL/ESP), post-crosslinking with EDC/NHS (20N−COL/ESP+CL), and post-functionalization with ICOS−Fc (20N−COL/ICOS−Fc).

Based on the literature, the features of the following absorption bands were considered: amide I at 1650 cm^{-1} (C=O stretching), amide II at 1555 cm^{-1} (N-H bending), amide III at 1239 cm^{-1} (CN stretching and NH bending), and carboxylate groups of proline at 1450 cm^{-1} (COO$^-$ vibration) [34–36].

FTIR spectra showed for all samples the bands ascribed to the amide I (1650 cm^{-1}), the amide II (1555 cm^{-1}), and the proline stretch (1450 cm^{-1}). The amide II band did not suffer significant alterations [34,37] while the amide III band demonstrated a gradual widening when collagen is processed by electrospinning and further crosslinked and functionalized. In details, immediately after electrospinning the band is less evident, with a restoration of higher intensity upon crosslinking. These variations in the amide III band suggest a potential change in the protein orientation following the processing steps as suggested by different authors in the literature [13,38]. Overall, the spectra indicate that no significant alterations occurred to the collagen tertiary structure since all the main characteristic peaks of the protein were preserved without registering evident shifts.

The structural variations generated by the crosslinking process were also evaluated by TGA (Figure 7A,B). For collagen there are three ranges of temperature where the main weight losses are shown: I (50–200 °C), II (200–450 °C), and III (450–700 °C) [39,40].

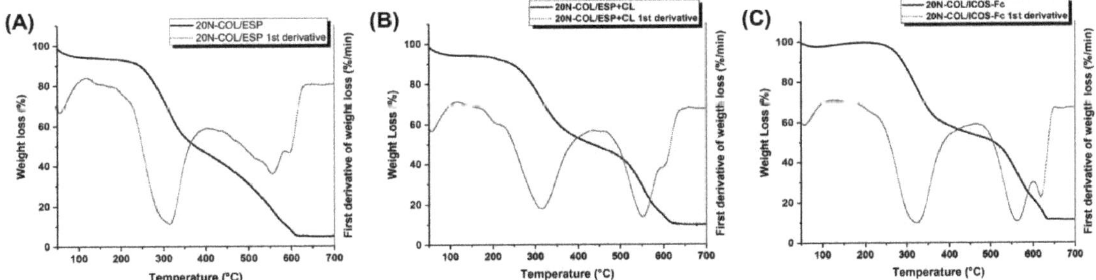

Figure 7. TGA analysis and first derivative of samples produced with (**A**) N-COL after ESP (20N-COL ESP), (**B**) post-crosslinking with EDC/NHS without ICOS-Fc addition, and (**C**) post-crosslinking, functionalized with ICOS-Fc.

The first loss relates to the desorption of physiosorbed water from collagen samples' both pre- and post-crosslinking, and it is identified by the first negative peak in their derivative curves (green line). The 20N-COL/ESP (Figure 7A) presents a slightly higher percentage of weight loss as visible from the first derivative, suggesting larger amount of retained molecular water, compared to 20N-COL/ESP+CL and 20N-COL/ICOS-Fc (Figure 7B,C), which due to consumption of amine groups during the crosslinking reaction results less prone to engage the H-bonding with water molecules. The second stage, between 200 °C and 400 °C, indicates the release of water bound to collagen and degradation products of the collagen chains. The electrospun collagen before crosslinking (Figure 7A) depicts most of the weight loss between 250 and 300 °C, as clearly shown by the first derivative curve. The crosslinked collagen (Figure 7B) and the functionalized one (Figure 7C) also present a less intense loss at 300 °C compared to the non-crosslinked collagen, implying that it suffers less degradation as a result from the successful crosslinking reaction. After 400 °C, the non-crosslinked collagen showed a minor weight loss related to the degradation of the residual organic components, in contrast with the crosslinked and functionalized samples, which presented a significant additional loss around 500 °C. This indicated that the structure did not fully decompose at lower temperatures. In general, before 500 °C the non-crosslinked sample lost 68% of the initial weight, while the crosslinked and functionalized ones 55% and 53%, respectively, with a difference of more than 10%. This difference was maintained up to 600 °C, the point at which all samples had lost over 80% of the total weight.

3.3. Cytocompatibility of Functionalized Membranes and Influence on Osteosarcoma Motility

To evaluate cytotoxicity, U2OS human osteosarcoma cells were seeded on 20N-COL/ESP+CL or 20N-COL/ICOS-Fc samples. 3, 5, and 7 days after seeding, cell viability was assessed by using XTT reagent. As reported in Figure 8A, the registered values did not evidence significant differences in cell viability compared to cells seeded on tissue culture plastic (TCP) over time, meaning the membranes are not cytotoxic.

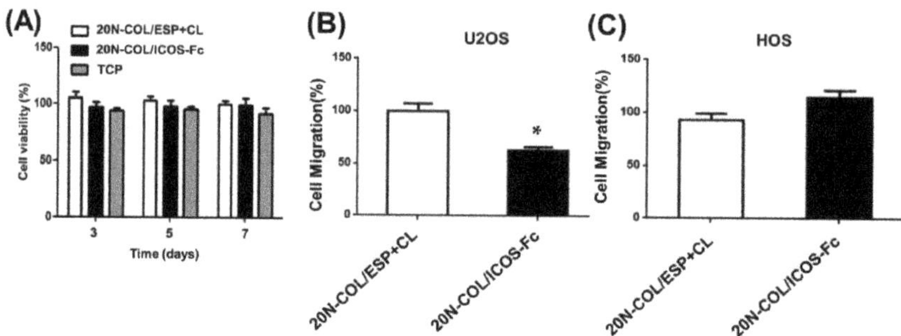

Figure 8. Cell viability and migration studies performed on electrospun collagen membranes, with and without ICOS-Fc. (**A**) Viability of U2OS cells when in contact with 20N-COL/ESP+CL and 20N-COL/ICOS-Fc samples, tissue culture plastic (TCP), at different timepoints: 3, 5, and 7 days. The graph shows the cell viability (%) as mean and standard error obtained from five independent experiments. (**B**) U2OS (ICOSL positive) and (**C**) HOS (ICOSL negative) cells migration after contact with collagen membranes functionalized with ICOS-Fc (20N-COL/ICOS-Fc) or not (20N-COL/ESP+CL). Data are expressed as mean $\pm$ SEM (n = 5) of the percentage of migration versus control migration in the absence of any collagen scaffold. * $p < 0.05$.

The retention of the ICOS-Fc ability to inhibit cell migration [21] was assessed through the Boyden chamber migration assay with either the ICOSL positive cell line U2OS (Figure 8B) or the ICOSL negative cell line HOS (Figure 8C). Results showed that the exposure of U2OS cells to 20N-COL/ICOS-Fc membranes inhibited their migration by 40%, compared to 20N-COL/ESP+CL membranes. This confirmed the proven biological inhibitory effect of ICOS-Fc on cell migration [22,41]. By contrast, the migration of the ICOSL negative HOS cells was not affected by the contact with 20N-COL/ICOS-Fc scaffolds, which was predictable as these cells are not responsive to its inhibitory action. No differences were found between control samples (TCP and 20N-COL/ESP+CL).

4. Discussion

Collagen, as one of the main constituents of bone, is a common choice as a base material for the development of scaffolds aiming at BTE. The combination of ESP with collagen can boost the degree of biomimicry of a device as it allows the creation of structures that are similar to the ECM, at both compositional and architectural level [6].

In this work, an aqueous solution of acetic acid was used as mild solvent for the dissolution of collagen in order to avoid the protein denaturation and allow the electrospinning process [16,42]. To investigate the effects of the solubilization and ESP process on collagen's structural integrity, CD and SDS-PAGE analysis were performed (Figure 2), both confirming the presence of the triple helical structure. At the molecular level, the triple helix of collagen type I is composed of three identical α-chains (two α_1 chains and one α_2), each one composed of a repeating amino acid sequence of glycine-X-Y, where typically X is a proline and Y is an hydroxyproline [28,29]. The three α chains then assemble into a triple helix by coiling around each other in a rope-like fashion, forming tropocollagen. In SDS-PAGE analysis, these chains are represented in an electrophoretic profile as bands. The analysis performed on N-COL, 20N-COL, and the commercial reference Roche (Figure 2A) shows the α_1 chains at 180 kDa and the α_2 at 130 kDa. The representation of α_1 and α_2-chains together, or two α_1-chains, is seen by the presence of the β-band, a dimer, which is seen at 250 kDa. Finally, the confirmation that the three α-chains are together, possibly arranged as a triple helix, is given by the γ-band, which was present for all samples. The data from SDS-PAGE was further confirmed by the CD analysis (Figure 2B), where the strong positive peak at 220 nm indicates the presence of a triple helix conformation [30]. Altogether these results show that the used solvent system allowed to preserve the protein structure ensuring the full retention of its bioactivity.

ATR-FTIR spectroscopy provided further insights on collagen structure upon each process step. The collected spectra (Figure 6) show that all samples presented the expected amide bands, with exception of 20N-COL/ESP which did not present the amide III signal. This was associated with a slight loss of molecular structure [36], specifically to β-sheet secondary structures, associated with a band at 1239 cm^{-1} [34]. The loss of this band can be ascribed to the fast solvent evaporation and fibre assembly occurring during ESP, which together with the dissolution in the solvent, can affect to some extent the structural conformation of the protein [36]. Similar results are reported in the studies by Sizeland et al. [10], where the results of the ATR-FTIR of electrospun membranes suggested that the alteration occurred, although the SDS-PAGE of their membranes evidenced that the α chains were intact. Their study concluded that the protein was not degraded, but the triple helices did not redevelop after ESP. The spectrum registered after crosslinking shows that the amide III band reappears, highlighting the effect of crosslinking in promoting the reconstitution and stabilization of the collagen molecular structure.

Despite the positive effects in terms of collagen stability, crosslinking treatments are often associated with loss of morphology (e.g., fibre merging and increase in fibre diameter). Therefore, minimizing the post-processing steps and optimizing the crosslinking strategy is key to ensure that the desired microstructure is preserved. In this work, this was achieved by combining the crosslinking and functionalization in a *one-step* reaction, by the simultaneous activation via EDC/NHS of the carboxylic groups exposed both by collagen and by ICOS-Fc molecule [17]. The successful outcome of the functionalization step was confirmed by ELISA-like assays which showed a reduction in ICOS-Fc in the supernatant collected from the crosslinking reaction (Figure 4). This was seen for all the three concentrations tested (50, 75, and 100 μg/mL), however, due to the high costs of ICOS-Fc (200 EUR/mg), in this instance experiments were performed with 50 μg/mL, to attain a functionalization that is both efficient and easily translated commercially. The UV-Vis analysis (Figure 5), performed on the samples exposed to 50 μg/mL of ICOS-Fc, confirmed the obtained results for crosslinking and functionalization through a significant decrease in the amount of free amines after crosslinking, and significantly lower after the grafting with ICOS-Fc.

To further investigate how crosslinking improved collagen's stability, a TGA analysis was performed (Figure 7), showing that the process led to the increase in the denaturation temperature of ca 10 °C for crosslinked membranes. UV-Vis and TGA results clearly evidenced a high degree of collagen crosslinking, which is expected to provide enhanced biodegradation kinetics and bioactivity (angiogenesis [43], osteogenesis [44]).

The crosslinked membranes remained intact for 7 days during the cytotoxicity assay, confirming that crosslinking reaction provided a significant improvement in the overall stability and that the electrospun membranes would be able to support cell migration and proliferation.

The produced electrospun collagen fibrous membranes are expected to provide multiple biologicals and topological cues that can modulate cell adhesion, proliferation and/or differentiation and aims to provide an effective alternative strategy to the more common combination with growth factors and cells to enhance and support the process of bone formation [45,46]. In this study, with the aim to widen the exerted biological functions, the collagen-based scaffolds have been further biofunctionalized with ICOS-Fc molecule [17,21,22]. The target of the followed approach is the combination in a single multifunctional platform of several abilities to support osteoblast growth and function, whilst temporarily inducing the inhibition of osteoclasts activity through the peculiar biological properties of ICOS-Fc. The resulting multifunctional device is expected to actively contribute to the process of bone regeneration, which is key when the physiological remodelling mechanism is delayed or even altered, as in the case of elderly people or patients affected by osteoporosis.

The biological assays demonstrated that the electrospun membranes are fully cytocompatible, confirming that neither the electrospinning process nor the chemicals of the cross-linking/functionalization step have altered the overall biocompatibility.

Since the effect of free ICOS-Fc on cell migratory activity was previously reported by the authors [22] the retention of this essential biological effect was also assessed for ICOS-Fc grafted on collagen membranes by using the Boyden chamber migration assay, both with ICOSL-positive and ICOSL-negative cell lines, as a *proof of concept* of the efficacy of the developed approach. The results of this assay evidenced a 40% inhibition of U2OS (ICOSL-positive cells) migratory activity after only 30 min of contact between cells and ICOS-Fc functionalized membranes. This finding fully confirmed the retention of the inhibitory effect of ICOS-Fc anchored to electrospun membranes, in analogy to its free form [21,22] and when grafted onto the surface of bioactive glass particles [17]. ICOSL-negative cells (HOS) were used as a control, and exhibited no changes in their migration behaviour, attesting once more the specificity of the inhibitory effect derived from the ICOS:ICOSL binding at the collagen surface.

Further in vitro studies will aim at exploring the action of the functionalized membranes on osteoclast-precursor cells to evaluate the inhibitory effect on cell differentiation and the downregulation of osteoclast differentiation genes.

5. Conclusions

The work presented reports the successful development of *one step* strategy to achieve simultaneously the crosslinking and biofunctionalization of electrospun collagen membranes. The ICOS-Fc molecule, chosen for its ability to reversibly inhibit osteoclast function by binding its ligand ICOSL, has been effectively grafted on the collagen membranes to impart multifunctional biological effects and thus promoting the remodelling process of bone tissue in compromised clinical situations.

The stability of the ICOS-Fc binding was assessed by an *in house*-developed ELISA-like assay, revealing a functionalization yield higher than 95%, with a full retention of functionality by the grafted biomolecules.

After 7 days in culture, cells showed high viability regardless of the presence of ICOS-Fc, suggesting that neither the crosslinking nor the functionalization have altered the cytocompatibility of the electrospun collagen scaffolds. The contact of U2OS, chosen as ICOSL-positive cells, with the collagen membranes exposing ICOS-Fc at their surface resulted in the inhibition of cell migration, confirming once more the successful binding to the collagen fibres and the retention of ICOS-Fc biological properties (*proof of efficacy*). In contrast, the ICOSL-negative cell line (HOS) did not show inhibitory effects, confirming the specificity of the ICOS-Fc effect that was mediated by binding to ICOSL.

By inhibiting the migration of ICOSL-positive cells, e.g., osteoclasts, the developed membranes can play an active role on bone remodelling, placing this strategy in the category of future therapies based on cell behaviour modulation to achieve improved regeneration.

The results of this study highlight the high potential of the developed multifunctional platform (i.e., osteoconductive, pro-osteogenic, anti-clastogenic) for treating delayed bone healing and pave the way to further in vivo studies to implement minimally invasive clinical solutions (e.g., injection via cannulated instruments at the fracture site).

Author Contributions: For this research paper, C.V.-B. and S.F. formulated the research ideas; P.M. and G.M. developed the materials and interpreted the results under the supervision of C.V.-B., S.F. and U.D.; P.M. and G.M. synthesized and characterized the materials; E.B. and C.L.G. created the home made ELISA-Like assay and performed the biological assessment under the supervision of U.D.; C.D. performed the migration assay; P.M. wrote a draft of the article that was implemented by S.F. and all other authors revised the manuscript and contributed to the discussion of the results. Conceptualization, S.F. and C.V.-B.; Data curation, P.M. and G.M.; Formal analysis, P.M., G.M., E.B., C.L.G. and C.D.; Funding acquisition, C.V.-B.; Investigation, P.M., G.M., E.B., and C.L.G.; Methodology, P.M., G.M., S.F., E.B.,C.L.G. and C.D.; Project administration, C.V.-B.; Supervision, S.F., U.D. and C.V.-B.; Validation, S.F., P.M., G.M., E.B. and C.L.G.; Visualization, S.F. and C.V.-B.; Writing—original draft, P.M., G.M. and S.F.; Writing—review and editing, U.D. and C.V.-B. All authors have read and agreed to the published version of the manuscript.

Funding: This project has received funding from the European Union's Horizon 2020 research and innovation program under grant agreement No 814410 (GIOTTO).

Data Availability Statement: The data presented in this study are openly available in ZENODO at https://doi.org/10.5281/zenodo.7063972.

Conflicts of Interest: Authors Elena Boggio and Casimiro Luca Gigliotti are, respectively, CTO and CEO of the company NOVAICOS s.r.l.s. The remaining authors declare that the research was conducted in the absence of any commercial or financial relationships that could be construed as a potential conflict of interest.

References

1. Dimitriou, R.; Jones, E.; McGonagle, D.; Giannoudis, P.V. Bone Regeneration: Current Concepts and Future Directions. *BMC Med.* **2011**, *9*, 66. [CrossRef] [PubMed]
2. Schlundt, C.; Bucher, C.H.; Tsitsilonis, S.; Schell, H.; Duda, G.N.; Schmidt-Bleek, K. Clinical and Research Approaches to Treat Non-Union Fracture. *Curr. Osteoporos. Rep.* **2018**, *16*, 155–168. [CrossRef]
3. Brown, J.L.; Laurencin, C.T. 2.6.6—Bone Tissue Engineering. In *Biomaterials Science*, 4th ed.; Wagner, W.R., Sakiyama-Elbert, S.E., Zhang, G., Yaszemski, M.J., Eds.; Academic Press: Cambridge, MA, USA, 2020; pp. 1373–1388. ISBN 978-0-12-816137-1.
4. Wu, A.-M.; Bisignano, C.; James, S.L.; Abady, G.G.; Abedi, A.; Abu-Gharbieh, E.; Alhassan, R.K.; Alipour, V.; Arabloo, J.; Asaad, M.; et al. Global, Regional, and National Burden of Bone Fractures in 204 Countries and Territories, 1990–2019: A Systematic Analysis from the Global Burden of Disease Study 2019. *Lancet Heal. Longev.* **2021**, *2*, e580–e592. [CrossRef]
5. Ye, G.; Bao, F.; Zhang, X.; Song, Z.; Liao, Y.; Fei, Y.; Bunpetch, V.; Heng, B.C.; Shen, W.; Liu, H.; et al. Nanomaterial-Based Scaffolds for Bone Tissue Engineering and Regeneration. *Nanomedicine* **2020**, *15*, 1995–2017. [CrossRef] [PubMed]
6. Sofi, H.S.; Ashraf, R.; Beigh, M.A.; Sheikh, F.A. Scaffolds Fabricated from Natural Polymers/Composites by Electrospinning for Bone Tissue Regeneration. *Adv. Exp. Med. Biol.* **2018**, *1078*, 49–78. [CrossRef]
7. Lee, J.C.; Pereira, C.T.; Ren, X.; Huang, W.; Bischoff, D.; Weisgerber, D.W.; Yamaguchi, D.T.; Harley, B.A.; Miller, T.A. Optimizing Collagen Scaffolds for Bone Engineering: Effects of Cross-Linking and Mineral Content on Structural Contraction and Osteogenesis. *J. Craniofac. Surg.* **2015**, *26*, 1992–1996. [CrossRef]
8. Ramakrishna, S.; Fujihara, K.; Teo, W.-E.; Lim, T.-C.; Ma, Z. *An Introduction to Electrospinning and Nanofibers*; World Scientific: Singapore, 2005, ISBN 978-981-256-415-3.
9. Sharifi, E.; Azami, M.; Kajbafzadeh, A.-M.; Moztarzadeh, F.; Faridi-Majidi, R.; Shamousi, A.; Karimi, R.; Ai, J. Preparation of a Biomimetic Composite Scaffold from Gelatin/Collagen and Bioactive Glass Fibers for Bone Tissue Engineering. *Mater. Sci. Eng. C* **2016**, *59*, 533–541. [CrossRef]
10. Sizeland, K.H.; Hofman, K.A.; Hallett, I.C.; Martin, D.E.; Potgieter, J.; Kirby, N.M.; Hawley, A.; Mudie, S.T.; Ryan, T.M.; Haverkamp, R.G.; et al. Nanostructure of Electrospun Collagen: Do Electrospun Collagen Fibers Form Native Structures? *Materialia* **2018**, *3*, 90–96. [CrossRef]
11. Geng, X.; Kwon, O.H.; Jang, J. Electrospinning of Chitosan Dissolved in Concentrated Acetic Acid Solution. *Biomaterials* **2005**, *26*, 5427–5432. [CrossRef]
12. Zhou, Y.; Yao, H.; Wang, J.; Wang, D.; Liu, Q.; Li, Z. Greener Synthesis of Electrospun Collagen/Hydroxyapatite Composite Fibers with an Excellent Microstructure for Bone Tissue Engineering. *Int. J. Nanomed.* **2015**, *10*, 3203–3215. [CrossRef]
13. Zeugolis, D.; Khew, S.; Yew, E.; Ekaputra, A.; Tong, Y.; Yung, L.-Y.; Hutmacher, D.; Sheppard, C.; Raghunath, M. Electrospinning of Pure Collagen Nano-Fibres—Just an Expensive Way to Make Gelatin? *Biomaterials* **2008**, *29*, 2293–2305. [CrossRef] [PubMed]
14. Jiang, Q.; Reddy, N.; Zhang, S.; Roscioli, N.; Yang, Y. Water-Stable Electrospun Collagen Fibers from a Non-Toxic Solvent and Crosslinking System. *J. Biomed. Mater. Res. A* **2013**, *101*, 1237–1247. [CrossRef] [PubMed]
15. Ribeiro, N.; Sousa, S.R.; Van Blitterswijk, C.A.; Moroni, L.; Monteiro, F.J. A Biocomposite of Collagen Nano Fi Bers and Nanohydroxyapatite for Bone Regeneration. *Biofabrication* **2014**, *6*, 035015. [CrossRef] [PubMed]

16. Montalbano, G.; Tomasina, C.; Fiorilli, S.; Camarero-Espinosa, S.; Vitale-Brovarone, C.; Moroni, L. Biomimetic Scaffolds Obtained by Electrospinning of Collagen-Based Materials: Strategies to Hinder the Protein Denaturation. *Materials* **2021**, *14*, 4360. [CrossRef]

17. Fiorilli, S.; Pagani, M.; Boggio, E.; Gigliotti, C.L.; Dianzani, C.; Gauthier, R.; Pontremoli, C.; Montalbano, G.; Dianzani, U.; Vitale-Brovarone, C. Sr-Containing Mesoporous Bioactive Glasses Bio-Functionalized with Recombinant ICOS-Fc: An in Vitro Study. *Nanomaterials* **2021**, *11*, 321. [CrossRef] [PubMed]

18. Zhao, X.; Komatsu, D.E.; Hadjiargyrou, M. Delivery of RhBMP-2 Plasmid DNA Complexes via a PLLA/Collagen Electrospun Scaffold Induces Ectopic Bone Formation. *J. Biomed. Nanotechnol.* **2016**, *12*, 1285–1296. [CrossRef]

19. Miszuk, J.M.; Xu, T.; Yao, Q.; Fang, F.; Childs, J.D.; Hong, Z.; Tao, J.; Fong, H.; Sun, H. Functionalization of PCL-3D Electrospun Nanofibrous Scaffolds for Improved BMP2-Induced Bone Formation. *Appl. Mater. Today* **2018**, *10*, 194–202. [CrossRef]

20. Azari Matin, A.; Fattah, K.; Saeidpour Masouleh, S.; Tavakoli, R.; Houshmandkia, S.A.; Moliani, A.; Moghimimonfared, R.; Pakzad, S.; Dalir Abdolahinia, E. Synthetic Electrospun Nanofibers as a Supportive Matrix in Osteogenic Differentiation of Induced Pluripotent Stem Cells. *J. Biomater. Sci. Polym. Ed.* **2022**, *33*, 1–25. [CrossRef]

21. Gigliotti, C.L.; Boggio, E.; Clemente, N.; Shivakumar, Y.; Toth, E.; Sblattero, D.; D'Amelio, P.; Isaia, G.C.; Dianzani, C.; Yagi, J.; et al. ICOS-Ligand Triggering Impairs Osteoclast Differentiation and Function In Vitro and In Vivo. *J. Immunol.* **2016**, *197*, 3905–3916. [CrossRef]

22. Dianzani, C.; Minelli, R.; Gigliotti, C.L.; Occhipinti, S.; Giovarelli, M.; Conti, L.; Boggio, E.; Shivakumar, Y.; Baldanzi, G.; Malacarne, V.; et al. B7h Triggering Inhibits the Migration of Tumor Cell Lines. *J. Immunol.* **2014**, *192*, 4921–4931. [CrossRef]

23. Doillon, C.J.; Mantovani, D.; Rajan, N.; Habermehl, J.; Cote, M.; Coté, M.-F.; Doillon, C.J.; Mantovani, D. Preparation of Ready-to-Use, Storable and Reconstituted Type I Collagen from Rat Tail Tendon for Tissue Engineering Applications. *Nat. Protoc.* **2006**, *1*, 2753–2758. [CrossRef]

24. Di Niro, R.; Ziller, F.; Florian, F.; Crovella, S.; Stebel, M.; Bestagno, M.; Burrone, O.; Bradbury, A.R.M.; Secco, P.; Marzari, R.; et al. Construction of Miniantibodies for the in Vivo Study of Human Autoimmune Diseases in Animal Models. *BMC Biotechnol.* **2007**, *7*, 46. [CrossRef] [PubMed]

25. Habeeb, A.F.S.A. Determination of Free Amino Groups in Proteins by Trinitrobenzenesulfonic Acid. *Anal. Biochem.* **1966**, *14*, 328–336. [CrossRef]

26. Tronci, G.; Russell, S.J.; Wood, D.J. Photo-Active Collagen Systems with Controlled Triple Helix Architecture. *J. Mater. Chem. B* **2013**, *1*, 3705–3715. [CrossRef]

27. Róisín Holmes, X.B.Y.; Dunne, A.; Florea, L.; Wood, D.; Tronci, G. Thiol-Ene Photo-Click Collagen-PEG Hydrogels: Impact of Water-Soluble Photoinitiators on Cell Viability, Gelation Kinetics and Rheological Properties. *Polymers* **2017**, *9*, 226. [CrossRef]

28. Li, Y.; Qiao, C.; Shi, L.; Jiang, Q.; Li, T. Viscosity of Collagen Solutions: Influence of Concentration, Temperature, Adsorption, and Role of Intermolecular Interactions. *J. Macromol. Sci.* **2014**, *53*, 893–901. [CrossRef]

29. Rabotyagova, O.S.; Cebe, P.; Kaplan, D.L. Collagen Structural Hierarchy and Susceptibility to Degradation by Ultraviolet Radiation. *Mater. Sci. Eng. C Mater. Biol. Appl.* **2008**, *28*, 1420–1429. [CrossRef]

30. Usha, R.; Ramasami, T. The Effects of Urea and N-Propanol on Collagen Denaturation: Using DSC, Circular Dicroism and Viscosity. *Thermochim. Acta* **2004**, *409*, 201–206. [CrossRef]

31. Meng, L.; Arnoult, O.; Smith, M.; Wnek, G.E. Electrospinning of in Situ Crosslinked Collagen Nanofibers. *J. Mater. Chem.* **2012**, *22*, 19412–19417. [CrossRef]

32. Dong, B.; Arnoult, O.; Smith, M.E.; Wnek, G.E. Electrospinning of Collagen Nanofiber Scaffolds from Benign Solvents. *Macromol. Rapid Commun.* **2009**, *30*, 539–542. [CrossRef]

33. Lopez Marquez, A.; Gareis, I.E.; Dias, F.J.; Gerhard, C.; Lezcano, M.F. Methods to Characterize Electrospun Scaffold Morphology: A Critical Review. *Polymers* **2022**, *14*, 467. [CrossRef] [PubMed]

34. Stani, C.; Vaccari, L.; Mitri, E.; Birarda, G. FTIR Investigation of the Secondary Structure of Type I Collagen: New Insight into the Amide III Band. *Spectrochim. Acta Part A Mol. Biomol. Spectrosc.* **2020**, *229*, 118006. [CrossRef] [PubMed]

35. Luo, X.; Guo, Z.; He, P.; Chen, T.; Li, L.; Ding, S.; Li, H. Study on Structure, Mechanical Property and Cell Cytocompatibility of Electrospun Collagen Nanofibers Crosslinked by Common Agents. *Int. J. Biol. Macromol.* **2018**, *113*, 476–486. [CrossRef] [PubMed]

36. Fiorani, A.; Gualandi, C.; Panseri, S.; Montesi, M.; Marcacci, M.; Focarete, M.L.; Bigi, A. Comparative Performance of Collagen Nanofibers Electrospun from Different Solvents and Stabilized by Different Crosslinkers. *J. Mater. Sci. Mater. Med.* **2014**, *25*, 2313–2321. [CrossRef]

37. Lee, J.; Lee, S.Y.; Jang, J.; Jeong, Y.H.; Cho, D.W. Fabrication of Patterned Nanofibrous Mats Using Direct-Write Electrospinning. *Langmuir* **2012**, *28*, 7267–7275. [CrossRef] [PubMed]

38. Sell, S.A.; McClure, M.J.; Garg, K.; Wolfe, P.S.; Bowlin, G.L. Electrospinning of Collagen/Biopolymers for Regenerative Medicine and Cardiovascular Tissue Engineering. *Adv. Drug Deliv. Rev.* **2009**, *61*, 1007–1019. [CrossRef]

39. León-Mancilla, B.H.; Araiza-Téllez, M.A.; Flores-Flores, J.O.; Piña-Barba, M.C. Physico-Chemical Characterization of Collagen Scaffolds for Tissue Engineering. *J. Appl. Res. Technol.* **2016**, *14*, 77–85. [CrossRef]

40. Sionkowska, A.; Skopinska-Wisniewska, J.; Gawron, M.; Kozlowska, J.; Planecka, A. Chemical and Thermal Cross-Linking of Collagen and Elastin Hydrolysates. *Int. J. Biol. Macromol.* **2010**, *47*, 570–577. [CrossRef]

41. Boggio, E.; Gigliotti, C.L.; Moia, R.; Scotta, A.; Crespi, I.; Boggione, P.; De Paoli, L.; Deambrogi, C.; Garzaro, M.; Vidali, M.; et al. Inducible T-Cell Co-Stimulator (ICOS) and ICOS Ligand Are Novel Players in the Multiple-Myeloma Microenvironment. *Br. J. Haematol.* **2022**, *196*, 1369–1380. [CrossRef]

42. Estévez, M.; Montalbano, G.; Gallo-Cordova, A.; Ovejero, J.G.; Izquierdo-Barba, I.; González, B.; Tomasina, C.; Moroni, L.; Vallet-Regí, M.; Vitale-Brovarone, C.; et al. Incorporation of Superparamagnetic Iron Oxide Nanoparticles into Collagen Formulation for 3D Electrospun Scaffolds. *Nanomaterials* **2022**, *12*, 181. [CrossRef]
43. Yao, C.; Markowicz, M.; Pallua, N.; Noah, E.M.; Steffens, G. The Effect of Cross-Linking of Collagen Matrices on Their Angiogenic Capability. *Biomaterials* **2008**, *29*, 66–74. [CrossRef] [PubMed]
44. Grosso, A.; Burger, M.G.; Lunger, A.; Schaefer, D.J.; Banfi, A.; Di Maggio, N. It Takes Two to Tango: Coupling of Angiogenesis and Osteogenesis for Bone Regeneration. *Front. Bioeng. Biotechnol.* **2017**, *5*, 68. [CrossRef] [PubMed]
45. De Oliveira Lomelino, R.; Castro-Silva, I.I.; Linhares, A.B.R.; Alves, G.G.; de Albuquerque Santos, S.R.; Gameiro, V.S.; Rossi, A.M.; Granjeiro, J.M. The Association of Human Primary Bone Cells with Biphasic Calcium Phosphate (BTCP/HA 70:30) Granules Increases Bone Repair. *J. Mater. Sci. Mater. Med.* **2012**, *23*, 781–788. [CrossRef]
46. Von der Mark, K.; Park, J.; Bauer, S.; Schmuki, P. Nanoscale Engineering of Biomimetic Surfaces: Cues from the Extracellular Matrix. *Cell Tissue Res.* **2009**, *339*, 131. [CrossRef] [PubMed]

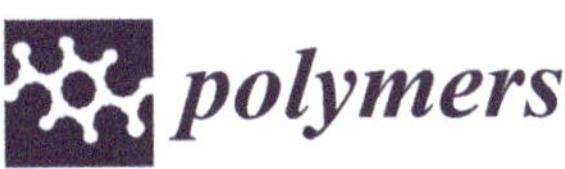 *polymers*

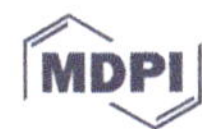

Article

Aquaponics-Derived Tilapia Skin Collagen for Biomaterials Development

Nunzia Gallo [1,*], Maria Lucia Natali [1,2], Alessandra Quarta [3], Antonio Gaballo [3], Alberta Terzi [4], Teresa Sibillano [4], Cinzia Giannini [4], Giuseppe Egidio De Benedetto [5], Paola Lunetti [6], Loredana Capobianco [6], Federica Stella Blasi [1], Alessandro Sicuro [6], Angelo Corallo [1], Alessandro Sannino [1] and Luca Salvatore [1,2]

[1] Department of Engineering for Innovation, University of Salento, Via Monteroni, 73100 Lecce, Italy; marialucia.natali@unisalento.it (M.L.N.); federicastella.blasi@unisalento.it (F.S.B.); angelo.corallo@unisalento.it (A.C.); alessandro.sannino@unisalento.it (A.S.); luca.salvatore@unisalento.it (L.S.)

[2] Typeone Biomaterials Srl, Via Vittorio Veneto, 73036 Lecce, Italy

[3] CNR Nanotec, Institute of Nanotechnology, Via Monteroni, 73100 Lecce, Italy; alessandra.quarta@nanotec.cnr.it (A.Q.); antonio.gaballo@nanotec.cnr.it (A.G.)

[4] Institute of Crystallography, National Research Council, 70125 Bari, Italy; alberta.terzi@ic.cnr.it (A.T.); teresa.sibillano@ic.cnr.it (T.S.); cinzia.giannini@ic.cnr.it (C.G.)

[5] Department of Cultural Heritage, University of Salento, Via Monteroni, 73100 Lecce, Italy; giuseppe.debenedetto@unisalento.it

[6] Department of Biological and Environmental Sciences and Technologies, University of Salento, Via Monteroni, 73100 Lecce, Italy; paola.lunetti@unisalento.it (P.L.); loredana.capobianco@unisalento.it (L.C.); alessandro.sicuro@unisalento.it (A.S.)

* Correspondence: nunzia.gallo@unisalento.it

Citation: Gallo, N.; Natali, M.L.; Quarta, A.; Gaballo, A.; Terzi, A.; Sibillano, T.; Giannini, C.; De Benedetto, G.E.; Lunetti, P.; Capobianco, L.; et al. Aquaponics-Derived Tilapia Skin Collagen for Biomaterials Development. *Polymers* **2022**, *14*, 1865. https://doi.org/10.3390/polym14091865

Academic Editor: Dan Cristian Vodnar

Received: 31 March 2022
Accepted: 29 April 2022
Published: 2 May 2022

Publisher's Note: MDPI stays neutral with regard to jurisdictional claims in published maps and institutional affiliations.

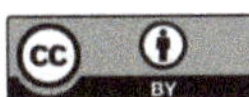

Copyright: © 2022 by the authors. Licensee MDPI, Basel, Switzerland. This article is an open access article distributed under the terms and conditions of the Creative Commons Attribution (CC BY) license (https://creativecommons.org/licenses/by/4.0/).

Abstract: Collagen is one of the most widely used biomaterials in health-related sectors. The industrial production of collagen mostly relies on its extraction from mammals, but several issues limited its use. In the last two decades, marine organisms attracted interest as safe, abundant, and alternative source for collagen extraction. In particular, the possibility to valorize the huge quantity of fish industry waste and byproducts as collagen source reinforced perception of fish collagen as eco-friendlier and particularly attractive in terms of profitability and cost-effectiveness. Especially fish byproducts from eco-sustainable aquaponics production allow for fish biomass with additional added value and controlled properties over time. Among fish species, *Oreochromis niloticus* is one of the most widely bred fish in large-scale aquaculture and aquaponics systems. In this work, type I collagen was extracted from aquaponics-raised Tilapia skin and characterized from a chemical, physical, mechanical, and biological point of view in comparison with a commercially available analog. Performed analysis confirmed that the proprietary process optimized for type I collagen extraction allowed to isolate pure native collagen and to preserve its native conformational structure. Preliminary cellular studies performed with mouse fibroblasts indicated its optimal biocompatibility. All data confirmed the eligibility of the extracted Tilapia-derived native type I collagen as a biomaterial for healthcare applications.

Keywords: type I collagen; tilapia; skin; aquaponic; biomaterials

1. Introduction

Type I collagen is the predominant structural component of vertebrates' connective tissues that accounts for approximately 70% of the total collagens found in the human body [1,2]. Being one of the major extracellular matrix (ECM) components, it is intrinsically bioactive, biodegradable, and particularly low immunogenic and weak antigenic [2–7]. Therefore, its employment as a biomaterial in the food, pharmaceutical, cosmetic, and biomedical industries is not surprising. Particularly high is its request in the health-related sector that makes extensive use of type I collagen for the manufacture of several kinds of formulations for tissue restoration/regeneration [2].

Collagen used in the biomedical field is usually derived from animal tissues. Large terrestrial mammals (i.e., bovine, porcine, equine, ovine) are currently the preferred sources for collagen extraction, for the high sequence homology with human collagen (>90%) [3] as well as for the possibility of accessing large quantities of raw materials. However, the application potential of mammalian-derived collagen is limited by issues such as triggering immune reactions (about 3% of the population), zoonosis transmission risks (i.e., the foot and mouth disease and the group of the bovine spongiform encephalopathies), besides cultural and religious concerns [3,8,9].

In this perspective, in the last two decades, marine organisms have attracted interest as safe, alternative, and abundant sources for collagen extraction [10–12]. Apart from owing biocompatibility, bioactivity, and biodegradability, fish collagen revealed an intrinsically lower threat of transmissible diseases, freedom from religious concerns [9], and weak antigenicity [13]. Marine collagen and its derivates (i.e., gelatin) were revealed to be easily processed in different types of formulations (i.e., injectable hydrogels, implantable temporary scaffolds, orally administrable pills) and relative properties tunable to suit diverse applications in a variety of biomedical fields [14–18].

Moreover, the possibility of developing waste recovery technologies to obtain high added value products from the abundant discards (e.g., skin, bones, fins, heads, guts, and scales) of the fish processing industry (70–85% of the total weight of catch) is of large scientific and industrial interest [10,19,20]. In particular, Nile Tilapia (*Oreochromis niloticus*), one of the World's most representative species of the fisheries and aquaculture food sector, attracted interest as a byproduct source for collagen extraction. Tilapia skin was demonstrated to provide for 28–40% dry weight yield of acid-soluble collagen (ASC) or pepsin soluble collagen (PSC) [21–24]. The fast growth speed, adaptability to a wide range of environmental conditions, ability to grow and reproduce in captivity, easy feeding at low trophic level, and easy processing to fish fillets [25] made Tilapia the second most important group of farmed fish after carps [22,26], with a global production of 6.5 million tons in 2018 and an aquaculture production increasing 11% per year [27]. The possibility to tune growth conditions and produce hazardous-free commercial products with controlled and reproducible final properties through, e.g., the aquaponics farming method, gives to Tilapia fillets and byproducts a high added value. Aquaponics is, in fact, known as a form of sustainable aquaculture, because it imitates natural systems, where aquatic organisms and plants grow symbiotically (the latter using nutrients from the fish waste processed by nitrifying bacteria) [28]. As a result, it proves to have higher water use efficiency than conventional aquaculture and agriculture, it does not use pesticides, and even the use of fertilizers is reduced, which makes aquaponics greener and more sustainable than conventional techniques [28]. For this reason, the valorization of aquaponics Tilapia-waste polluting byproducts as sources of collagen makes the derived biomaterial not only eco-friendlier but also particularly attractive in terms of profitability and cost-effectiveness [29].

In this study, the physical, chemical, and biological properties of a fibrillar type I collagen isolated from an aquaponics-derived Tilapia skin were extensively assessed and compared with those of a commercially available isoform from the same species and tissue. The identity and the nativeness of the extracted protein were assessed by Poly-Acrylamide Gel Electrophoresis in the presence of Sodium Dodecyl Sulphate (SDS-PAGE). The collagen secondary structure was investigated by Fourier Transform Infrared Spectroscopy (FT-IR), while its ultrastructure by Wide-angle X-ray scattering (WAXS). The amino acid composition was investigated by Gas Chromatography coupled with Mass Spectrometry (GC-MS). The thermal behavior was determined by Differential Scanning Calorimetry (DSC). Static contact angle measurements were conducted to achieve information about the surface hydrophobic character. The collagen mechanical response was assessed by the uniaxial tensile test. Lastly, the cytocompatibility was assessed by two standard assays, 3-[4,5-dimethylthiazol-2-yl]-2,5 diphenyl tetrazolium bromide (MTT) test and Live/Dead.

The viability, the morphology, and the distribution of 3T3 mouse fibroblasts seeded over collagen films were followed up for 12 days.

2. Materials

Type I collagen (T) was extracted from the skin of Nile Tilapia (*Oreochromis niloticus*) bred in the pilot aquaponics plant inside the Dept. of Innovation Engineering's Urban Farming Lab of the (University of Salento, Lecce, Italy). This plant consists of 3 cooperating subsystems (the recirculating aquaculture systems, the biofilter, and the hydroponic cultivation system), which ensure that the nutrients contained in the fish feed and feces are used to grow plants without wasting water. Both the fish biomass and the environmental parameters are constantly checked through an innovative ICT monitoring, control, and implementation system, based on IoT (Internet of Things) technologies, ensuring that the whole aquaponics system is managed efficiently. Nile Tilapia was fed tailored commercial feed EFICO Cromis 832F 3 (BioMar SAS, Nersac, France). Tilapia specimens of about 16–17 months with a mean weight of about 301 $\pm$ 48 g, 25.4 $\pm$ 1.3 $\times$ 8.4 $\pm$ 0.5 cm (l $\times$ h) sized, were selected for collagen extraction.

Collagen extraction was performed according to a proprietary process developed by Typeone Biomaterials Srl (Lecce, Italy) and provided in dry flakes. An analogous suspension of a commercial type I collagen (N) from Tilapia skin was provided in dry flakes from Nippi Inc. (Tokyo, Japan) and used for comparative analysis. Aqueous suspensions (10 mg/mL) were obtained by slowly hydrating collagen dry flakes in acetic acid 0.2 M for 3 h under magnetic stirring at 4°C in order to avoid collagen denaturation. Distilled water was obtained from the Millipore Milli-U10 water purification facility from Merck KGaA (Darmstadt, Germany). Standard proteins for SDS-PAGE of precise molecular weights ranging from 10 to 250 kDa were provided by Bio-Rad Laboratories Inc (Hercules, CA, USA). N, N-dimethylformamide was provided by VWR International PBI S.r.l. (Milan, Italy). Acetic acid, norleucine, and *N*-tert-butyldimethylsilyl-*N*-methyltrifluoroacetamide (MTBSTFA) were purchased by Sigma-Aldrich (Milan, Italy). For the cellular assays, culture media, supplements, trypsin and MTT were purchased from Sigma-Aldrich (Milan, Italy). The Live/Dead assay was purchased from Thermo Fisher Scientific Inc. (Waltham, MA, USA). If not otherwise stated, all other chemicals used were of analytical grade and purchased by Sigma-Aldrich (Milan, Italy).

3. Methods

3.1. Extracts Purity and Integrity

T and N purity and molecular weight were firstly assessed by SDS-PAGE using a Mini-Protean Tetra Cell system from Bio-Rad Laboratories, Inc. (Hercules, CA, USA). Hand cast gels (5% stacking gel, 7% resolving gel) were prepared using acrylamide/bisacrylamide solution with a ratio of 37.5:1. About 0.3 g of T and N collagen gels (10 mg/mL) were dissolved in 0.5 mL of reducing solution (Urea 2 M, Laemmli buffer: 62.5 mM Tris-HCl pH 6.8, 10% glycerol, 2% SDS, 0.01% bromophenol blue, 5% β-mercaptoethanol) and heated at 50 °C for 1 h [30–34]. Native type I collagen from horse tendon was also subjected to the reducing treatment to provide an example of protein integrity and purity [33,34]. After 1 min at max speed centrifugation, a few µL of supernatants were withdrawn and subjected to the electrophoretic run at 70 V for about 10 min in the stacking gel and at 120 V for about 2 h within the resolving gel in the presence of protein standards of precise molecular weights ranging from 10 to 250 kDa. At the end of the run, the gel was rapid Coomassie stained and acquired [34,35]. Then, the revealed protein bands were analyzed by mean of GelAnalyzer 19.1 (www.gelanalyzer.com, accessed on the 4 November 2021) by Istvan Lazar Jr., PhD and Istvan Lazar Sr., PhD, CSc for protein subunits ratio and molecular weight determination.

3.2. Amino Acid Composition

The amino acid composition of T and C was investigated by mean of GC-MS as described elsewhere [36,37], with slight modifications. Briefly, after hydrolysis in 6 N hydrochloric acid for 2 h at 120 °C, samples were transferred into a glass vial; norleucine was added as an internal standard (5 µL of a 100 ng/µL norleucine solution) and freeze-dried [36,37]. After lyophilization, the residues were reconstituted with 70 µL of *N, N*-dimethylformamide, and 20 µL of MTBSTFA. Derivatization with MTBSTFA was performed at 100 °C for 60 min. After cooling the solution at room temperature for 5 min, 1 µL of the solutions was injected in spit mode (split ratio 10:1). Samples were run on a GC-QqQ-MS (Bruker 456 gas chromatograph coupled to a triple quadrupole mass spectrometer Bruker Scion TQ) equipped with an autosampler (GC PAL, CTC Analytics AG). The GC was operated at a constant flow of 1.0 mL/min, and analytes were separated on an HP 5 MS capillary column (50 m with a 2 m guard column, inner diameter 250 µm, and film thickness 0.25 µm). The oven was kept at 60 °C for 1 min after injection, then a temperature gradient of 10 °C/min was employed until 320 °C was reached. The oven was then held at 320 °C for 10 min. The total run time was 37 min. The mass detector was operated at 70 eV in the electron impact (EI) ionization mode scanning the mass range 50–550 Da. The ion source and transfer line temperatures were 230 °C and 280 °C, respectively. Bruker MS Workstation 8.2 software was used to acquire chromatograms, process the data, and quantify amino acids. Samples were run thrice.

3.3. Structural Analysis

FT-IR was performed by means of FTIR-6300 from Jasco GmbH (Pfungstadt, Germany) in order to investigate the protein identity and the triple helical structure integrity. Briefly, T and N aqueous suspensions (5 mg/mL) were under vacuum degassed, casted into Petri dishes and air-dried for 72 h in a laminar flow hood. Films were then 1×1 cm cut and placed in the reading area. Absorption spectra were recorded in the range 1800–800 cm^{-1} at a resolution of 4 cm^{-1}, smoothed according to the Savitsky–Golay method, and analyzed by mean of the Origin software from OriginLab Corporation (Northampton, MA, USA) [34]. Peak positions were designated according to the spectrum shapes to make sure that all the wavelength ranges of the β-sheet (1610–1642 cm^{-1}), random coil (1642–1650 cm^{-1}), α-helix (1650–1660 cm^{-1}), β-turn (1660–1680 cm^{-1}), and β-antiparallel (1680–1700 cm^{-1}) had the designated peak positions. Then, the area of the deconvoluted secondary structures detected were calculated. The secondary structures percentage was calculated by dividing the peak area of each secondary structure by the whole peak area of all the secondary structures [38]. Additionally, the relative number of triple helices (ca. 1630 cm^{-1}) with respect to α-helices was calculated as the percentage of the total amide I peak area ascribable to the triple helix peak [33,39]. Four samples for each sample type were scanned, and each spectrum was collected as the average of 64 scans.

3.4. X-rays Structural Analysis

WAXS experiments were performed on T and N at the X-ray Micro Imaging Laboratory (XMI-LAB) [40], which is equipped with a Fr-E+ SuperBright copper anode MicroSource (λ = 0.154 nm, 2475 W) coupled through a focusing multilayer optics ConfocalMax-Flux (CMF 15–105) to a 3-pinholes camera for X-ray microscopy. The beam size was about 0.5×0.5 mm^2. In order to have access to a range of scattering vector moduli (q = 4 psinϑ/λ) from 0.3 to 3.5 Å^{-1}, corresponding to a 1.8 ÷ 21 Å range in the direct space, an Image Plate (IP) detector (250 $\times$ 160 mm^2, 100µm effective pixel size) placed at ~10 cm distance from the sample was employed for WAXS data collection. All measurements were digitally transformed by an off-line RAXIA reader. The data were elaborated by SAXSGUI and SUNBIM software [41]. All the samples were placed in the Ultralene® sachet for the measurement.

3.5. Thermal Properties

DSC allows measuring protein thermal behavior along with their denaturation temperature (T_d). Thermograms of T and N were determined using a Q2000 Series DSC from TA Instruments (New Castle, DE, USA). T and N gels were accurately weighed (5–10 mg) into aluminum pans, hermetically sealed, and scanned from 5 °C to 80 °C at 5 °C/min in an inert nitrogen atmosphere (50 mL min^{-1}) [34,42]. An empty aluminum pan was used as a reference probe. The T_d was measured as the mid-point of the corresponding endothermic peak [33,34,43]. The area under the peak allowed for estimating the enthalpy required for the transition [33,43]. Each sample was run in triplicate.

3.6. Wettability

Static contact angle measurements were performed by dropping 10 µL milli-Q water on 10 × 10 mm T and C films using the sessile-drop method using a FTA 1000 analysis system (First Ten Angstroms, Newark, NJ, USA) [34]. An average of three drops was conducted for each sample type.

3.7. Mechanical Properties

The constitutive bond of Tilapia skin-derived collagens was evaluated in a hydrated state using a ZwickiLine universal testing machine (Zwick/Roell, Ulm, Germany) equipped with a loading cell of 1 kN. Samples of T and N (5 × 20 mm) were hydrated in 0.01 M PBS at room temperature for 1 h, clamped and tensile tested under displacement-control until failure with a preload of 0.1 N and a load speed of 0.1 mm/s [34]. The Young modulus (E), the stress at break (σmax), and the strain at break (εr) were measured. In particular, E was calculated as the slope of the linear elastic region of the stress–strain curve at low strain values (in the range 1–5%). The thickness and width of wet specimens were measured using a Dino-Lite digital microscope (AnMo Electronics Corporation, New Taipei City, Taiwan). The experiment was performed in triplicate for each sample type.

3.8. Biocompatibility

Mouse fibroblasts, namely 3T3, were purchased from ATCC (Manassas, VA, USA) and cultured in high glucose Dulbecco's Modified Eagle Medium (DMEM) supplemented with 10% Fetal Bovine Serum (FBS), 100 U mL^{-1} penicillin and 100 µg mL^{-1} streptomycin at 37 °C in an atmosphere of 5% CO_2. To assess the cytocompatibility of T and N, fibroblasts were seeded into cell culture plates previously coated with T or N gels. In brief, prior to cell seeding, T and N gels (0.3 mL with a concentration equal to 5 mg/mL) were casted at the bottom of 24-well culture plates and let dry for 72 h; upon casting, plates were exposed to UV light irradiation for 2 h and then equilibrated overnight in cell culture medium at 37 °C. Then, 2×10^4 cells in 1 mL of culture medium were seeded into each well. Cells seeded directly into the multiwells were used as control samples. At 3, 6, and 12 days after seeding the medium was removed from the plates, and the samples were washed twice with phosphate buffer saline (PBS) prior to proceeding with the assays. Two kinds of tests were performed, the Live/Dead assay kit and the standard MTT assay.

In the case of the Live/Dead assay, a PBS solution containing calcein and ethidium homodimer was prepared according to the manufacturer's indications, added to the cell culture plated, and incubated at 37 °C for 1 h. The activity of intracellular esterase induces non-fluorescent, cell-permeant calcein acetoxymethyl ester to become fluorescent after hydrolysis, giving a green fluorescence to the viable cells. Conversely, ethidium homodimer enters only into damaged cells and binds to nucleic acids producing a red fluorescence that indicates dead cells. Finally, the solution was replaced with fresh PBS before imaging under the Fluorescence Microscope EVOS FLoid Cell Imaging Station (ThermoFisher, Waltham, MA, USA). To obtain a quantitative estimation of cell viability, the fluorescent pixels of both the green channel (live cells) and the red channel (dead cells) of 3 independent images for each type of sample were quantified with ImageJ Software (Rasband, W.S., ImageJ, U. S.

National Institutes of Health, Bethesda, MD, USA) and averaged. Then, the percentage of living cells over the number of total cells was estimated as follows:

$$\text{Viability (\%)} = \frac{\text{Average pixels of the green channel}}{(\text{Average pixels of the green channel} + \text{Average pixels of the red channel})} * 100$$

To perform the MTT assay, at 3, 6, and 12 days after cell seeding, MTT was dissolved into a culture medium without serum (final concentration $500\,\mu g/mL$). Then, 1 mL of the medium was added to each plate and incubated for 2 h at 37 °C. Subsequently, it was removed, and the dark-blue formazan crystals produced by MTT metabolization were solubilized by dimethyl sulfoxide. Finally, the absorbance of the obtained solutions was measured using the CLARIO star Plus microplate reader (BMG Labtech, Ortenberg, Germany), ($\lambda = 570$ nm) and was considered proportional to cell proliferation. The assay was also performed on blank film samples (i.e., T and N gels without cells) to assess colorimetric interference by the gels themselves. For each sample, an average value derived from $n = 3$ independent replicates were calculated and expressed as a percentage of viable cells over control cells (i.e., cells seeded on the standard well surface and considered as 100% viable).

The percentage of cell viability was determined according to the following formula:

$$\text{Viability (\%)} = \frac{\text{Absorption of the treated sample}}{\text{Absorption of the control sample}} * 100$$

3.9. Statistical Analysis

All data were expressed as mean $\pm$ the standard deviation. Statistical significance of experimental data was determined using t-Student test. Differences were considered significant at $p < 0.05$.

4. Results

4.1. Extracts Purity and Integrity

The electrophoretic patterns of T and N are shown in Figure 1 and were characterized by protein bands attributable to the two type I collagen $\alpha1$ and $\alpha2$ chains of about 120 kDa and 110 kDa respectively, as reported in the literature for collagen obtained from Tilapia skin [23,38,44–53]. In particular the $\alpha1$ chain was found at 120 ± 3 kDa for T and 116 ± 2 kDa for N, while $\alpha2$ chain was found at about 110 ± 2 kDa for T and 106 ± 1 kDa for N ($\alpha1$, $p = 0.02$; $\alpha2$, $p = 0.03$). High molecular weight components, including γ chains (trimers) and β chains (dimers) were present. In particular, β chains were found at about 242 ± 12 kDa for T and at 226 ± 8 kDa for N (γ, $p = 0.03$) [23,45,46,52,54–56]. Furthermore, no non-collagenous protein bands were observed, indicating the purity of both collagens and the preservation of their native structure after the extraction process. As expected, the band intensity of $\alpha1$ was higher than that of $\alpha2$ by approximately 2-fold, confirming that the extracted collagens contained two identical subunits of $\alpha1$ and only one $\alpha2$, which was consistent with the molecular composition of type I collagen $(\alpha1)_2\alpha2$. The band intensity ratio of cross-linked chains ($\beta + \gamma$) to non-cross-linked monomer chains ($\alpha1 + \alpha2$) was calculated to evaluate the efficacy of the extraction method in disassembling fibril units [23]. The $(\beta + \gamma)/(\alpha1 + \alpha2)$ ratio was found to be 0.28 ± 0.11 for T and 0.77 ± 0.16 for N ($p = 0.002$). In T more β and γ chains were converted to monomer chains ($\alpha1$ and $\alpha2$), suggesting how the extraction process optimized for T was more effective in collagen fibrils disassembly [23].

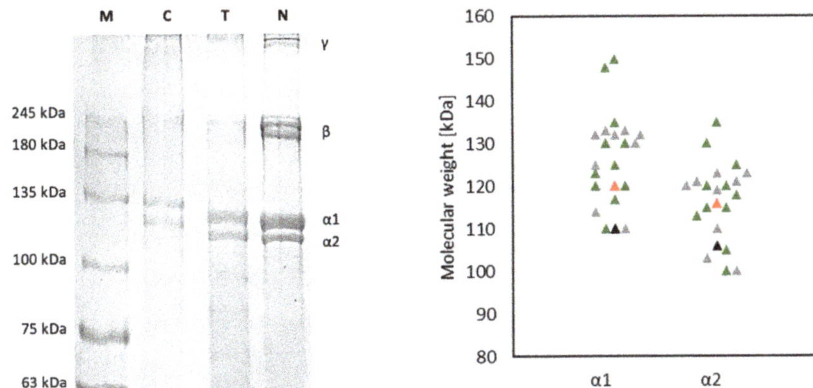

Figure 1. On the **left**: Comparison of electrophoretic pattern of T and N; proteins were separated by SDS-PAGE and Coomassie stained; high molecular weight protein markers (MW) ranging from 10 to 250 kDa were used to estimate the molecular weight of the proteins, type I collagen from horse tendon (C) was used as an example of integrity and purity. On the **right**: comparison of the molecular weight of α1 and α2 chains of T (red) and N (black) with literature data about α1 and α2 of ASC (green) and PSC (grey) isolated from Tilapia skin [23,38,44–46,49–55,57].

4.2. Amino Acid Composition

The amino acid composition of T, expressed as number of residues per 1000 total amino acid residues, was reported in Table 1 and was found to be comparable to N. Moreover, it was found to be in line with literature data on Tilapia skin-derived collagen (Figure 2) [22–24,44,45,50–52,54,57–59], common aquatic organisms [9], and very similar to land mammals [3]. Collagens are typically characterized by a repetitive tripeptide (Glycine-X-Y)n structure, where X and Y positions are usually occupied by a residue of proline and hydroxyproline, respectively. As expected, both T and N samples were found to be rich in glycine, proline, alanine, and hydroxyproline. Glycine, which accounts for about one-third of the total residues, is the most abundant species with 325 and 345 residues in T and N, respectively. The X position of the (Glycine-X-Y)n repetition is often occupied by proline, which is consistent with results reported in Table 1 (112 and 127 proline residues in T and N). The Y position is usually occupied by hydroxyproline, with a content of about 56 residues for both. The hydroxyproline content, although it was found to be lower than the literature data, is known to be correlated with living conditions [60] and feeding. However, to the best of our knowledge, it is not possible to correlate with certainty the low hydroxyproline content to specific species features and breeding conditions. The imino acid content of T and N was found to be about 168 and 184 residues/1000 amino acid residues for T and N, respectively. The higher imino acid content of N reflected its greater structural rigidity since a higher pyrrolidine rings content imposes more restrictions on the polypeptide chain conformation.

Table 1. Amino acid composition of T and N and comparison with the literature data on type I collagen (ASC and PSC) isolated from Tilapia skin [22–24,44,45,50–52,54,57–59]. Results are expressed as residues/1000 total amino acid residues.

Amino Acids	T	N	ASC										PSC						
			[22]	[54]	[50]	[23]	[24]	[52]	[45]	[58]	[59]	[59]	[23]	[51]	[24]	[52]	[57]	[45]	[44]
Alanine	123	142	119	122	141	104	126	171	87	98	123	127	104	118	124	180	124	85	98
Glycine	325	345	356	333	287	252	338	230	322	332	354	360	256	319	333	230	343	343	216
Valine	20	18	17	26	33	19	21	20	22	26	19	18	17	16	19	20	18	25	23
Leucine	23	19	20	26	24	27	24	20	22	22	23	22	23	2	23	20	21	20	28
Isoleucine	10	8	8	16	11	13	10	10	11	7	9	9	9	8	10	10	9	16	14
Proline	112	127	128	115	127	110	110	120	106	112	132	136	111	113	119	121	125	115	122

Polymers **2022**, 14, 1865

Table 1. *Cont.*

Amino Acids	T	N	ASC										PSC						
			[22]	[54]	[50]	[23]	[24]	[52]	[45]	[58]	[59]	[59]	[23]	[51]	[24]	[52]	[57]	[45]	[44]
Methionine	2	1	5	23	14	14	3	8	9	34	10	9	15	6	2	7	6	10	4
Serine	32	32	32	32	19	31	35	21	31	32	35	35	26	33	35	20	31	28	32
Threonine	18	25	22	24	27	26	23	20	15	24	25	25	28	24	23	20	23	17	23
Phenylalanine	16	11	13	20	18	18	14	11	10	16	13	12	12	12	14	11	12	16	23
Aspartate	61	56	42	44	56	60	47	50	40	47	45	45	60	41	46	50	42	37	51
Glutamate	72	69	69	67	51	96	78	91	98	71	71	69	97	68	76	91	70	93	93
Lysine	29	28	20	26	52	35	24	41	32	28	25	25	37	24	23	31	23	22	34
Histidine	1	0	6	3	14	8	8	10	10	7	6	5	6	5	8	10	6	12	12
Tyrosine	4	1	3	3	5	5	4	3	9	1	4	2	2	2	3	4	3	6	6
Cysteine	0	0	0	4	1	0	2	0	0	2	0	0	0	0	3	0	0	0	9
Hydroxyproline	56	57	82	62	70	84	79	80	86	83	50	49	85	77	86	70	86	70	134
Arginine	27	35	58	51	41	82	55	40	90	52	53	52	96	52	51	40	58	85	78
Imino acids	168	184	210	177	197	194	189	200	192	195	182	185	196	190	205	191	211	185	256
Tot.	1000	1000	1000	1000	1000	1000	1000	1000	1000	1000	1000	1000	1000	1000	1000	1000	1000	1000	1000

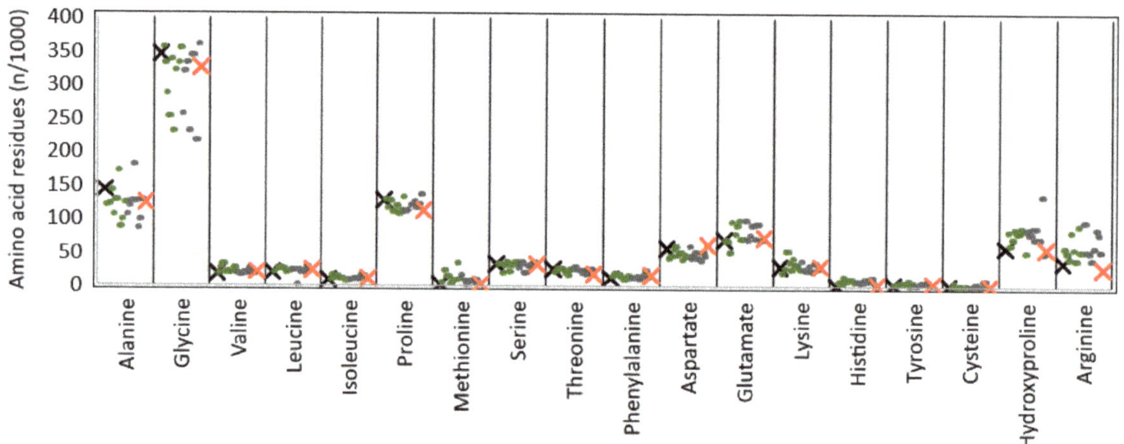

Figure 2. Comparison of the amino acid relative abundance of T (red) and N (black) with the literature data from ASC (green) and PSC (grey) isolated from Tilapia skin [22–24,44,45,50–52,54,57–59].

4.3. Structural Analysis

FT-IR spectra of T and N were both characterized by the presence of the three typical peaks of type I collagen (Figure 3) from land animals [32,33,61,62] and from Tilapia skin [12,21,24,38,44,45,49,50,52,53,55–57,63]. The amides contributes (amide I, amide II and amide III) are fundamental for collagen identification and for secondary structure studies [21,32,33,57].

The amide III band (ca. 1230–1250 cm^{-1}), which resulted from C-N stretching of the peptide group, was found at 1241 cm^{-1} for T and 1243 cm^{-1} for N. The greater band intensity of T suggested the formation of more intermolecular interactions compared to N [24]. The amide II band (ca. 1540–1560 cm^{-1}), which resulted from N-H bending vibration, was found at about 1541 cm^{-1} for T and 1551 cm^{-1} for N. The shift of N to a higher frequency indicated a higher content of ordered molecules compared to T [64]. The amide I (ca. 1630–1680 cm^{-1}), which resulted from the stretching vibrations of the C=O bond along with polypeptide backbone or hydrogen bond coupled with the –COOH groups, was found at about 1644 cm^{-1} for T and 1652 cm^{-1} for N. The decrease of T band intensity indicated that the carbonyl groups were involved more in the cross-linking to form new bands. Thus, the amide I and II shift suggested that T had stronger hydrogen bonds and a lower degree of molecular order than N, because the shift of these peaks to higher frequencies is related to the increased hydrogen bonding in the triple helical structure [50,57].

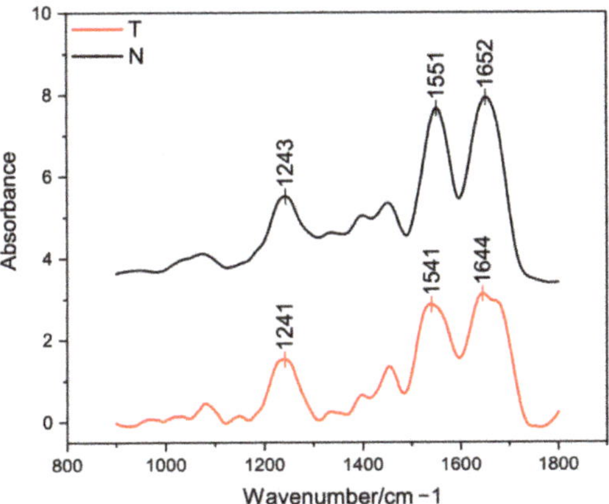

Figure 3. FT-IR spectra of T (red) and N (black) samples (A).

In order to in-depth investigate collagen secondary structure, the amide I peak was further analyzed. According to the literature [38,55], five contributions were identified and analyzed in terms of peak center and relative area under the peak. The β-sheet (peak center: 1610–1642 cm^{-1}), random coil (peak center: 1642–1650 cm^{-1}), α-helix (peak center: 1650–1660 cm^{-1}), β-turn (peak center 1660–1680 cm^{-1}), and β-antiparallel (peak center 1680–1700 cm^{-1}) contributes were identified and compared to the literature (Table 2). While ASC is usually found to be rich in β-sheet [53,55], PSC was revealed to have a more homogeneous distribution of contributes, with a lower β-sheet and a higher α-helix content [55]. Contributes distribution of T and N were found to have a lower β-sheet and a higher α-helix content compared to the literature data [38,53,55]. In particular, N was found to have a higher α-helix content (54%) than T (35%), suggesting its higher structural order. Additionally, according to Terzi et al. [39], the asymmetrical amide I band was deconvoluted in order to separate the contribute arising from single α-helices (ca. 1660 cm^{-1}) from the one related to the triple helix organization (ca. 1630 cm^{-1}) and to evaluate the relative number of triple helices for the investigated collagens. Thus, the percentage of the total amide I peak area ascribable to the triple helix peak was found to be higher for N but not statistically different from T (T: 55 ± 7 %, N: 59 ± 2%, $p = 0.3$).

Table 2. Secondary structure percentage (%) analysis of T and N in the 1600–1700 cm^{-1} spectral range in comparison with the literature data [38,53,55].

Collagen	β-Sheet 1610–1642 cm^{-1}	Random Coil 1642–1650 cm^{-1}	α-Helix 1650–1660 cm^{-1}	β-Turn 1660–1680 cm^{-1}	β-Antiparallel 1680–1700 cm^{-1}
T	7	36	35	16	5
N	4	19	54	19	4
[55] ASC	30	25	24	21	-
[55] PSC	26	26	30	17	-
[38] ASC	24	14	20	33	9
[53] ASC	52	16	14	13	5

4.4. X-rays Structural Analysis

As reported in the literature [32,39,65] type I collagen has a typical 2D diffraction pattern characterized by the presence of the equatorial diffraction signal $q_2 = 0.56$ Å $d_2 = 11.21$ Å (Figure 4, along the black arrow) ascribable to the lateral packing of collagen molecules inside the fibrillary structure, and the meridional diffraction signals $q_1 = 2.24$ Å $d_1 = 2.8$ Å (Figure 4, along the red arrow) related to the axial distance between amino acid residues in the triple helical conformation.

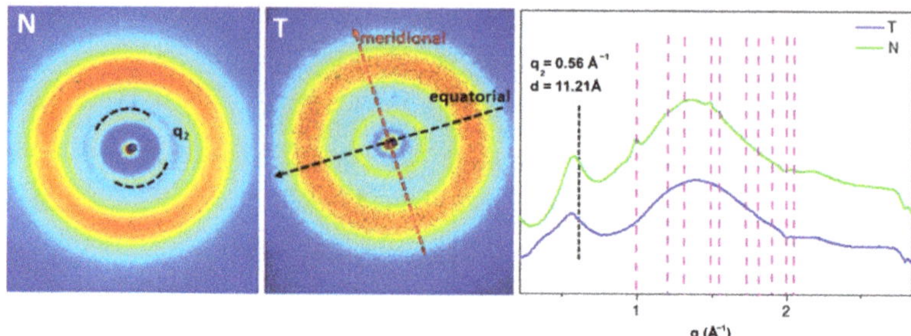

Figure 4. On the **left** the 2D WAXS patterns on N and T samples. The black and the red arrows show the directions along which the equatorial and the meridional diffraction signals, respectively. On the **right** the 1D diffraction profiles of both samples. The equatorial peak (q_2) is marked with the black line. The magenta lines show the peak positions of Ultralene sachet.

On fish skin collagen, in both T and N patterns, the meridional diffraction peak was no longer visible. In N, a preferential orientation of the equatorial signal (q_2), marker of the molecular lateral packing retention, was clearly detectable as two small arcs with high signal intensity distributed along the same direction marked with the dashed arc, the equator (Figure 4, N). In the diffraction pattern of T (Figure 4, T), the observed equatorial q_2 signal along the black arrow was characterized by signal intensity distributed as a continuous ring, marker of no preferential orientation, and, therefore, of a reduced packing order in the molecule. Comparing the 1D WAXS diffraction profiles, it was observed that the equatorial diffraction peaks at $q_2 \sim 0.56 \pm 0.03$ Å^{-1} corresponded to the average value of d-spacing of 11 Å in both samples. However, as shown in Table 3, the FWHM of the q_2 in T is higher than in N ones, leading to a lower extent of the crystalline domain in T (37 ± 3 Å) that in N collagen (52 ± 6 Å), thus a reduced lateral packing and molecular order in T.

Table 3. Mean values of lateral packing (q_2) of collagen molecules in the samples in the reciprocal space (Å^{-1}) and the corresponding values in the direct space (Å). The FWHM value of the analyzed diffraction peaks is also shown, and the relative value of the crystalline domain for the lateral packing. The mean values were obtained from the mean of the experimental values measured for each sample.

Sample	Reciprocal Space (Å^{-1})		Direct Space (Å)	
	q_2 Equatorial	FWHM	d_2 Equatorial	Cristalline Domain
T	0.55 ± 0.03	0.169 ± 0.002	11	37 ± 3
N	0.57 ± 0.03	0.120 ± 0.001	11	52 ± 6

4.5. Thermal Properties

Representative thermograms of T and N are shown in Figure 5. While heating, the inter-chain hydrogen bonds of the right-handed superhelix break and the triple helix unfolds in random chains. The endothermal peak present within the temperature range of 0–100 °C was attributed to the T_d of collagen [33] that was about 32.6 ± 0.2 °C for T and of 35.5 ± 0.1 °C for N ($p = 0.00006$) [66]. According to the literature, T_d was found to be lower than that of land animals [9,34] and comparable to that of Tilapia skin derived collagen (Figure 6) [12,13,22–24,44,45,51,52,54,56–59,66]. The higher T_d value of N reflected its higher native structure preservation compared to T, confirmed also by the higher enthalpy necessary for the transition (T: 0.33 ± 0.05 J/g, N: 0.53 ± 0.06 J/g, $p = 0.01$) and by the higher amount of cross-linked β+γ chains (see Section 4.1) [67].

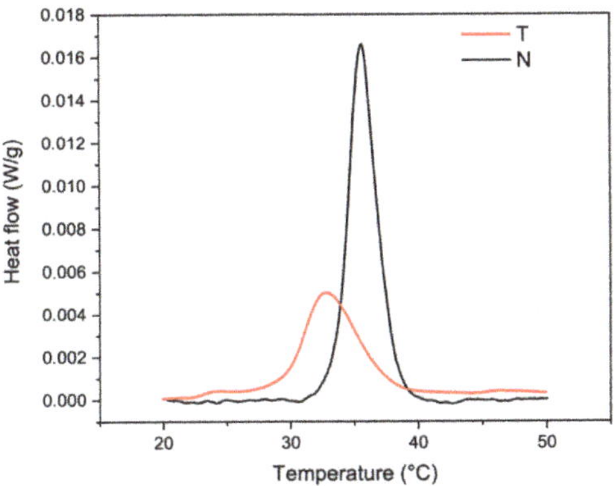

Figure 5. Representative DSC thermograms of T (red) and N (black) samples showing the endothermic phenomena of type I collagen denaturation.

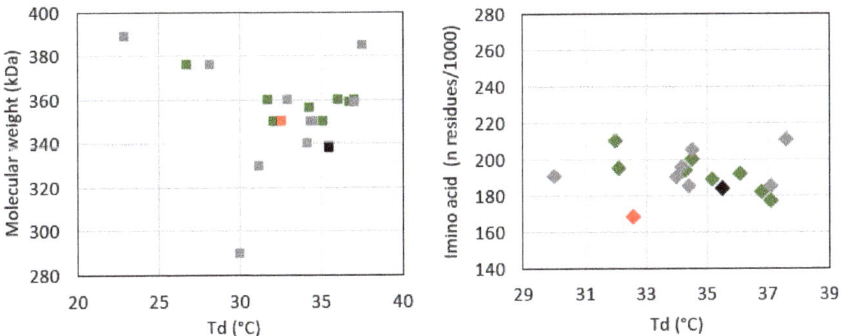

Figure 6. Correlation of the denaturation temperature with the hydroxyproline content (**left**) and the molecular weight (**right**), and comparison of T (red) and N (black) data with literature data on ASC (green) and PSC (grey) [12,13,22–24,44,45,51,52,54,56–59,66].

According to several studies, there is a direct correlation between the thermal stability of the proteins and their amino acid content [18,67,68]. In particular, the T_d is directly related to the imino acid content [22] and the non-helical region extent, which are responsible of the order and the structural compactness of the protein [59]. In this sense, the higher hydroxyproline and imino acid content of N (184 residues/1000) compared to T (168 residues/1000) might contribute to explaining its higher T_d value. Concerning the molecular weight, though SDS-PAGE revealed a higher molecular weight of T compared to N, this did not correspond to higher thermal resistance. Despite these experimental pieces of evidence, the analysis of the literature data did not show any clear correlation between protein molecular weight and T_d (Figure 6, left) on the one hand and between the protein amino acid composition and T_d (Figure 6, right) on the other. Reasonably, other parameters, such as growing conditions, extraction procedures (e.g., working temperature, acid treatment, pepsin-based treatment, mechanical fragmentation), and analytical techniques, may affect protein denaturation temperature [9,33,60,69,70].

4.6. Wettability

It is known that cell-material interactions are affected by surface properties and a moderate wettability is optimal for cell adhesion and proliferation [71]. The contact angle instantly recorded on T and N film was of $77 \pm 5°$ and $86 \pm 4°$, respectively ($p = 0.025$) (Figure 7). The slightly higher hydrophilicity of T samples might contribute to different cell responses.

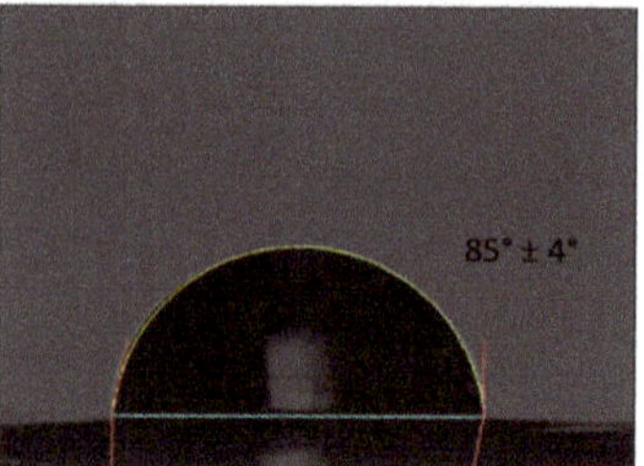

Figure 7. Instant contact angle on T (**left**) and N (**right**) substrates.

4.7. Mechanical Properties

Tensile tests were performed to investigate the mechanical properties of T and N substrates. As expected, tensile curves were characterized by a linear elastic region, followed by a non-elastic region and a rupture region (Figure 8). Although both formulations are composed only of native type I collagen, the slight differences found in their molecular structure strongly affected their mechanical behavior. The constitutive bond of T was found to be statistically different from N in terms of E, σ_{max}, and ε_r. In particular, while E and σ_{max} values of T (E_T: 0.5 ± 0.1 MPa, $\sigma_{max,T}$: 0.8 ± 0.1 MPa) were found to be about three times lower than N (E_N: 1.6 ± 0.2 MPa, $\sigma_{max,N}$: 2.5 ± 0.7 MPa) (p = 0.002 and p = 0.01, respectively), ε_r was found to be about 1.5 times higher than that of N ($\varepsilon_{r,T}$: 85 ± 12 %, $\varepsilon_{r,N}$: 59 ± 6 %, p = 0.02). These results suggest that the N-based substrate is characterized by higher stiffness, likely due to the broad conservation of its native structure and too strong inter-chain interactions of collagen molecules. However, a lower ε_r corresponds to a higher E value of N collagen. On the other hand, the T-based substrate displays greater elasticity as it reaches higher ε_r values but lower E. This behavior might be associated with the lower structural conservation degree that promotes the formation of inter- and intra-chain interactions between collagen molecules.

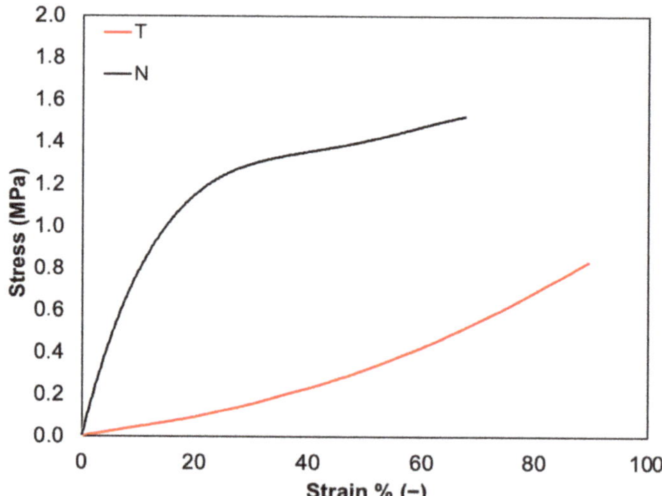

Figure 8. Representative stress-strain curves of T film (red) compared to N film (black).

4.8. Biocompatibility

Two cellular assays, MTT and Live/Dead, were performed to assess the cytocompatibility of the two materials. The two assays provide a collective estimation of the health status of the cells upon colorimetric evaluation of the activity of cytoplasmic and mitochondrial enzymes and of the integrity of the cell membrane. Thin collagen films were casted into culture plates, and 3T3 mouse fibroblasts were seeded over them. In both tests, cells seeded into standard multiwell plates were used as a control. Figure 9 reported cells viability percentage over time for both T and N. After 3 days, it looks that the viability of the cells grown over the two substrates was much lower than that of control cells, being equal to 54% and 29% in the case of T and N, respectively. At 6 and 12 days, the viability raised up to 100% for cells grown over the T substrates, while it reached 66% and 92% in the case of cells seeded over N collagen, respectively. From day 6, cells recovered their viability reaching values close to control samples. This cellular resilience likely indicates that the substrates do not exert a toxic effect, but rather the topography and structural features of the collagen films affect the adhesion and the replication phase of the cells, as already reported [72–74]. Interestingly, the differences between the metabolic response of cells grown on T and N at days 3 and 6, respectively, were statistically significant, supporting the evidence of a different affinity between materials and cells. To shed light on the interactions between the substrates and the cells, optical images of cells seeded over T, N and standard plates, respectively, were acquired (Figure S1). After 1 and 3 days, the fibroblasts grown over the T film showed the typical elongated morphology of these cells while the density was slightly lower than control samples. On the other hand, after 1 day, cells seeded on N film looked spherical, an indication of weak adhesion, while after 3 days, as cell density increased, both elongated and spherical cell clusters coexisted. This heterogeneous cell culture was maintained up to day 6, while at day 12 cell distribution was similar to that of the control.

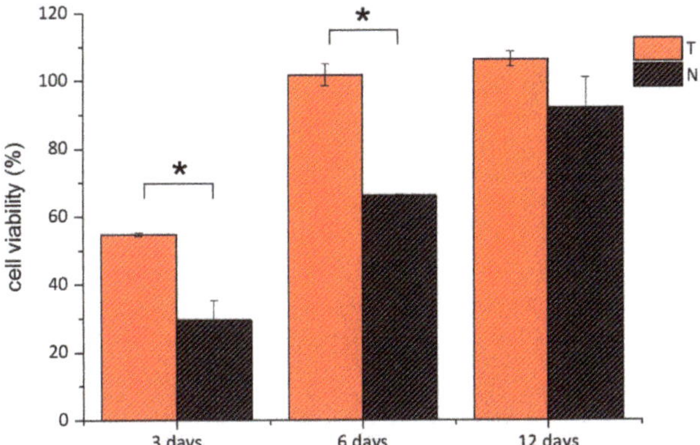

Figure 9. MTT viability assay of 3T3 cells grown over T (red bars) and N (black bars) was performed after 3, 6, and 12 days. Data were reported as the percentage viability of the samples over the control cells (i.e., cells grown on standard plates). (*) indicates statistical significance with $p < 0.01$.

Live/Dead assay was performed under the same experimental conditions. As shown in Figure 10, fibroblasts looked viable in both samples and at all the imaged times (Figures S2–S4). Few dead cells were detected, as reported in the inset of Figure 10. The morphology and the distribution of the cells were in agreement with the previous images and confirmed that the results of the MTT assay did not indicate inherent toxicity of the biomaterials but a delayed replication time as compared to the control.

The quantitative analysis of the fluorescent pixels by the Image J Software 1.52t (NIH, USA) allowed us to estimate the number of living cells. The histograms in Figure 11 showed that the percentage number of viable cells over the total cells was very similar in all the samples. Based on these findings, we concluded that the T and N were biocompatible but presented different surface topography that affected cellular adhesion and replication time.

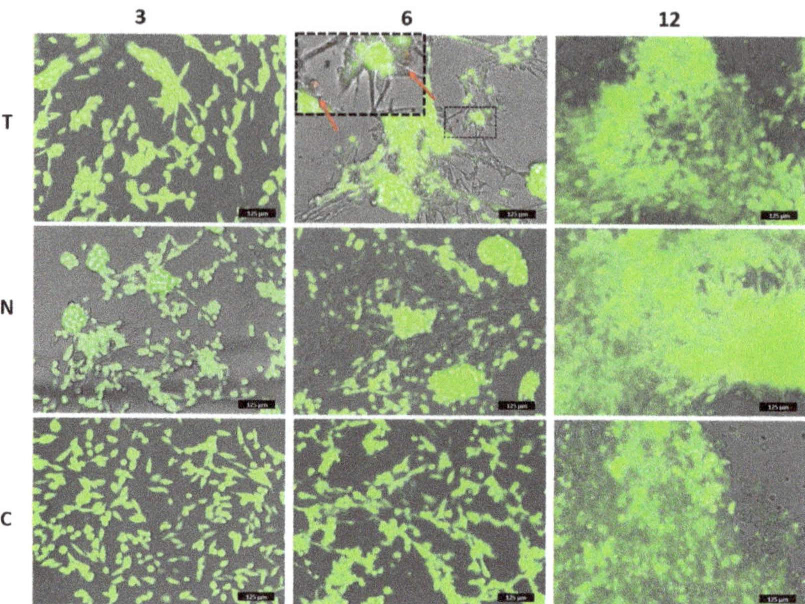

Figure 10. Live/Dead assay of 3T3 cells grown over T and N was performed after 3, 6, and 12 days. The images correspond to the overlapped fluorescent channels (green for calcein signal and red for ethidium homodimer) and the bright field. The inset in the upper-central panel shows some dead cells among the live ones. Note: in the panels in which cells are localized on different focal lanes (elongated on the bottom plane and clustered on the upper plane), the green fluorescent channel has been slightly reduced to allow the detection of the dead cells. Please, refer to the images of Figures S2–S4 for the original signal intensity for each fluorescent channel. Scale bar is 125 μm.

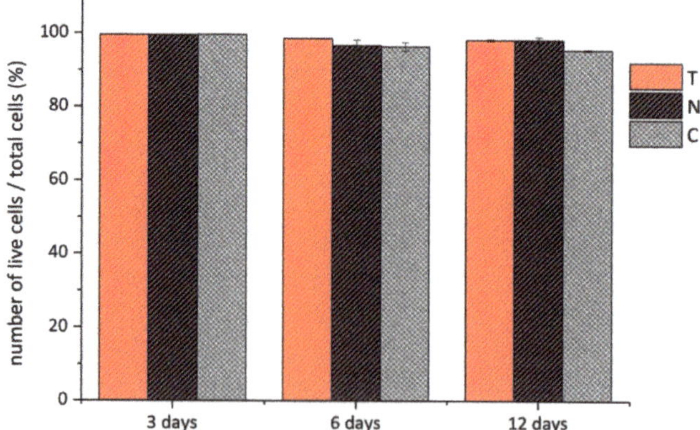

Figure 11. Live/Dead assay of 3T3 cells grown over T (red bars) and N (black bars) substrates performed after 3, 6, and 12 days. The data are presented as the average percentage of live cells over the number of total cells. The analysis was performed through Image J Software over three different fluorescent images for each sample and measuring the green (i.e., live cells) and red (i.e., dead cells) pixels of each image.

5. Discussion

Collagen is the most abundant structural protein of animal tissues that provides strength and structural stability on the one hand and performs highly specialized regulatory functions on the other. The interesting structural and biological properties of collagen, besides its biodegradability, high biocompatibility, and low immunogenicity [2–7], made it one of the most widely required biomaterials for food and healthcare applications, including medical care, pharmaceutics, and cosmetics [75].

The increasing demand for collagen brought to the examination of several extraction sources, including mammals (i.e., bovine, swine, equine, ovine, rodents), birds, and marine organisms (i.e., fish and invertebrates), with the aim of finding the optimal one in term of biocompatibility, safety, and availability [9]. The best extraction source is represented by mammals for the high sequence homology with human collagen [3]. However, mammals-derived collagen use is limited because of issues such as the high immune response rate, zoonosis transmission risks, and religious/cultural constraints [3,8,9]. Due to these restrictions, alternative safer sources were investigated.

In this perspective, marine organisms seemed to be free from all the aforementioned limitations [9,13] and attracted interest as safe and abundant sources for collagen extraction [9,11,12]. In particular, among fish species, Nile tilapia (*Oreochromis niloticus*) and its byproducts (i.e., skin, scale, bone) are emerging as alternative sources for collagen isolation. Being one of the World's most representative species of the fisheries and aquaculture food sector for its fast growth speed, adaptability, reproducibility in captivity, easy feed, and easy processing [22,25,26] it offers a huge quantity of byproducts (70–85% of the total weight of catch) that could be exploited to develop waste recovery technologies to obtain high added-value products and at the same time to reduce the environmental pollution related to their breeding and processing [10,19,20]. Additionally, eco-sustainable aquaponic systems give the possibility to obtain hazardous-free Tilapia biomass with an additional added value and controlled properties over time. Thus, the possibility to valorize the huge quantity of fish industry waste and byproducts as collagen source makes Tilapia-derived collagen eco-friendlier and particularly attractive in terms of profitability and cost-effectiveness.

In this work, type I collagen extracted according to a proprietary process from the skin of aquaponics-derived Tilapia was characterized from a chemical, physical, mechanical, and biological point of view and compared with a commercially available isoform. Particular attention was paid to its native structure preservation since it is widely known that it not only influences bioengineering parameters but also cell-biomaterial interaction and thus cell processes [65,76–78].

First of all, the protein integrity and the presence of other protein species were evaluated. The revealed electrophoretic pattern confirmed the purity of the extracts and the extraction process accuracy since there were only two bands visible of about 120 kDa and 110 kDa attributable to $\alpha1(I)$ and $\alpha2(I)$ chain of type I collagen [23,45,46,52,54–56]. In particular, T was found to have a molecular weight slightly higher than N (T: $\alpha1 = 120 \pm 3$ kDa, $\alpha2 = 110 \pm 2$ kDa; N: $\alpha1 = 116 \pm 2$ kDa, $\alpha2 = 106 \pm 1$ kDa) and a content of high molecular weight components lower than N (T: 0.28 ± 0.11; N: 0.77 ± 0.16). The conversion of more cross-linked chains (β, γ) into non-cross-linked monomer chains ($\alpha1$, $\alpha2$) directly indicated a greater efficacy of T extraction method in disassembling fibril units [23].

The integrity of T secondary structure and its ultrastructure was evaluated by means of FT-IR and WAXS. The presence of the three amide contributes (amide I: 1644 cm^{-1} for T, 1652 cm^{-1} for N; amide II: 1541 cm^{-1} for T, 1551 cm^{-1} for N; amide III: 1241 cm^{-1} for T, 1243 cm^{-1} for N) allowed to confirm the protein identity, that was attributable to type I collagen, comparable to N and according to literature data about Tilapia skin derived collagen [12,21,24,38,44,45,49,50,52,53,55–57,63]. The amides shift suggested that T had a lower degree of molecular order than N, besides a lower α-helix content (T: 35%; N: 54%). However, from the deconvolution of the amide I came out a slightly lower but not statistically different triple helix content of T from N (T: 55 ± 7%, N: 59 ± 2%), suggesting the employment of less tightened extraction conditions and better preservation of native collagen structure of N. Higher partial preservation of the native lateral packing of collagen molecules in N with respect to T was observed through WAXs measurements. However, the presence of a clear equatorial signal in T collagen allowed us to identify the presence of native structure, although it is less organized than the N one. Indeed, the continuous ring intensity distribution of the equatorial diffraction signal in T, associated with the decrease of the extension of the crystalline domain, obtained by the peak analyses, is a clear marker of the presence of lateral packing arrangement of triple helices. While in N collagen triple helices are arranged by a preferential orientation in a larger crystalline domain.

In order to ascribe protein structural differences to compositional variations, protein amino acid composition was also investigated. The amino acid composition of T was found to be comparable to N, and the literature data on Tilapia skin collagen [22–24,44,45,50–52,54,57–59], common aquatic organisms [3,9], and to be very similar to land mammals [3]. Thus, both T and N were found to be rich in glycine (T: 325/1000 residues; N: 345/1000 residues), proline (T: 112/1000 residues; N: 127/1000 residues), alanine (T: 123/1000 residues; N: 142/1000 residues), and hydroxyproline (T: 56/1000 residues; N: 57/1000 residues). The imino acid content of T (168/1000 residues) and N (184/1000 residues) revealed a greater N structural rigidity since a higher pyrrolidine rings content imposes more restrictions on the polypeptide chain conformation.

To investigate how the collagen isolation procedure affects its thermal stability, thermal behavior was investigated. Thermograms revealed a T_d value of T (32.6 ± 0.2 °C) that was similar to that one of N (35.5 ± 0.1 °C) and according to literature data about Tilapia skin-derived collagen [12,13,22–24,44,45,51,52,54,56–59,66]. In addition, the lower denaturation enthalpy value of T compared to N (T: 0.33 ± 0.05 J/g; N: 0.53 ± 0.06 J/g) indicated that lower energy is required to start the protein unfolding process in T collagen, likely due to slightly lower preservation of the native structure than N. This result is accordance with the SDS-PAGE, FT-IR and WAXS findings. According to several studies, there is a direct correlation between protein thermal stability and their imino acid content [18,67,68] and non-helical region extent [59]. While the imino acid content might contribute to explain protein T_d value, any correlation with protein molecular weight was found. Additionally, literature data analysis did not show any clear correlation between protein T_d, amino acid composition, and molecular weight. Reasonably, other parameters, such as growing conditions, extraction procedures, and analytical techniques, may strongly affect protein features [9,33,69] and deeply affect data comparative analysis. Anyhow, T_d is key parameter to validate Tilapia-derived collagen as a raw biomaterial for healthcare applications, and its lower value than that of land animals [9,34] restricted its use. Nevertheless, various strategies have been developed for improving fish collagen thermal stability. Among these, recalling to chemical cross-linking (e.g., carbodiimides, genipine) [79] allowed to successfully increase fish collagen T_d up to body temperature and thus to show great promise for biomedical or clinical use.

Cellular studies indicate that T substrates are highly biocompatible and support the adhesion, growth, and spreading of fibroblasts. In addition, the topography of the substrate looks to play a crucial role in determining the interactions among the substrate and the cells. The comparison of the two collagen substrates shows that adhesion of the fibroblasts over T occurs faster than over N rapidly. On the other hand, the tensile tests showed that T substrates are softer than N, and several literature studies evidenced that fibroblasts generally prefer stiffer surfaces [80,81]. Interestingly, the experimental evidence suggests that beyond surface stiffness, the structure and the organization of collagen-based substrates affect the interaction with the cells.

6. Conclusions

Type I collagen is one of the most widely used biomaterials for healthcare applications for its well-known advantages. Its increasing demand brought to the examination of several extraction sources, with the aim of finding the optimal one in term of biocompatibility, safety, and availability. Although the discovery of numerous alternatives, the best extraction source is currently represented by mammals. However, several issues limited their use. In this circumstance, marine organisms seemed to be free from many limitations and promising raw materials sources for collagen extraction. Among fish species, Nile tilapia byproducts emerged as an alternative source for collagen isolation because of their abundance from fisheries and aquaculture plants. The recovery from eco-sustainable aquaponic systems gave the possibility to obtain hazardous-free Tilapia biomass with additional added value and controlled properties.

In this perspective, type I collagen was characterized from a chemical, physical, mechanical, and biological point of view and compared with a commercially available isoform. Particular attention was paid to its native structure preservation since it is widely known that it influences not only bioengineering parameters but also cell-biomaterial interaction and thus cell processes. All analyses confirmed that the proprietary process optimized for type I collagen extraction allowed to isolate pure native collagen and preserve its native conformational structure. The slight differences observed between T collagen and the commercial preparation may be due to different breeding conditions, besides extraction and purification procedures, resulting in collagen molecular organization alteration and thus in its bioactivity modification. These evidence, in combination with the positive feedback of the cellular studies, suggested that type I collagen from aquaponics-raised Tilapia skin could be a suitable high-controlled alternative biomaterial for healthcare application. The bioactivity of fish collagen makes its use in multiple forms (including native, gelatin, and peptide form) in rapid expansion for specific biomedical pharmaceutical, cosmetics, nutraceutical, nutricosmetic, and food applications. Although fish collagen has been proposed as an alternative biomaterial for tissue engineering applications, there is a lack of literature data about its immunogenicity. The host immunologic response is a critical aspect when considering it for clinical implementation since the success of a biomaterial-based formulation for healthcare applications is directly related to the immune response to the selected material. Based on these findings, further studies should be performed to evaluate the immunogenicity response triggered by the isolated type I collagen. Additionally, to the best of our knowledge, no studies were available on the effective lower cost of fish-derived collagen compared to mammalian-derived collagen, an accurate cost-effectiveness study should be performed.

Supplementary Materials: The following supporting information can be downloaded at: https://www.mdpi.com/article/10.3390/polym14091865/s1, Figure S1: optical images acquired after 1-, 3-, 6-, and 12-days growth of 3T3 cells over T, N substrates and standard plates -control samples- (C). Figure S2. Live/dead assay of 3T3 cells performed after 3 days growth over T and N substrates. Control samples are reported as well (C). The first column refers to the overlaid channels, while the others correspond to the bright field, to the green channel of calcein and to the red channel of ethidium homodimer, respectively. Figure S3. Live/dead assay of 3T3 cells performed after 6 days growth over T and N substrates. Control samples are reported as well (C). The first column refers to the overlaid channels, while the others correspond to the bright field, to the green channel of calcein and to the red channel of ethidium homodimer, respectively. Figure S4. Live/dead assay of 3T3 cells performed after 12 days growth over T and N substrates. Control samples are reported as well (C). The first column refers to the overlaid channels, while the others correspond to the bright field, to the green channel of calcein and to the red channel of ethidium homodimer, respectively.

Author Contributions: Conceptualization, N.G., and L.S.; methodology, N.G., A.Q., A.G., A.T.; validation, M.L.N., and L.S.; formal analysis, N.G., A.Q., A.T.; investigation, N.G., A.Q., A.G., A.T., G.E.D.B., and P.L.; resources, A.S. (Alessandro Sannino), A.C.; data curation, N.G., A.T., A.Q., A.S. (Alessandro Sicuro); writing—original draft preparation, N.G., A.T., A.Q., G.E.D.B., and F.S.B.; writing—review and editing, L.S., A.G., T.S., C.G., L.C., A.C., A.S. (Alessandro Sannino); visualization, N.G. and L.S.; supervision, L.C., C.G., A.S. (Alessandro Sannino), and L.S.; project administration, A.C., and F.S.B.; funding acquisition, A.C. All authors have read and agreed to the published version of the manuscript.

Funding: This work was supported by the project "ISEPA-Improving Sustainability, Efficiency and Profitability of Large Scale Aquaponics (CUP: B37H17004760007)" funded by Regione Puglia in the frame-work of "InnoNetwork-Sostegno alle attività di R&S per lo sviluppo di nuove tecnologie sostenibili, di nuovi prodotti e servizi".

Institutional Review Board Statement: Not applicable.

Informed Consent Statement: Not applicable.

Acknowledgments: R. Lassandro is acknowledged for his support in the XMI-Lab at CNR-IC.

Conflicts of Interest: The authors declare no conflict of interest.

References

1. Gelse, K.; Pöschl, E.; Aigner, T. Collagens—Structure, function, and biosynthesis. *Adv. Drug Deliv. Rev.* **2003**, *55*, 1531–1546. [CrossRef] [PubMed]
2. Salvatore, L.; Gallo, N.; Natali, M.L.; Terzi, A.; Sannino, A.; Madaghiele, M. Mimicking the Hierarchical Organization of Natural Collagen: Toward the Development of Ideal Scaffolding Material for Tissue Regeneration. *Front. Bioeng. Biotechnol.* **2021**, *9*, 644595. [CrossRef] [PubMed]
3. Gallo, N.; Natali, M.L.; Sannino, A.; Salvatore, L. An overview of the use of equine collagen as emerging material for biomedical applications. *J. Funct. Biomater.* **2020**, *11*, 79. [CrossRef] [PubMed]
4. Bianchini, P.; Parma, B. Immunological safety evaluation of a horse collagen haemostatic pad. *Arzneim. Forsch./Drug Res.* **2001**, *51*, 414–419. [CrossRef] [PubMed]
5. Lynn, A.; Yannas, I.; Bonfield, W. Antigenicity and immunogenicity of collagen. *J. Biomed. Mater. Res. Part B Appl. Biomater.* **2004**, *71*, 343–354. [CrossRef]
6. Delgado, L.M.; Bayon, Y.; Pandit, A.; Zeugolis, D.I. To Cross-Link or Not to Cross-Link? Cross-Linking Associated Foreign Body Response of Collagen-Based Devices. *Tissue Eng. Part B Rev.* **2015**, *21*, 298–313. [CrossRef]
7. Delgado, L.M.; Shologu, N.; Fuller, K.; Zeugolis, D.I. Acetic acid and pepsin result in high yield, high purity and low macrophage response collagen for biomedical applications. *Biomed. Mater.* **2017**, *12*, 065009. [CrossRef]
8. Silvipriya, K.S.; Kumar, K.K.; Bhat, A.R.; Kumar, B.D.; John, A.; Lakshmanan, P. Collagen: Animal sources and biomedical application. *J. Appl. Pharm. Sci.* **2015**, *5*, 123–127. [CrossRef]
9. Salvatore, L.; Gallo, N.; Natali, M.L.; Campa, L.; Lunetti, P.; Madaghiele, M.; Blasi, F.S.; Corallo, A.; Capobianco, L.; Sannino, A. Marine collagen and its derivatives: Versatile and sustainable bio-resources for healthcare. *Mater. Sci. Eng. C* **2020**, *113*, 110963. [CrossRef]
10. Felician, F.F.; Xia, C.; Qi, W.; Xu, H. Collagen from Marine Biological Sources and Medical Applications. *Chem. Biodivers.* **2018**, *15*, e1700557. [CrossRef]
11. Berillis, P. Marine Collagen: Extraction and Applications. In *Research Trends Biochemistry, Molecular Biology and Microbiology*; SM Group Open Access eBook; SM Group: Kolkata, India, 2015; pp. 1–13.
12. Valenzuela-Rojo, D.R.; López-Cervantes, J.; Sánchez-Machado, D.I. Tilapia (*Oreochromis aureus*) Collagen for Medical Biomaterials. *Seaweed Biomater.* **2018**, *4*, 48–66. [CrossRef]
13. Zhang, J.; Wenhui, W.; Elango, J. Antigen Response Properties of Tilapia Skin Type I Collagen. *Food Sci. (Biol. Eng.)* **2015**, *36*, 79–83. [CrossRef]
14. Lv, L.-C.; Huang, Q.-Y.; Ding, W.; Xiao, X.-H.; Zhang, H.-Y.; Xiong, L.-X. Fish gelatin: The novel potential applications. *J. Funct. Foods* **2019**, *63*, 103581. [CrossRef]
15. Yoon, H.J.; Shin, S.R.; Cha, J.M.; Lee, S.-H.; Kim, J.-H.; Do, J.T.; Song, H.; Bae, H. Cold water fish gelatin methacryloyl hydrogel for tissue engineering application. *PLoS ONE* **2016**, *11*, e0163902. [CrossRef] [PubMed]
16. Wang, Z.; Tian, Z.; Menard, F.; Kim, K. Comparative study of gelatin methacrylate hydrogels from different sources for biofabrication applications. *Biofabrication* **2017**, *9*, 044101. [CrossRef]
17. León-López, A.; Morales-Peñaloza, A.; Martínez-Juárez, V.M.; Vargas-Torres, A.; Zeugolis, D.I.; Aguirre-Álvarez, G. Hydrolyzed collagen-sources and applications. *Molecules* **2019**, *24*, 4031. [CrossRef]
18. Lim, Y.-S.; Ok, Y.-J.; Hwang, S.-Y.; Kwak, J.-Y.; Yoon, S. Marine Collagen as A Promising Biomaterial for Applications. *Mar. Drugs* **2019**, *17*, 467. [CrossRef]
19. Pal, G.K.; Suresh, P. Sustainable valorisation of seafood by-products: Recovery of collagen and development of collagen-based novel functional food ingredients. *Innov. Food Sci. Emerg. Technol.* **2016**, *37*, 201–215. [CrossRef]
20. Martins, M.E.O.; Sousa, J.R.; Claudino, R.L.; Lino, S.C.O.; Vale, D.A.D.; Silva, A.L.C.; Morais, J.P.S.; Filho, M.D.S.M.D.S.; De Souza, B.W.S. Thermal and Chemical Properties of Gelatin from Tilapia (*Oreochromis niloticus*) Scale. *J. Aquat. Food Prod. Technol.* **2018**, *27*, 1120–1133. [CrossRef]
21. Ge, B.; Wang, H.; Li, J.; Liu, H.; Yin, Y.; Zhang, N.; Qin, S. Comprehensive Assessment of Nile Tilapia Skin (Oreochromis niloticus) Collagen Hydrogels for Wound Dressings. *Mar. Drugs* **2020**, *18*, 178. [CrossRef]
22. Zeng, S.-K.; Zhang, C.-H.; Lin, H.; Yang, P.; Hong, P.-Z.; Jiang, Z. Isolation and characterisation of acid-solubilised collagen from the skin of Nile tilapia (*Oreochromis niloticus*). *Food Chem.* **2009**, *116*, 879–883. [CrossRef]
23. Potaros, T.; Raksakulthai, N.; Runglerdkreangkrai, J.; Worawattanamateekul, W. Characteristics of collagen from nile tilapia (*Oreochromis niloticus*) skin isolated by two different methods. *Kasetsart J. Nat. Sci.* **2009**, *43*, 584–593.

24. Sun, L.; Hou, H.; Li, B.; Zhang, Y. Characterization of acid- and pepsin-soluble collagen extracted from the skin of Nile tilapia (*Oreochromis niloticus*). *Int. J. Biol. Macromol.* **2017**, *99*, 8–14. [CrossRef] [PubMed]

25. El-Sayed, A.F.M. *Tilapia Culture*; CABI: Wallingford, UK, 2006.

26. LWang, L.; Jiang, Y.; Wang, X.; Zhou, J.; Cui, H.; Xu, W.; He, Y.; Ma, H.; Gao, R. Effect of oral administration of collagen hydrolysates from Nile tilapia on the chronologically aged skin. *J. Funct. Foods* **2018**, *44*, 112–117. [CrossRef]

27. Barroso, R.M.; Pizarro Munoz, A.E.; Cai, J. *Social and Economic Performance of Tilapia Farming in Brazil*; FAO Fisheries and Aquaculture Circular: Rome, Italy, 2019.

28. Yep, B.; Zheng, Y. Aquaponic trends and challenges—A review. *J. Clean. Prod.* **2019**, *228*, 1586–1599. [CrossRef]

29. Liu, D.; Zhang, X.; Li, T.; Yang, H.; Zhang, H.; Regenstein, J.M.; Zhou, P. Extraction and characterization of acid- and pepsin-soluble collagens from the scales, skins and swim-bladders of grass carp (*Ctenopharyngodon idella*). *Food Biosci.* **2015**, *9*, 68–74. [CrossRef]

30. Falini, G.; Fermani, S.; Foresti, E.; Parma, B.; Rubini, K.; Sidoti, M.C.; Roveri, N. Films of self-assembled purely helical type I collagen molecules. *J. Mater. Chem.* **2004**, *14*, 2297–2302. [CrossRef]

31. Ruozi, B.; Tosi, G.; Leo, E.; Parma, B.; Vismara, S.; Forni, F.; Vandelli, M.A. Intact collagen and atelocollagen sponges: Characterization and ESEM observation. *Mater. Sci. Eng. C* **2007**, *27*, 802–810. [CrossRef]

32. Terzi, A.; Gallo, N.; Bettini, S.; Sibillano, T.; Altamura, D.; Campa, L.; Natali, M.L.; Salvatore, L.; Madaghiele, M.; De Caro, L.; et al. Investigations of processing–induced structural changes in horse type-I collagen at sub and supramolecular levels. *Front. Bioeng. Biotechnol.* **2019**, *7*, 203. [CrossRef]

33. Salvatore, L.; Gallo, N.; Aiello, D.; Lunetti, P.; Barca, A.; Blasi, L.; Madaghiele, M.; Bettini, S.; Giancane, G.; Hasan, M.; et al. An insight on type I collagen from horse tendon for the manufacture of implantable devices. *Int. J. Biol. Macromol.* **2020**, *154*, 291–306. [CrossRef]

34. Gallo, N.; Natali, M.L.; Curci, C.; Picerno, A.; Gallone, A.; Vulpi, M.; Vitarelli, A.; Ditonno, P.; Cascione, M.; Sallustio, F.; et al. Analysis of the physico-chemical, mechanical and biological properties of crosslinked type-i collagen from horse tendon: Towards the development of ideal scaffolding material for urethral regeneration. *Materials* **2021**, *14*, 7648. [CrossRef] [PubMed]

35. Lawrence, A.-M.; Besir, H. Staining of proteins in gels with Coomassie G-250 without organic solvent and acetic acid. *J. Vis. Exp.* **2009**, *30*, e1350. [CrossRef] [PubMed]

36. Lunetti, P.; Damiano, F.; De Benedetto, G.; Siculella, L.; Pennetta, A.; Muto, L.; Paradies, E.; Marobbio, C.M.T.; Dolce, V.; Capobianco, L. Capobianco, Characterization of Human and Yeast Mitochondrial Glycine Carriers with Implications for Heme Biosynthesis and Anemia. *J. Biol. Chem.* **2016**, *291*, 19746–19759. [CrossRef] [PubMed]

37. Fico, D.; Margapoti, E.; Pennetta, A.; De Benedetto, G.E. An enhanced GC/MS procedure for the identification of proteins in paint microsamples. *J. Anal. Methods Chem.* **2018**, *2018*, 6032084. [CrossRef]

38. Shi, C.; Bi, C.; Ding, M.; Xie, J.; Xu, C.; Qiao, R.; Wang, X.; Zhong, J. Polymorphism and stability of nanostructures of three types of collagens from bovine flexor tendon, rat tail, and tilapia skin. *Food Hydrocoll.* **2019**, *93*, 253–260. [CrossRef]

39. Terzi, A.; Storelli, E.; Bettini, S.; Sibillano, T.; Altamura, D.; Salvatore, L.; Madaghiele, M.; Romano, A.; Siliqi, D.; Ladisa, M.; et al. Effects of processing on structural, mechanical and biological properties of collagen-based substrates for regenerative medicine. *Sci. Rep.* **2018**, *8*, 1429. [CrossRef]

40. Altamura, D.; Lassandro, R.; Vittoria, F.A.; Decaro, L.; Siliqi, D.; Ladisa, M.; Giannini, C. X-ray microimaging laboratory (XMI-LAB). *J. Appl. Crystallogr.* **2012**, *45*, 869–873. [CrossRef]

41. Siliqi, D.; De Caro, L.; Ladisa, M.; Scattarella, F.; Mazzone, A.; Altamura, D.; Sibillano, T.; Giannini, C. SUNBIM: A package for X-ray imaging of nano- and biomaterials using SAXS, WAXS, GISAXS and GIWAXS techniques. *J. Appl. Crystallogr.* **2016**, *49*, 1107–1114. [CrossRef]

42. Salvatore, L.; Calò, E.; Bonfrate, V.; Pedone, D.; Gallo, N.; Natali, M.L.; Sannino, A.; Madaghiele, M. Exploring the effects of the crosslink density on the physicochemical properties of collagen-based scaffolds. *Polym. Test.* **2021**, *93*, 106966. [CrossRef]

43. Kodre, K.; Attarde, S.; Yendhe, P.; Patil, R.; Barge, V. Differential Scanning Calorimetry: A Review. *Res. Rev. J. Pharm. Anal.* **2014**, *3*, 11–22.

44. Bao, Z.; Sun, Y.; Rai, K.; Peng, X.; Wang, S.; Nian, R.; Xian, M. The promising indicators of the thermal and mechanical properties of collagen from bass and tilapia: Synergistic effects of hydroxyproline and cysteine. *Biomater. Sci.* **2018**, *6*, 3042–3052. [CrossRef] [PubMed]

45. Song, W.-K.; Liu, D.; Sun, L.-L.; Li, B.-F.; Hou, H. Physicochemical and Biocompatibility Properties of Type I Collagen from the Skin of Nile Tilapia (*Oreochromis niloticus*) for Biomedical Applications. *Mar. Drugs* **2019**, *17*, 137. [CrossRef] [PubMed]

46. Pan, B.-Q.; Su, W.-J.; Cao, M.-J.; Cai, Q.-F.; Weng, W.-Y.; Liu, G.-M. IgE reactivity to type i collagen and its subunits from tilapia (*Tilapia zillii*). *Food Chem.* **2012**, *130*, 127–133. [CrossRef]

47. Tang, J.; Saito, T. Biocompatibility of Novel Type i Collagen Purified from Tilapia Fish Scale: An in Vitro Comparative Study. *BioMed Res. Int.* **2015**, *2015*, 139476. [CrossRef]

48. Yan, M.; Li, B.; Zhao, X.; Qin, S. Effect of concentration, pH and ionic strength on the kinetic self-assembly of acid-soluble collagen from walleye pollock (*Theragra chalcogramma*) skin. *Food Hydrocoll.* **2012**, *29*, 199–204. [CrossRef]

49. Zhang, Q.; Wang, Q.; Lv, S.; Lu, J.; Jiang, S.; Regenstein, J.M.; Lin, L. Comparison of collagen and gelatin extracted from the skins of Nile tilapia (*Oreochromis niloticus*) and channel catfish (*Ictalurus punctatus*). *Food Biosci.* **2016**, *13*, 41–48. [CrossRef]

50. Chen, J.; Li, L.; Yi, R.; Xu, N.; Gao, R.; Hong, B. Extraction and characterization of acid-soluble collagen from scales and skin of tilapia (*Oreochromis niloticus*). *LWT Food Sci. Technol.* **2016**, *66*, 453–459. [CrossRef]
51. Zhou, T.; Wang, N.; Xue, Y.; Ding, T.; Liu, X.; Mo, X.; Sun, J. Development of biomimetic tilapia collagen nanofibers for skin regeneration through inducing keratinocytes differentiation and collagen synthesis of dermal fibroblasts. *ACS Appl. Mater. Interfaces* **2015**, *7*, 3253–3262. [CrossRef]
52. Li, J.; Wang, M.; Qiao, Y.; Tian, Y.; Liu, J.; Qin, S.; Wu, W. Extraction and characterization of type I collagen from skin of tilapia (*Oreochromis niloticus*) and its potential application in biomedical scaffold material for tissue engineering. *Process Biochem.* **2018**, *74*, 156–163. [CrossRef]
53. Bi, C.; Li, X.; Xin, Q.; Han, W.; Shi, C.; Guo, R.; Shi, W.; Qiao, R.; Wang, X.; Zhong, J. Effect of extraction methods on the preparation of electrospun/electrosprayed microstructures of tilapia skin collagen. *J. Biosci. Bioeng.* **2019**, *128*, 234–240. [CrossRef]
54. Tang, L.; Chen, S.; Su, W.; Weng, W.; Osako, K.; Tanaka, M. Physicochemical properties and film-forming ability of fish skin collagen extracted from different freshwater species. *Process Biochem.* **2015**, *50*, 148–155. [CrossRef]
55. Yan, M.; Qin, S.; Li, J. Study on the self-assembly property of type I collagen prepared from tilapia (*Oreochromis niloticus*) skin by different extraction methods. *Int. J. Food Sci. Technol.* **2015**, *50*, 2088–2096. [CrossRef]
56. Thuanthong, M.; Sirinupong, N.; Youravong, W. Triple helical structure of acid-soluble collagen derived from Nile tilapia skin as affected by extraction temperature. *J. Sci. Food Agric.* **2016**, *96*, 3795–3800. [CrossRef] [PubMed]
57. Liao, W.; Guanghua, X.; Li, Y.; Shen, X.R.; Li, C. Comparison of characteristics and fibril-forming ability of skin collagen from barramundi (*Lates calcarifer*) and tilapia (*Oreochromis niloticus*). *Int. J. Biol. Macromol.* **2018**, *107*, 549–559. [CrossRef] [PubMed]
58. Le, T.M.T.; Nguyen, V.M.; Tran, T.T.; Takahashi, K.; Osako, K. Comparison of acid-soluble collagen characteristic from three important freshwater fish skins in Mekong Delta Region, Vietnam. *J. Food Biochem.* **2020**, *44*, e13397. [CrossRef] [PubMed]
59. Song, Z.; Liu, H.; Chen, L.; Chen, L.; Zhou, C.; Hong, P.; Deng, C. Characterization and comparison of collagen extracted from the skin of the Nile tilapia by fermentation and chemical pretreatment. *Food Chem.* **2021**, *340*, 128139. [CrossRef] [PubMed]
60. Fujii, K.K.; Taga, Y.; Takagi, Y.K.; Masuda, R.; Hattori, S.; Koide, T. The Thermal Stability of the Collagen Triple Helix Is Tuned According to the Environmental Temperature. *Int. J. Mol. Sci.* **2022**, *23*, 2040. [CrossRef]
61. Gallo, N.; Lunetti, P.; Bettini, S.; Barca, A.; Madaghiele, M.; Valli, L.; Capobianco, L.; Sannino, A.; Salvatore, L. Assessment of physico-chemical and biological properties of sericin-collagen substrates for PNS regeneration. *Int. J. Polym. Mater. Polym. Biomater.* **2021**, *70*, 403–413. [CrossRef]
62. Masullo, U.; Cavallo, A.; Greco, M.R.; Reshkin, S.J.; Mastrodonato, M.; Gallo, N.; Salvatore, L.; Verri, T.; Sannino, A.; Cardone, R.A.; et al. Semi-interpenetrating polymer network cryogels based on poly(ethylene glycol) diacrylate and collagen as potential off-the-shelf platforms for cancer cell research. *J. Biomed. Mater. Res. Part B Appl. Biomater.* **2021**, *109*, 1313–1326. [CrossRef]
63. Tian, H.; Ren, Z.; Shi, L.; Hao, G.; Chen, J.; Weng, W. Self-assembly characterization of tilapia skin collagen in simulated body fluid with different salt concentrations. *Process Biochem.* **2021**, *108*, 153–160. [CrossRef]
64. Yan, M.; Wang, X. Study on the kinetic self-assembly of type I collagen from tilapia (Oreochromis niloticus) skin using the fluorescence probe thioflavin T. *Spectrochim. Acta Part A Mol. Biomol. Spectrosc.* **2018**, *203*, 342–347. [CrossRef] [PubMed]
65. Terzi, A.; Gallo, N.; Bettini, S.; Sibillano, T.; Altamura, D.; Madaghiele, M.; De Caro, L.; Valli, L.; Salvatore, L.; Sannino, A.; et al. Sub- and Supramolecular X-Ray Characterization of Engineered Tissues from Equine Tendon, Bovine Dermis and Fish Skin Type-I Collagen. *Macromol. Biosci.* **2020**, *20*, 2000017. [CrossRef] [PubMed]
66. Yamamoto, K.; Igawa, K.; Sugimoto, K.; Yoshizawa, Y.; Yanagiguchi, K.; Ikeda, T.; Yamada, S.; Hayashi, Y. Biological safety of fish (tilapia) collagen. *BioMed Res. Int.* **2014**, *2014*, 630757. [CrossRef] [PubMed]
67. Oliveira, V.D.M.; Assis, C.R.D.; Costa, B.D.A.M.; Neri, R.C.D.A.; Monte, F.T.D.; Freitas, H.M.S.D.C.V.; França, R.C.P.; Santos, J.F.; Bezerra, R.D.S.; Porto, A.L.F. Physical, biochemical, densitometric and spectroscopic techniques for characterization collagen from alternative sources: A review based on the sustainable valorization of aquatic by-products. *J. Mol. Struct.* **2021**, *1224*, 129023. [CrossRef]
68. Välimaa, A.-L.; Mäkinen, S.; Mattila, P.; Marnila, P.; Pihlanto, A.; Mäki, M.; Hiidenhovi, J. Fish and fish side streams are valuable sources of high-value components. *Food Qual. Saf.* **2019**, *3*, 209–226. [CrossRef]
69. Rodrigues Menezes, M.d.L.L.; Ribeiro, H.L.; da Silva Abreu, F.d.O.M.; de Andrade Feitosa, J.P.; de Souza Filho, M.d.S.M. Optimization of the collagen extraction from Nile tilapia skin (*Oreochromis niloticus*) and its hydrogel with hyaluronic acid. *Colloids Surf. B: Biointerfaces* **2020**, *189*, 110852. [CrossRef]
70. Meyer, M. Processing of collagen based biomaterials and the resulting materials properties. *BioMedical Eng. Online* **2019**, *18*, 24. [CrossRef]
71. Bose, S.; Narayan, R.; Bandyopadhyay, A. *Biomaterials Science: Processing, Properties and Applications III*; John Wiley & Sons, Inc.: Hoboken, NJ, USA, 2013.
72. Plant, A.L.; Bhadriraju, K.; Spurlin, T.A.; Elliott, J.T. Cell response to matrix mechanics: Focus on collagen. *Biochim. Biophys. Acta Mol. Cell Res.* **2009**, *1793*, 893–902. [CrossRef]
73. Cai, S.; Wu, C.; Yang, W.; Liang, W.; Yu, H.; Liu, L. Recent advance in surface modification for regulating cell adhesion and behaviors. *Nanotechnol. Rev.* **2020**, *9*, 971–989. [CrossRef]
74. Kanta, J. Collagen matrix as a tool in studying fibroblastic cell behavior. *Cell Adhes. Migr.* **2015**, *9*, 308–316. [CrossRef]
75. Lee, C.H.; Singla, A.; Lee, Y. Biomedical applications of collagen. *Int. J. Pharm.* **2001**, *221*, 1–22. [CrossRef]

Polymers **2022**, *14*, 1865

76. Masci, V.L.; Taddei, A.R.; Gambellini, G.; Giorgi, F.; Fausto, A.M. Ultrastructural investigation on fibroblast interaction with collagen scaffold. *J. Biomed. Mater. Res. Part A* **2016**, *104*, 272–282. [CrossRef] [PubMed]
77. Croce, M.A.; Silvestri, C.; Guerra, D.; Carnevali, E.; Boraldi, F.; Tiozzo, R.; Parma, B. Adhesion and Proliferation of Human Dermal Fibroblasts on Collagen Matrix. *J. Biomater. Appl.* **2004**, *18*, 209–222. [CrossRef] [PubMed]
78. Böhm, S.; Strauß, C.; Stoiber, S.; Kasper, C.; Charwat, V. Charwat, Impact of Source and Manufacturing of Collagen Matrices on Fibroblast Cell Growth and Platelet Aggregation. *Materials* **2017**, *10*, 1086. [CrossRef] [PubMed]
79. Subhan, F.; Ikram, M.; Shehzad, A.; Ghafoor, A. Marine Collagen: An Emerging Player in Biomedical applications. *J. Food Sci. Technol.* **2015**, *52*, 4703–4707. [CrossRef]
80. Dokukina, I.V.; Gracheva, M.E. A model of fibroblast motility on substrates with different rigidities. *Biophys. J.* **2010**, *98*, 2794–2803. [CrossRef]
81. Lo, C.-M.; Wang, H.-B.; Dembo, M.; Wang, Y.-L. Cell movement is guided by the rigidity of the substrate. *Biophys. J.* **2000**, *79*, 144–152. [CrossRef]

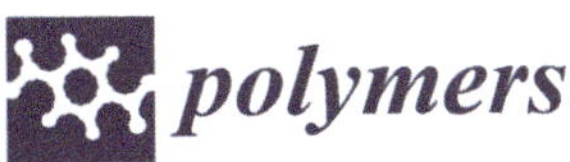

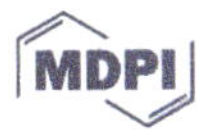

Article

The *Dosidicus gigas* Collagen for Scaffold Preparation and Cell Cultivation: Mechanical and Physicochemical Properties, Morphology, Composition and Cell Viability

Veronika Anohova [1], Lyudmila Asyakina [1], Olga Babich [1], Olga Dikaya [1], Aleksandr Goikhman [1], Ksenia Maksimova [1], Margarita Grechkina [2], Maxim Korobenkov [1], Diana Burkova [2], Aleksandr Barannikov [1], Anton Narikovich [1], Evgeny Chupakhin [1,3], Anatoly Snigirev [1] and Sergey Antipov [1,2,*]

1 Immanuel Kant Baltic Federal University, Nevskogo 14, Kaliningrad 236006, Russia
2 Voronezh State University, 1, University Square, Voronezh 394063, Russia
3 Saint Petersburg State University, Saint Petersburg 199034, Russia
* Correspondence: ss.antipov@gmail.com; Tel.: +7-(960)118-56-70

Abstract: Directed formation of the structure of the culture of living cells is the most important task of tissue engineering. New materials for 3D scaffolds of living tissue are critical for the mass adoption of regenerative medicine protocols. In this manuscript, we demonstrate the results of the molecular structure study of collagen from *Dosidicus gigas* and reveal the possibility of obtaining a thin membrane material. The collagen membrane is characterized by high flexibility and plasticity as well as mechanical strength. The technology of obtaining collagen scaffolds, as well as the results of studies of its mechanical properties, surface morphology, protein composition, and the process of cell proliferation on its surface, are shown in the given manuscript. The investigation of living tissue culture grown on the surface of a collagen scaffold by X-ray tomography on a synchrotron source made it possible to remodel the structure of the extracellular matrix. It was found that the scaffolds obtained from squid collagen are characterized by a high degree of fibril ordering and high surface roughness and provide efficient directed growth of the cell culture. The resulting material provides the formation of the extracellular matrix and is characterized by a short time to living tissue sorption.

Keywords: collagen scaffolds; mechanical properties; physicochemical properties; morphology; composition; cell viability; molecular structure; *Dosidicus gigas*; X-ray tomography; SynchrotronLike

Citation: Anohova, V.; Asyakina, L.; Babich, O.; Dikaya, O.; Goikhman, A.; Maksimova, K.; Grechkina, M.; Korobenkov, M.; Burkova, D.; Barannikov, A.; et al. The *Dosidicus gigas* Collagen for Scaffold Preparation and Cell Cultivation: Mechanical and Physicochemical Properties, Morphology, Composition and Cell Viability. *Polymers* **2023**, *15*, 1220. https://doi.org/10.3390/polym15051220

Academic Editors: Nunzia Gallo, Marta Madaghiele, Alessandra Quarta, Amilcare Barca and Alberto Romero García

Received: 6 December 2022
Revised: 19 January 2023
Accepted: 30 January 2023
Published: 28 February 2023

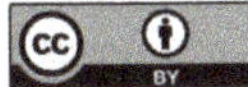

Copyright: © 2023 by the authors. Licensee MDPI, Basel, Switzerland. This article is an open access article distributed under the terms and conditions of the Creative Commons Attribution (CC BY) license (https://creativecommons.org/licenses/by/4.0/).

1. Introduction

Collagen is the main protein of connective tissue, which consists of three subunits in the form of an alpha helix [1–3]. The size of the turns of the fibrillar structure of collagen is 67 nm (D-period). There are 20 types of collagen proteins; the main type is type I collagen (collagen I) [4]. Collagen proteins have the property of self-structuring in solution and in the process of drying and lyophilization [5], which makes it possible to obtain collagen materials, particularly matrices, which have an ordered structure and are similar to the connective tissues of the human body [6–8]. Self-assembly of collagen molecules into supramolecular structures—fibrils—is the main process of collagen matrix formation [9]. Collagen I is used in medicine for early healing, skin buildup [10], as suture material, and as artificial skin [11]. Implantable materials obtained from collagen type I do not induce an immunological rejection; such materials are highly biocompatible and capable of controlled degradation [12]. Collagen scaffold materials can be obtained from collagen I solutions by casting, lyophilization, electrospinning, and coagulation. The use of this technology makes it possible to obtain collagen materials with an adjustable fiber size, which is used to obtain substrates in cell technologies [13]. The formation of structures similar to native collagen is difficult for the technologies that are available today. Electrospinning and deposition technologies cannot establish the long-range orientation of collagen fibers [14]. Collagen films obtained by lyophilization are not able to copy the extracellular matrix of living biological systems [15,16]. Today, the investigation of tissue proliferation processes and cell differentiation is carried out by real-time X-ray tomography technology [17–20]. At the same time, investigations of scaffolds' surface topography for tissue engineering based on collagens of various origins are known [21,22]. The results of investigations of collagen molecules' surface topography have made it possible to estimate the value of the D-period of fibrils, which is 68 ± 0.8 nm for collagen proteins [23]. Parameters of X-rays generated by synchrotrons are of particular importance for the research fields of regenerative medicine and cell and tissue engineering, as well as for the investigation of atomic and electron environments of composite bioorganic macromolecules [24–28]. Previously, we studied the molecular structure features of collagen from *Dosidicus gigas* [29]. At the same time, there exist results giving evidence that materials based on collagen proteins of hydrobionts inhabiting the South Atlantic are highly durable and biocompatible [30,31]. We focused our attention on the study of the living cell proliferation process on the surface of scaffolds obtained from *Dosidicus gigas* collagens, because the high availability of raw materials for obtaining collagen will allow the introduction of tissue engineering technique as a generally available method of therapy. We have investigated the characteristics of collagen proteins, their molecular structure features, amino acid sequences of their peptides, the strength of the surface and prepared collagen matrix morphology, as well as the proliferation process with the identification of the tissue formation area using soft X-ray radiation generated by a synchrotron source.

2. Materials and Methods

Commercially available reagents, nutrient media, and cell cultures were used in this research according to standard protocol. Cell imaging reagents were from Thermo Fisher and used according to the manufacturer's protocols.

2.1. Extraction of Collagen

Extraction of acid-soluble collagen was carried out according to the method published in [32]. The skin of the hydrobiont *Dosidicus gigas* was separated from the mantle and lyophilized at $-20\ ^\circ$C and a pressure of 0.03 mbar. Lyophilized skin was homogenized on an IKA mechanical disperser at 2600 rpm. The powder weighing 50 g was placed in a flat-bottomed flask. For the extraction of non-collagen proteins and lipids, 250 mL of PBS buffer solution, pH 8.4, containing 2000 U of trypsin and 2500 U phospholipase A was added. The mixture was sonicated (2.4 kHz, 200 W) for 1 min every hour at room temperature for 6 h. Collagen proteins were separated by centrifugation at 2500 rpm and transferred to a 500 mL flat-bottomed flask containing 300 mL of 0.2 M NaOH and mixed for 6 h. Next, collagen proteins were precipitated by centrifugation at 2500 rpm and the resulting precipitate was used to isolate acid-soluble collagen. To obtain 300 mL of acid-soluble collagen, a 3% solution of acetic acid was added to the precipitate and mixed for 3 h under periodic sonication of ultrasound with the same parameters as above. The insoluble fraction was separated by centrifugation at 1500 rpm. The resulting colloidal solution was neutralized by 0.2 M NaOH to pH 7.4, and the precipitate of type I collagen was isolated by centrifugation at 3500 rpm. The precipitate washed by three portions of distilled water until the acid reaction disappeared, and then the obtained sample was lyophilized.

2.2. Preparation Collagen Scaffold

The technology for obtaining collagen material was developed. Collagen weighing 10 g was suspended in 50 mL of a 3% glycerol solution in distilled water under ultrasound treatment. The suspension was placed on a Teflon substrate and air dried at $120\ ^\circ$C in a convection dryer chamber until the moisture content in the sample was less than 3% under constant conditions. Moisture content was controlled by the standard gravimetric method. The sample was dried to a constant weight and the mass fraction of moisture was calculated as the difference in the masses of the sample before and after drying. The measurements were carried out in two repeats. Additionally, the moisture content was monitored using near-infrared spectroscopy. After scaffold drying, it was sterilized in UV at a wavelength of 280 nm and a temperature of 40 °C. The resulting collagen sheets were used to obtain ready-to-use cell scaffolds.

2.3. Mechanical Properties of Collagen Scaffold Investigation

The mechanical properties of the collagen scaffolds were estimated according to [33]. Tensile properties of 3D collagen matrices were measured using a modified Minimat 2000 mini-materials tester (Rheometric Scientific, Inc. (https://www.ssgca.com/), Piscataway, NJ, USA) and by standard testing procedures for matrices of low mechanical strength. One end of each specimen was attached to a stepper motor-controlled linear actuator and the other end was attached to a load cell. For these experiments, a load cell designed with a sensitivity of 0.0003 N was utilized. Clamps offset the loading axis and allowed the matrix to be submerged longitudinally within a bath of PBS, pH 7.4, at approximately 37 °C. For most experiments, the extension speed was 10 mm/min and the strain rate was 38.5 percent/min.

2.4. Atomic Force Microscopy

The study of the topography of the fibrillar structure and surface of collagen matrices was carried out according to [34]. AFM imaging and indentation of collagen fibrils were performed using a Nanowizard AFM (JPK Instruments, Berlin, Germany) and SOLVER P47 (NT-MDT, Russia). All measurements were taken in air at room temperature. Aluminum-coated silicon AFM cantilevers (resonance frequency up to 150 kHz and nominal spring constant up to 4.5 N/m (NSC12 tip-C, MikroMasch, Tallinn, Estonia)) and gold-coated silicon AFM cantilevers (resonance frequency up to 150 kHz and nominal spring constant up to 6.1 N/m (NSG 03, NT-MDT, Moscow, Russia)) were used. These cantilevers were chosen to match the stiffness of collagen for optimizing the sensitivity and signal/noise ratio (SNR). For imaging collagen fibrils without damage, the relatively high stiffness of the cantilevers required the use of intermittent contact mode (also known as tapping mode). After taking a topographic image of the fibril, the force mapping mode (also known as force volume mode) was used to perform quasi-static indentations. The 64×64 indentation curves, consisting of 256 data points each, were taken on a square area. The area's dimensions were 1.5×1.5 mm $\pm$ 0.5 mm, optimized in each experiment to balance approximately the number of data points taken on the fibril and on the substrate. The time for both the approach and retraction of the cantilevers was set to 0.2 s (5 Hz), with zero delay in between.

2.5. Scanning Electron Microscopy

Collagen scaffolds were fixed overnight at 4 °C with 3% glutaraldehyde in 0.05 M phosphate buffer (PB) at pH 7.2. Following extensive rinsing with the same buffer at 4 °C, blocks were soaked for 1 h in 0.5% tannic acid in PB at 4 °C. Then, they were rinsed four times in the same buffer for 15 min at 4 °C and post-fixed with 1% osmium tetroxide in PB for 1 h at 4 °C. Samples were washed in distilled water, dehydrated in a graded series of ethanol, and freeze-dried in a Balzers Union CPD 020 (Balzers, Liechtenstein) using the procedure of critical point drying. Images of collagen scaffolds were obtained with scanning electron microscopy (SEM) in the bright field mode by Jeol JSM-6390 (Japan) with an accelerating voltage of 5 kV (low vacuum mode). As SEM demands a conductive surface to obtain an image, samples were covered with a platinum thin film (calibrated 30 nm) sputtered by the magnetron set-up Jeol JFC-1600 (Japan).

2.6. Amino Acid Content by HPLC

For the preparation of dabsyl-cloride derivatized amino acids (dabsyl-AA), each amino acid mixture was dissolved in 0.1 N HCl solution . Dabsyl-Cl (26 mg) was dissolved in 20 mL of acetonitrile. A 0.1 M $NaHCO_3$ solution (pH 8.3) and a 0.05 M Na_2HPO_4 solution (pH 7.0) were separately mixed with an equal volume of ethanol. A 0.5 mL aliquot of amino acid solution was placed in a test tube and mixed well with 0.5 mL of $NaHCO_3$ solution and 2 mL of dabsyl-Cl solution. The test tube was incubated in a 70 °C water bath for 15 min before 3 mL Na_2HPO_4/ethanol solution was added to stop the reaction. Dabsyl-AA mixtures were resolved with a LiChroCART 125-2 Superspher 100 RP-18 column (Merck) end detection on a UV/VIS detector. The sample size was 10 μL. The flow rate was 0.5 mL/min. Both solvent A (H_2O) and solvent B (acetonitrile) contained 0.1% (*v/v*) formic acid. The gradient was programmed as follows: 15% B for 3 min, linear gradient from 15% to 85% B for 60 min, and 85% B for 7 min. The relationship of the responding peak area and the concentration of each dabsyl-AA was calculated with Excel software (Microsoft Co., Seattle, WA, USA). Next, 100 mg of the collagen matrix was hydrolyzed in 6 N HCl and sealed in hydrolysis tubes under nitrogen atmosphere and incubated in an oil bath at 108 °C for 24 h. For the hydrolysate of the collagen matrix used for dabsyl-AA derivates, the preparation was as described above, and amino acid content was determined on HPLC with a UV/Vis detector.

2.7. Size Exclusion Chromatography

Size exclusion chromatography was performed by following [35] on chromatography system (Biorad, NGC) equipped with a fraction collector and a photometric detector. Fractionation was carried out on the column (ENRICH SEC 650 10 × 300 mm, BioRad) using 25 mM of acetate buffer as an eluant and a flow rate of 1 mL/min. Detection was carried out at a wavelength of 210 nm. To the column was applied 5 mL of a collagen colloidal solution in 25 mM of acetate buffer by means of a constant flow pump to a site exclusion chromatography column, followed by fractionation.

2.8. SDS-PAGE

Electrophoresis under a denaturing condition in the presence of sodium dodecyl sulfate (SDS-PAGE) was carried out according to the modified Laemmli method [36] in the presence of 8% polyacrylamide. Powdered samples of collagen (5 mg) were dissolved in 1 mL of 0.02 M sodium phosphate buffer (pH 7.2) containing 1% (*w/v*) SDS and 3.5 M of freshly prepared urea at 1 mg/mL concentration. The samples were mixed gently at 4 °C for 2 h to dissolve collagen and placed on PAGE. Protein markers produced by Thermo Scientific in the range of 10–200 kDa (product number 26614) and 20–120 kDa (product number 26612) were used as standards.

2.9. FTIR Spectra Registration

FTIR spectra were obtained using an FT-IR ATR Alpha spectrometer equipped with an attenuated total reflectance unit (Bruker, Germany) and an InGAs detector. For FTIR spectra acquisition, the system was used in point mode (aperture of 250 × 250 μm) with a 2.0 cm^{-1} resolution and using 30 scans in transmittance mode (n = 35 spectra), and spectra acquisitions were performed under complete N2 purge of the analytical system.

2.10. MALDI-TOF

All mass spectra data were acquired by the MALDI-TOF mass spectrometer Autoflex (Bruker Daltonic, Germany). MALDI-TOF settings were as follows: high-voltage output on ion source - 19.5 and 18.45 kV; high voltage output on first reflector - 8 kV; frequency of Nd:YAG laser - 1 GHz (500 shots). The process of lyophilization of collagen was carried out in a freeze dryer (Labconco Triad) in standard mode.

2.11. Cell Culture

Cell cultivation was carried out in parallel with [37,38]. The collagen matrix was placed into the wells of an 18-well plate, and 2 mL of DMEM culture medium containing glutamine, ceftriaxone, and penicillin was added. A suspension of HEK cells in 1 mL of DMEM containing 500 units of cells was added to each well and incubated for 4 days in an incubator at 37 °C and 5% CO_2 partial pressure. The collagen matrix was removed, treated with appropriate dyes, and visualized using confocal microscopy.

2.12. MTT Assay for Toxic Effect Determination

The effects of the collagen matrix on cell viability were determined using the MTT colorimetric test. For the MTT test, collagen scaffold disks 30 mm in diameter and 60 μm thick were used. The MTT protocol was optimized to increase well volume from 200 μL to 2000 μL. The discs were cut from edge to center once to form a 5 mm high cone. The cone was placed on a culture plate with cells 60 mm in diameter. The culture medium containing the cells was added in a volume of 2 mL (so that the cones were completely submerged). Cultivation was carried out in an incubator in a CO_2 atmosphere. The culture plates were placed on an orbital shaker to simulate the movement of the culture fluid. HEK cells were diluted with the growth medium containing 100 μM of $CoCl_2$ for chemically induced hypoxia to 3.5×10^4 cells per mL, and the aliquots (7×10^3 cells per (200 μL) were placed in individual wells on 96-well multiplates (Eppendorf, Germany) and incubated for 24 h. The next day, the cells were treated with synthesized compounds separately at a concentration of 100 μM and incubated for 72 h at 37 °C in 5% CO_2 atmosphere. Each compound was tested in triplicate. After incubation, the cells were then treated with 40 μL of MTT solution (3-(4,5-dimethylthiazol-2-yl)-2,5-diphenyltetrazolium bromide, 5 mg mL^{-1} in PBS) and incubated for 4 h. After an additional 4 h of incubation, the medium with MTT was removed and DMSO (150 μL) was added to dissolve the formazan crystals. The plates were shaken for 10 min. The optical density of each well was determined at 560 nm using the ClarioStar microplate reader (BMG Labteh, Germany). The tested collagen matrix was evaluated for the antiproliferative action in three separate experiments.

2.13. Fluorescent Dying

Cells cultured on a collagen scaffold were fixed with a 4% paraformaldehyde solution in PBS, washed with PBS + 0.5% Triton X-100, and washed with PBS. Cells were incubated with Mitotracker Red, DAPI, and FITC for 30 min according to the manufacturer's protocol and washed with PBS. The obtained stained specimen was examined by confocal laser fluorescence microscopy.

2.14. Visualization of Extracellular Matrix

Unstained 3D matrices of type I collagen were polymerized on cover glasses and imaged using confocal refection microscopy as previously described [39], employing a direct Carl Zeiss LSM 800 confocal using either the 10× Plan-Neofluar (NA = 0.3), a 20× water immersion Plan-Apochromat (NA = 1.0) objective, or a 63× water immersion C-Apochromat (NA = 1.2).

2.15. Study of Cell Culture on the Surface of a Collagen Matrix at a Laboratory Complex, "SynchrotronLike"

The cells obtained on the surface of the collagen matrixes were fixed with a solution of the formalin and then studied by a high-resolution X-ray radiography technique on a scientific and educational multifunctional system for synchrotron studies called "SynchrotronLike" [40]. The main element of the system is the MetalJet D2+ 70 kV microfocus X-ray source from Excillum [41]. A liquid gallium–indium alloy with a characteristic line of 9.251 keV (Ga Kα1) is used as an anode in this source. The minimum size of the X-ray source is 5 μm, and the maximum power of the electron gun is 250 W. This results in a source brightness of 10^{10}–10^{11} photons/sec/mm^2/mrad^2/(0.1%$\Delta\lambda/\lambda$), which is an order of magnitude higher than for conventional solid anode X-ray tubes and comparable with the brightness of a bending magnet of the synchrotron sources. A collagen scaffold with cells was placed on a motorized stage with five degrees of freedom (X, Y, Z, θ, ω) located at a 60 cm distance from the X-ray source. To record the images, the Rigaku X Sight Micron LC CCD camera installed 5 cm behind the sample was used. This camera was equipped with a lens with an optical magnification of 10×, providing a pixel size of 0.55 μm and 1.5 μm spatial resolution.

2.16. Image Processing of High-Resolution X-ray Radiography and Microscopy

ImageJ software was used to overlay images and determine the relative position of cells [42].

3. Results

3.1. Scaffolds' Mechanical Properties, Surface Topography, and Composition

The scaffolds' mechanical properties and surface topography were investigated using three independent techniques. It was found that the thickness of the obtained matrix according to Section 2.2 was 100–150 μm, the tensile strength was 80–100 MPa, the elongation ability was up to 47%, and Young's modulus was 1.5 GPa (Figure 1(I)).

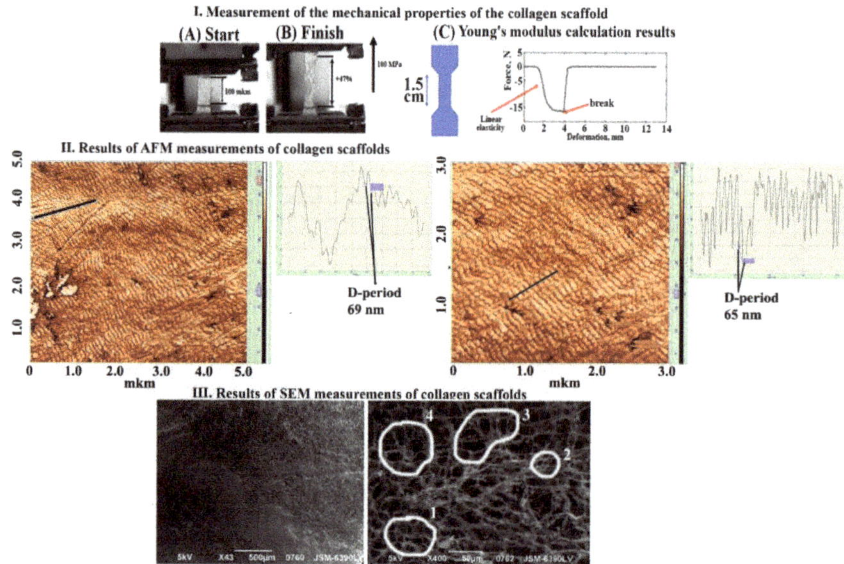

Figure 1. Mechanical and topography investigation results. **(I)** Measurement of the mechanical properties of the collagen scaffold: thickness, tensile strength, elongation ability, and Young's modulus **(A,B)**, and Young's modulus result calculation **(C)**. **(II)** Results of AFM measurements of collagen scaffolds and results of D-period calculation. **(III)** Results of SEM measurements of collagen scaffolds and results of analysis of developed pore structure and cell size: 1,2 (Panel **III**)—small-sized pores (5–12 mkm), 3,4 (Panel **III**) —large-sized pores (12–25 mkm).

Thus, the mechanical properties of the collagen matrix have evidenced the ability to use it as a potential model for cell scaffolds for surgery. The topography of the collagen matrix surface was studied by atomic force microscopy. The presence of a dense, self-structured fibrillar surface was observed. It was detected that the D-period of *Dosidicus gigas* collagen (Figure 1(II)) in the molecule's helix is 65–69 nm, which corresponds to the parameter of the helix of most proteins of the mammalian and bird collagen family. Examination of the collagen scaffold surface by scanning electron microscopy made it possible to detect a developed pore structure, the cell size of which varies within 5–25 μm, which is an effective size of the cellular matrix for the regeneration of connective tissue in surgery, as well as a barrier matrix in transplantology [43–45] (Figure 1(III)), and in the next step of this investigation, these possibilities were tested.

According to the literature, collagen types I, III, IV, and V have several characteristic FTIR regions located in the ranges of 1.700–1.600 cm^{-1}, 1.480–1.350 cm^{-1}, 1.300–1.180 cm^{-1}, and 1.100–1.005 cm^{-1}, respectively [46]. In addition, there is evidence that FTIR spectra of fish skin collagens demonstrate the presence of amides (3423 and 3337 cm^{-1} for amide A and 2928 and 2924 cm^{-1} for amide B, respectively). In addition, bands correspond to stretching vibrations of C-O of the polypeptide backbone in the region of 1600–1700 cm^{-1} and hydrogen bonding between the N-H and C-O (Gly) residues at 1654 and 1560 cm^{-1}. Signals for amide II and amide III in the structure of collagen were detected at 1240 cm^{-1} (48). At the same time, FTIR spectra obtained for collagen extracted from the skin of squid (*Doryteuthis singhalensis*) have similar characteristics [47].

FTIR investigations of the obtained scaffolds were carried out (Figure 2). The obtained data indicate the presence of bands in the regions of 3300 cm^{-1} and 2935 cm^{-1}, which may correspond to amide A and amide B; a band in the region of 1659 cm^{-1}, which can be correlated with the C-O backbone of the polypeptide chain; and a band in the region of 1538 cm^{-1}, which is consistent with regions characteristic of N-H and C-N. A band was also detected in the region of 1235 cm^{-1}, which can be correlated with amide II and amide III. In general, the shape of the obtained spectrum (Figure 2) correlates with the literature data [48–50]. Thus, the data obtained correlate with the literature data and the data of the European Directorate for the Quality of Medicines & HealthCare library [51], which confirms the assumption about the collagen nature of the resulting scaffold.

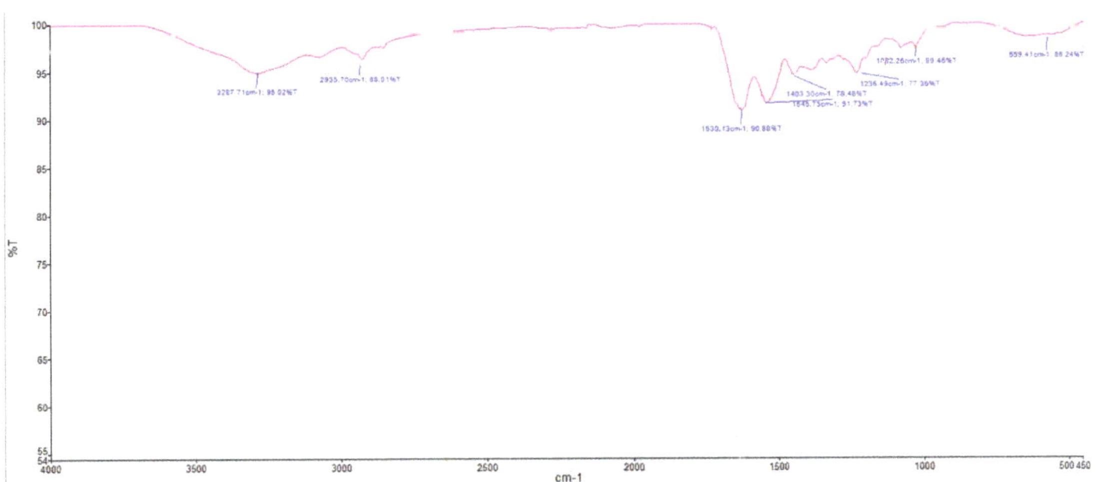

Figure 2. IR spectroscopy of collagen scaffold obtained from *Dosidicus gigas* Pink curve is the *Dosidicus gigas* collagen scaffold spectrum.

3.2. Fractional Composition Investigation of a Collagen Proteins Mixture

The fractional composition investigation was conducted in three steps: by size exclusion chromatography (Figure 3A), SDS-PAGE technique (Figure 3B,C), and MALDI-TOF (Figure 4). From the results of chromatography fractionation, we observed the presence of nine fractions in total with different migration rates. At the same time, more than 90% of the area of all peaks was accounted for by three fractions (Figure 3A, A/1, A/2, A/3). The elution rate of the most significant fractions corresponds to 0.4, 0.51, and 0.75–0.78 column volumes (CV). Typically, these elution rates correspond to collagen types I, II, and III.

The mixture of collagens isolated from the mantle of squid (*Dosidicus gigas*) was investigated in comparison to collagens from *Bos taurus* after collagenase treatment and trypsinolysis by SDS-PAGE (Figure 3B,C). The presence of proteins with molecular weight higher than 120 kDa was characteristic of the *Dosidicus gigas* collagen (Figure 3B, line N2), while the cattle (*Bos taurus*) collagen sample was enriched with the lower-molecular-weight proteins (Figure 3B, line N1). Next, we compared collagens from the different sources on SDS-PAGE after treatment with enzymes, collagenase (Figure 3B), and trypsin (Figure 3C) for 10, 30, and 30 min of reaction, respectively. Collagen from cattle demonstrates less sensitivity to collagenase as compared to collagen from hydrobionts (Figure 3B,C). Collagen from *Dosidicus gigas* likely has less sensitivity (higher resistivity) to trypsin, as the presence of higher-molecular-weight peptides after enzyme treatment was detected compared to *Bos taurus* collagen (Figure 3C, lanes 1 and 2, respectively).

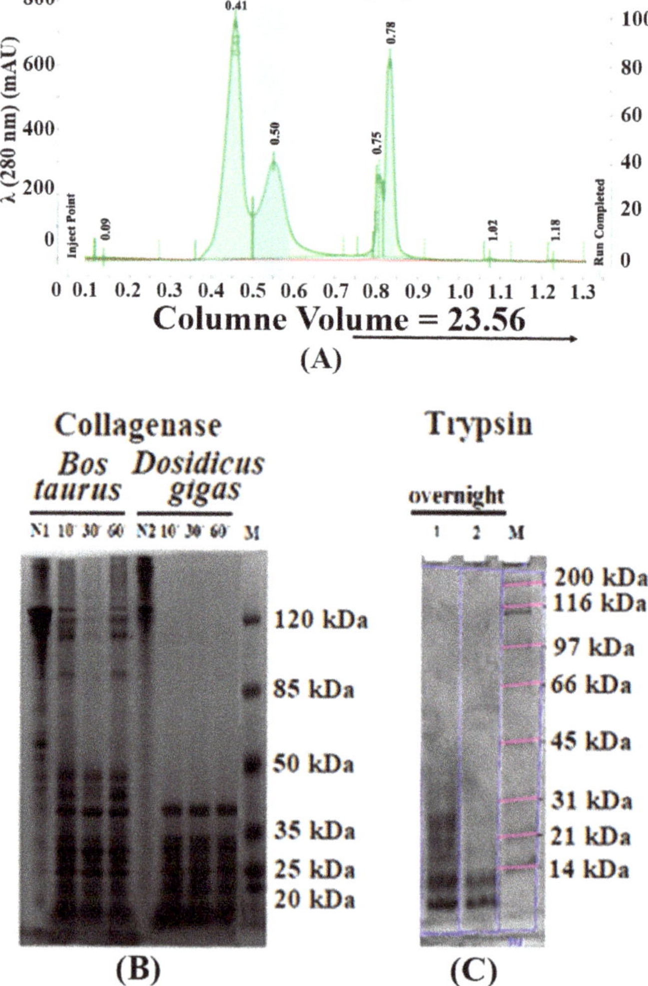

Figure 3. Results for hydrobionts collagen fractionation by SDS-PAGE in different conditions. (**A**) Size exclusion chromatography of hydrobionts collagen. (**B**) Results of hydrobionts collagen type I, II, and III fractionation by SDS-PAGE after collagenase treatment. (**C**) Results of hydrobionts collagen type I, II, and III fractionation by SDS-PAGE after trypsinolysis.

The amino acid compositions were investigated by HPLC (Table 1), and the sequence of products of hydrolysis in the presence of collagenase and trypsin was analyzed by MALDI-TOF (Figure 4). The results of determining the amino acid sequence by the Top-Dawn MALD-TOF method (Figure 4) made it possible to determine the belonging of the isolated collagen fractions to a certain type. It was found that the amino acid composition of *Dosidicus gigas* collagen is similar to mammalian collagen (Table 1), but given the conservatism of its protein family, this is not surprising. This is also consistent with the notion that collagens are poor in aromatic amino acids. Thus, the data obtained support the assumption that the resulting protein and material from it can be attributed to collagens.

Table 1. Amino acid content in collagen from *Dosidicus gigas*.

Amino Acid	%	Amino Acid	%
Hydroxyproline (OHPro)	10.13	Methionine (Met)	1.39
Asparagines (Asp)	7.49	Isoleucine (Ile)	1.64
Threonine (Thr)	2.97	Leucine (Leu)	3.47
Serine (Ser)	3.86	Threonine (Tyr)	1.04
Glutamine (Glu)	11.38	Phenylalanine (Phe)	1.64
Proline (Pro)	9.40	Hydroxy lysine (OH-L)	1.50
Glycine (Gly)	22.18	lysine (Lys)	1.83
Alanine (Ala)	6.87	histidine (His)	1.07
Cysteine (Cys)	0.74	arginine (Arg)	8.79
Valine (Val)	2.61		

Molecular profiles of peptides after proteolytic digestion of collagens from *Dosidicus gigas* and *Bos taurus* by two proteases using MALDI-TOF mass spectroscopy were investigated. Collagen proteins from *Dosidicus gigas* (Figure 3A,B) form more complex profiles of maximums corresponding to proteolytic peptides appearing upon splitting by any of the two proteases than does collagen from cattle (compare Figure 3B,C, Table 1). Treatment of the *Dosidicus gigas* collagen solution with collagenase gives peptides with molecular weights of 481, 916, 1493, 2231, 2554, and 3808 Da. The same treatment of cattle collagen solution gives a pattern of peaks corresponding to 567, 916, 2666, 4148, and 5119 Da peptides. Mass spectroscopic analysis of trypsin splitting products of the two collagens demonstrates differences in the sensitivity of the two collagens to trypsin. There were 481, 1654, 2231, 2554, and 3808 Da peptides detected in the hydrobionts collagen solution, and 567, 1042, 2599, and 5422 Da peptides in the mammalian collagen solution. There were 481, 2231, 2554, and 3808 Da peptides detected in the *Dosidicus gigas* collagen solution after treatment with two types of proteases, which could be used as a representative. No similar pattern was detected for the cattle collagen solution.

Amino acid sequences of collagen fractions isolated from *Dosidicus gigas* and *Bos taurus* are given in Table 1. Peptides characteristic of collagen types I, II, and III were identified (Table 2). Interestingly, the products of collagen hydrolysis are different when treated with trypsin and collagenase. It can be assumed that in the case of the hydrobionts collagen, the amino acid sequence is Gly-Pro-Gly-Hyp-Gly-Pro-Hyp-Gly-Gly-Lys (938.99 Da), which is formed by two fragments with a molecular weight of ~481 Da. The masses of the peptides are predominantly determined by the frequency of lysine or arginine residue occurrence [51], which means that the more lysine or arginine residues in the collagen molecule, the more short-chain peptides will be observed in the hydrolysis products. It was found that α-chains are formed by a repeating sequence which can be written as follows: (Gly-XY)n. The identification of the amino acid sequence of the isolated peptides was carried out using FlexAnalysis software. Basic amino acids such as proline, glycine, and lysine were identified automatically by the program. On the assumption that the hydroxylysine molecule has a monoisotopic mass of 144.103, it was identified from this mass. Moreover, hydroxyproline has a monoisotopic mass that is similar to the monoisotopic mass of leucine/isoleucine, 113.04–113.08 , and it was assumed that the amino acids with a mass of 113.061 to 114.083 would correspond to hydroxyproline. Moreover, the mass of valine is extremely close to the mass of acetylated glycine, but since glycine is the most likely amino acid in collagen, it was decided that a mass of 99.032 to 99.05 would correspond to acetylated glycine.

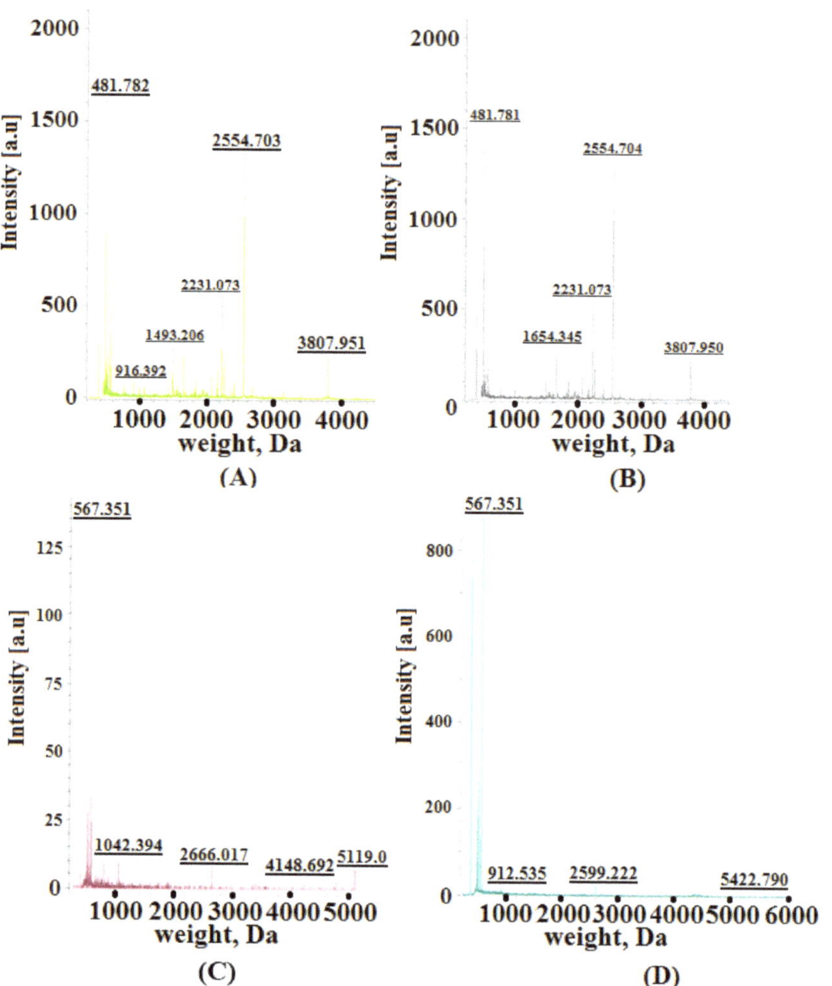

Figure 4. MALDI-TOF mass spectrogram of *Dosidicus gigas* collagen (**A,B**) and *Bos taurus* collagen (**C,D**) proteolytic digestion products by (**A,C**) collagenase and (**B,D**) trypsin. [a.u.]—absorption units.

Table 2. Amino acid sequences of collagen fractions isolated from *Dosidicus gigas*.

Collagen Type		
Collagen I	Collagen II	Collagen III
P*G	P*GPP*P*GE	P*GG*
KG	P*GI/LGE	KG
APTGGTTA	TAPP*	GHI/L
GPAG*AKDG*GYK*	P*HDP	I/LGCI/L
P*GDK*	P*P*EP*VG	CAG*I/L
PGMK*	P*P*EP*G*GGE	SMKG*PG
DK*I/LK*G*GG	P*P*EP*G*GEGM	SMMG*PG
	peptide - GVG P* M C PI/L	G*GP*G*
		P*G*GCK*

3.3. Visualization of Cell Compartments, Extracellular Matrix, and Estimation of Biocompatibility with Collagen Materials

As a result of the study of the suspension of HEK cells dyed by Mitotracker Red, DAPI, and FITC grown on the surface of the collagen scaffold, we observed the absence of cytotoxicity (Figure 5A). In the process of growth, cells probably actively use collagenous material as a source of amino acids, because they actively form intercellular contacts and a matrix. The obtained collagen scaffolds showed high cell viability, which suggests the possibility of biocompatibility of the resulting scaffold. A high cell survival rate was observed during the cultivation process (Figure 5B). Thereby, collagen matrix participates in the formation of a network of contacts and directs the process of tissue differentiation and participates in the formation of spatial morphology. In the MTT test, we found no toxicity from the collagen matrix, and cell survival was over 90%. The contribution of the collagen suspension was 3% in the pipetting medium.

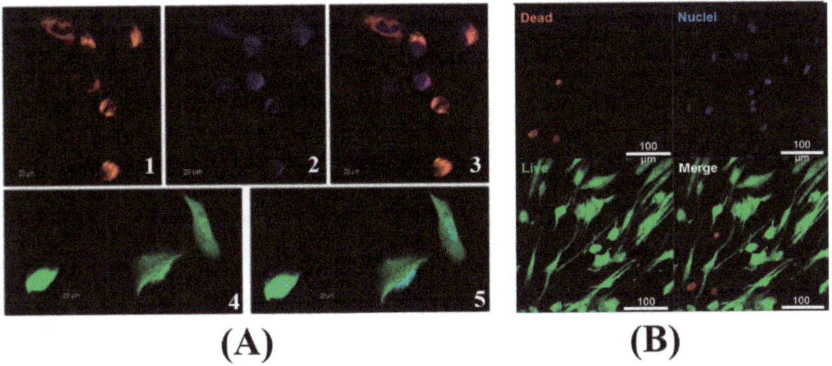

Figure 5. Results of confocal microscopy of collagen scaffold from *Dosidicus gigas* treated by cells stained by Mitotracker Red, DAPI, and FITC. (**A**) Fibroblasts, (**B**) viability estimation of cells. Mitochondria are stained in red; cell nuclei are stained in blue; matrix is stained in green.

3.4. High-Resolution X-ray Radiography on the Surface of the Collagen Matrix

High-resolution X-ray radiography on the laboratory complex "SynchrotronLike" made it possible to visualize the areas of the intercellular matrix forming on the surface of the collagen scaffold (Figure 6). The overlay of X-ray radiography and microscopy images of the area of the matrix with the nuclei of living cells stained with the DAPI dye made it possible to detect areas of the forming microenvironment of the connective tissue. The image shows separate areas of high density of the substance, which are associated with the formation of the extracellular matrix and the resulting living tissue. The method of high-resolution X-ray radiography was able to detect areas of high density coinciding with the structures of the extracellular matrix. Thus, this method can be applied to study the process of formation of the basal membrane and intercellular matrix on the surface of collagen matrices and to analyze their internal microstructure in laboratory conditions. The data obtained form the basis for the development of an optical scheme of experiments using coherent radiation from specialized sources of synchrotron radiation by the method of X-ray microtomography with a high time resolution.

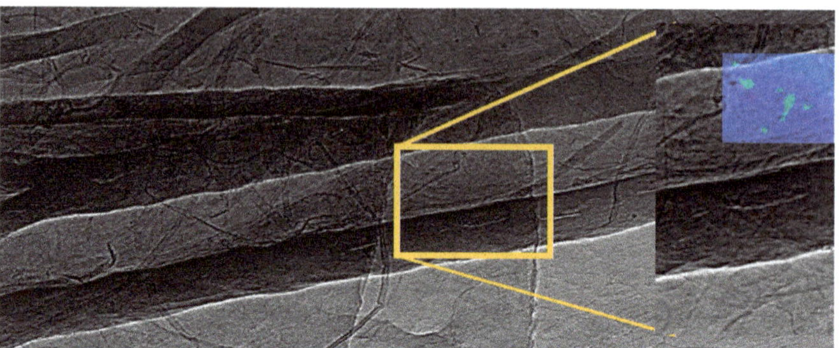

Figure 6. Radiographic image of a collagen matrix for a sample of proliferating cells with an overlaid optical image of a region of the matrix with stained nuclei of living cells.

4. Discussion

Collagen isolated from the mantle of the squid species *Dosidicus gigas* was used to create scaffolds for the cultivation of living cells. The protein fraction contains proteins that may correspond to collagen types I, II, and III. The technology for obtaining scaffolds based on collagen makes it possible to obtain this material on an industrial scale. In the process of forming scaffolds and thin films based on collagen, the self-structuring of fibrils occurs, while maintaining their tertiary structure. The topography of the collagen scaffold surface showed the presence of a developed rough surface, which ensures high cell adhesion. The mechanical properties of the obtained material make it possible to use it in surgical practice as a likely bioresorbable barrier material with a given sorption time and controlled biodegradation. The scaffolds obtained are not cytotoxic and have shown high biocompatibility. Direct visualization of the process of cell proliferation on the surface of the collagen scaffold using X-ray imaging made it possible to carry out remodeling of the spatial structure of the extracellular matrix, which is planned to be used in the future in the technology of printing 3D scaffolds to obtain living tissue with a given morphology and structure. The results of confocal microscopy indicate that the cell culture was growing on the surface of the studied collagen scaffold. Most likely, this can be explained by the high density of scaffold fibrils, which do not allow cells to penetrate inside. For 3D tissue prototyping, the obtained collagen should be reconstructed with the addition of a composite material (for example, polylysine). At the same time, the direction of surface cell growth is determined by the direction of the fibrils and can be used to provide controlled growth of connective tissue. The current results encourage the use of the resulting material as-is for a barrier scaffold. The resulting collagen scaffolds manifest themselves as a natural source of proteinogenic amino acids and provide a high rate of formation of the extracellular matrix.

Author Contributions: Conceptualization, E.C., O.B., A.S. and V.A.; methodology, M.K., K.M., A.S. and D.B.; software, A.N.; validation, A.B., S.A. and L.A.; formal analysis, O.B. and V.A.; investigation, V.A., M.G., D.B. and O.D.; resources, O.B. and A.G.; data curation, S.A.; writing—original draft preparation, E.C.; writing—review and editing, E.C.; visualization, S.A.; supervision, S.A.; project administration, A.S.; funding acquisition, S.A. All authors have read and agreed to the published version of the manuscript.

Funding: The study was supported by the Ministry of Science and Higher Education of Russia under agreement no. 075-15-2021-1351, concerning X-ray, SEM, AFM, and MALDI-TOF method. The reported study was funded by I. Kant Baltic Federal University, project number 877, concerning PAGE, HPLC, MTT, and biochemistry method.

Institutional Review Board Statement: Not applicable.

Informed Consent Statement: Not applicable.

Data Availability Statement: Not applicable.

Acknowledgments: We thank the Research Center for Nanotechnology and the Centre for Innovative Technologies of Composite Nanomaterials of Saint Petersburg State University Research Park for obtaining the analytical data, IR spectroscopy, AFM, and SEM.

Conflicts of Interest: The authors declare no conflict of interest.

References

1. Shoulders, M.D.; Raines, R.T. Collagen Structure and Stability. *Annu. Rev. Biochem.* **2009**, *78*, 929–958. [CrossRef] [PubMed]
2. Ricard-Blum, S. The Collagen Family. *Cold Spring Harb. Perspect. Biol.* **2011**, *3*, a004978. [CrossRef] [PubMed]
3. Goldberga, I.; Li, R.; Duer, M.J. Collagen Structure–Function Relationships from Solid-State NMR Spectroscopy. *Acc. Chem. Res.* **2018**, *51*, 1621–1629. [CrossRef]
4. Gordon, M.K.; Hahn, R.A. Collagens. *Cell Tissue Res.* **2009**, *339*, 247. [CrossRef]
5. Antipova, L.V.; Sukhov, I.V.; Slobodyanik, V.S.; Kotov, I.I.; Antipov, S.S. Improving the technology of collagen substance from raw fish materials for obtaining porous materials for cosmetology and medicine. *IOP Conf. Ser. Earth Environ. Sci.* **2021**, *640*, 32044. [CrossRef]
6. Sarkar, B.; O'Leary, L.E.R.; Hartgerink, J.D. Self-Assembly of Fiber-Forming Collagen Mimetic Peptides Controlled by Triple-Helical Nucleation. *J. Am. Chem. Soc.* **2014**, *136*, 14417–14424. [CrossRef] [PubMed]
7. Köster, S.; Evans, H.M.; Wong, J.Y.; Pfohl, T. An In Situ Study of Collagen Self-Assembly Processes. *Biomacromolecules* **2008**, *9*, 199–207. [CrossRef]
8. Revell, C.K.; Jensen, O.E.; Shearer, T.; Lu, Y.; Holmes, D.F.; Kadler, K.E. Collagen fibril assembly: New approaches to unanswered questions. *Matrix Biol. Plus* **2021**, *12*, 100079. [CrossRef]
9. Buehler, M.J. Nature designs tough collagen: Explaining the nanostructure of collagen fibrils. *Proc. Natl. Acad. Sci. USA* **2006**, *103*, 12285–12290. [CrossRef]
10. Antipova, L.V.A. *Study of the Use of Modified Collagen of Freshwater Fish as a Material for Personal Care Products*; Storublevtsev, S.A., Ed.; IntechOpen: Rijeka, Croatia, 2019; ISBN 978-1-78985-958-4.
11. Sionkowska, A.; Skrzyński, S.; Śmiechowski, K.; Kołodziejczak, A. The review of versatile application of collagen. *Polym. Adv. Technol.* **2017**, *28*, 4–9. [CrossRef]
12. Parenteau-Bareil, R.; Gauvin, R.; Berthod, F. Collagen-Based Biomaterials for Tissue Engineering Applications. *Materials* **2010**, *3*, 1863–1887. [CrossRef]
13. Belamie, E.; Mosser, G.; Gobeaux, F.; Giraud-Guille, M.M. Possible transient liquid crystal phase during the laying out of connective tissues: α-chitin and collagen as models. *J. Phys. Condens. Matter* **2006**, *18*, S115–S129. [CrossRef]
14. Castilla-Casadiego, D.A.; Rivera-Martínez, C.A.; Quiñones-Colón, B.A.; Almodóvar, J. *Electrospun Collagen Scaffolds BT—Electrospun Biomaterials and Related Technologies*; Almodovar, J., Ed.; Springer International Publishing: Cham, Switzerland, 2017; pp. 21–55. ISBN 978-3-319-70049-6.
15. Lowe, C.J.; Reucroft, I.M.; Grota, M.C.; Shreiber, D.I. Production of Highly Aligned Collagen Scaffolds by Freeze-drying of Self-assembled, Fibrillar Collagen Gels. *ACS Biomater. Sci. Eng.* **2016**, *2*, 643–651. [CrossRef] [PubMed]
16. Nitti, P.; Kunjalukkal Padmanabhan, S.; Cortazzi, S.; Stanca, E.; Siculella, L.; Licciulli, A.; Demitri, C. Enhancing Bioactivity of Hydroxyapatite Scaffolds Using Fibrous Type I Collagen. *Front. Bioeng. Biotechnol.* **2021**, *9*, 36. [CrossRef] [PubMed]
17. Appel, A.; Anastasio, M.A.; Brey, E.M. Potential for Imaging Engineered Tissues with X-Ray Phase Contrast. *Tissue Eng. Part B Rev.* **2011**, *17*, 321–330. [CrossRef]
18. Shearer, T.; Bradley, R.S.; Hidalgo-Bastida, L.A.; Sherratt, M.J.; Cartmell, S.H. Three-dimensional visualisation of soft biological structures by X-ray computed micro-tomography. *J. Cell Sci.* **2016**, *129*, 2483–2492. [CrossRef] [PubMed]
19. Rawson, S.D.; Maksimcuka, J.; Withers, P.J.; Cartmell, S.H. X-ray computed tomography in life sciences. *BMC Biol.* **2020**, *18*, 21. [CrossRef]
20. Papantoniou, I.; Sonnaert, M.; Geris, L.; Luyten, F.P.; Schrooten, J.; Kerckhofs, G. Three-Dimensional Characterization of Tissue-Engineered Constructs by Contrast-Enhanced Nanofocus Computed Tomography. *Tissue Eng. Part C Methods* **2013**, *20*, 177–187. [CrossRef] [PubMed]
21. Iturri, J.; Toca-Herrera, J.L. Characterization of Cell Scaffolds by Atomic Force Microscopy. *Polymers* **2017**, *9*, 383. [CrossRef]
22. Ahmed, M.; Ramos, T.A.d.S.; Damanik, F.; Quang Le, B.; Wieringa, P.; Bennink, M.; van Blitterswijk, C.; de Boer, J.; Moroni, L. A combinatorial approach towards the design of nanofibrous scaffolds for chondrogenesis. *Sci. Rep.* **2015**, *5*, 14804. [CrossRef]

23. Kukreti, U.; Belkoff, S.M. Collagen fibril D-period may change as a function of strain and location in ligament. *J. Biomech.* **2000**, *33*, 1569–1574. [CrossRef] [PubMed]
24. Liou, H.; Lin, H.; Chen, W.; Liou, W.; Hwu, Y. Tomography Observations of Osteoblast Seeding on 3-D Collagen Scaffold by Synchrotron Radiation Hard X-Ray. *J. Biomim. Biomater. Tissue Eng.* **2009**, *3*, 93–101. [CrossRef]
25. Mastrogiacomo, M.; Campi, G.; Cancedda, R.; Cedola, A. Synchrotron radiation techniques boost the research in bone tissue engineering. *Acta Biomater.* **2019**, *89*, 33–46. [CrossRef]
26. Duan, X.; Li, N.; Chen, X.; Zhu, N. Characterization of Tissue Scaffolds Using Synchrotron Radiation Microcomputed Tomography Imaging. *Tissue Eng. Part C Methods* **2021**, *27*, 573–588. [CrossRef]
27. Bukreeva, I.; Fratini, M.; Campi, G.; Pelliccia, D.; Spanò, R.; Tromba, G.; Brun, F.; Burghammer, M.; Grilli, M.; Cancedda, R.; et al. High-Resolution X-ray Techniques as New Tool to Investigate the 3D Vascularization of Engineered-Bone Tissue. *Front. Bioeng. Biotechnol.* **2015**, *3*, 133. [CrossRef] [PubMed]
28. Bailey, A.J.; Macmillan, J.; Shrewry, P.R.; Tatham, A.S.; Puxkandl, R.; Zizak, I.; Paris, O.; Keckes, J.; Tesch, W.; Bernstorff, S.; et al. Viscoelastic properties of collagen: Synchrotron radiation investigations and structural model. *Philos. Trans. R. Soc. London. Ser. B Biol. Sci.* **2002**, *357*, 191–197. [CrossRef]
29. Anokhova, V.D.; Chupakhin, E.G.; Pershina, N.A.; Storublevtsev, S.A.; Antipova, L.V.; Matskova, L.V.; Antipov, S.S. *Sensitivity of Different Collagens to Proteolytic Enzyme Treatment BT—Proceedings of the International Conference "Health and wellbeing in modern society" (ICHW 2020)*; Atlantis Press: Paris, France, 2020; pp. 44–49.
30. Xu, N.; Peng, X.-L.; Li, H.-R.; Liu, J.-X.; Cheng, J.-S.-Y.; Qi, X.-Y.; Ye, S.-J.; Gong, H.-L.; Zhao, X.-H.; Yu, J.; et al. Marine-Derived Collagen as Biomaterials for Human Health. *Front. Nutr.* **2021**, *8*, 493. [CrossRef] [PubMed]
31. Salvatore, L.; Gallo, N.; Natali, M.L.; Campa, L.; Lunetti, P.; Madaghiele, M.; Blasi, F.S.; Corallo, A.; Capobianco, L.; Sannino, A. Marine collagen and its derivatives: Versatile and sustainable bio-resources for healthcare. *Mater. Sci. Eng. C* **2020**, *113*, 110963. [CrossRef]
32. Jency, G.; Manjusha, W.A. Extraction and Purification of Collagen from Marine Squid Uroteuthis Duvauceli. *Int. J. Pharma Bio Sci.* **2020**, *10*. [CrossRef]
33. Roeder, B.A.; Kokini, K.; Sturgis, J.E.; Robinson, J.P.; Voytik-Harbin, S.L. Tensile Mechanical Properties of Three-Dimensional Type I Collagen Extracellular Matrices With Varied Microstructure. *J. Biomech. Eng.* **2002**, *124*, 214–222. [CrossRef]
34. Watanabe-Nakayama, T.; Itami, M.; Kodera, N.; Ando, T.; Konno, H. High-speed atomic force microscopy reveals strongly polarized movement of clostridial collagenase along collagen fibrils. *Sci. Rep.* **2016**, *6*, 28975. [CrossRef] [PubMed]
35. Toroian, D.; Lim, J.E.; Price, P.A. The Size Exclusion Characteristics of Type I Collagen: Implications for the role of noncollagenous bone constituents in mineralization *. *J. Biol. Chem.* **2007**, *282*, 22437–22447. [CrossRef] [PubMed]
36. Wu, J.; Li, Z.; Yuan, X.; Wang, P.; Liu, Y.; Wang, H. Extraction and isolation of type I, III and V collagens and their SDS-PAGE analyses. *Trans. Tianjin Univ.* **2011**, *17*, 111. [CrossRef]
37. Kanta, J. Collagen matrix as a tool in studying fibroblastic cell behavior. *Cell Adh. Migr.* **2015**, *9*, 308–316. [CrossRef] [PubMed]
38. Koohestani, F.; Braundmeier, A.G.; Mahdian, A.; Seo, J.; Bi, J.; Nowak, R.A. Extracellular Matrix Collagen Alters Cell Proliferation and Cell Cycle Progression of Human Uterine Leiomyoma Smooth Muscle Cells. *PLoS ONE* **2013**, *8*, e75844. [CrossRef]
39. Acuna, A.; Drakopoulos, M.A.; Leng, Y.; Goergen, C.J.; Calve, S. Three-dimensional visualization of extracellular matrix networks during murine development. *Dev. Biol.* **2018**, *435*, 122–129. [CrossRef]
40. Barannikov, A.; Shevyrtalov, S.; Zverev, D.; Narikovich, A.; Sinitsyn, A.; Panormov, I.; Snigireva, I.; Snigirev, A. Laboratory complex for the tests of the X-ray optics and coherence-related techniques. In Proceedings of the Proc.SPIE, Online, 19–29 April 2021; Volume 11776.
41. Hållstedt, J.; Espes, E.; Lundström, U.; Hansson, B. Liquid-metal-jet X-ray technology for nanoelectronics characterization and metrology. In Proceedings of the 2018 29th Annual SEMI Advanced Semiconductor Manufacturing Conference (ASMC), New York, NY, USA, 30 April 2018–3 May 2018; pp. 151–154.
42. Schneider, C.A.; Rasband, W.S.; Eliceiri, K.W. NIH Image to ImageJ: 25 years of image analysis. *Nat. Methods* **2012**, *9*, 671–675. [CrossRef]
43. Omar, O.; Elgali, I.; Dahlin, C.; Thomsen, P. Barrier membranes: More than the barrier effect? *J. Clin. Periodontol.* **2019**, *46*, 103–123. [CrossRef]
44. Sbricoli, L.; Guazzo, R.; Annunziata, M.; Gobbato, L.; Bressan, E.; Nastri, L. Selection of Collagen Membranes for Bone Regeneration: A Literature Review. *Materials* **2020**, *13*, 786. [CrossRef]
45. Montgomery, H.; Rustogi, N.; Hadjisavvas, A.; Tanaka, K.; Kyriacou, K.; Sutton, C.W. Proteomic Profiling of Breast Tissue Collagens and Site-specific Characterization of Hydroxyproline Residues of Collagen Alpha-1-(I). *J. Proteome Res.* **2012**, *11*, 5890–5902. [CrossRef]
46. Veeruraj, A.; Arumugam, M.; Ajithkumar, T.; Balasubramanian, T. Isolation and characterization of collagen from the outer skin of squid (*Doryteuthis singhalensis*). *Food Hydrocoll.* **2015**, *43*, 708–716. [CrossRef]
47. Rizk, M.A.; Mostafa, N.Y. Extraction and characterization of collagen from buffalo skin for biomedical applications. *Orient. J. Chem.* **2016**, *32*, 1601–1609. [CrossRef]
48. Krishnamoorthi, J.; Ramasamy, P.; Shanmugam, V.; Shanmugam, A. Isolation and partial characterization of collagen from outer skin of Sepia pharaonis (Ehrenberg, 1831) from Puducherry coast. *Biochem. Biophys. Rep.* **2017**, *10*, 39–45. [CrossRef] [PubMed]

49. Kim, S.H.; Park, H.S.; Lee, O.J.; Chao, J.R.; Park, H.J.; Lee, J.M.; Ju, H.W.; Moon, B.M.; Park, Y.R.; Song, J.E.; et al. Fabrication of duck's feet collagen–silk hybrid biomaterial for tissue engineering. *Int. J. Biol. Macromol.* **2016**, *85*, 442–450. [CrossRef]
50. Dogan, A.; Lasch, P.; Neuschl, C.; Millrose, M.K.; Alberts, R.; Schughart, K.; Naumann, D.; Brockmann, G.A. ATR-FTIR spectroscopy reveals genomic loci regulating the tissue response in high fat diet fed BXD recombinant inbred mouse strains. *BMC Genom.* **2013**, *14*, 386. [CrossRef] [PubMed]
51. Ortolani, F.; Giordano, M.; Marchini, M. A model for type II collagen fibrils: Distinctive D-band patterns in native and reconstituted fibrils compared with sequence data for helix and telopeptide domains. *Biopolymers* **2000**, *54*, 448–463. [CrossRef]

Disclaimer/Publisher's Note: The statements, opinions and data contained in all publications are solely those of the individual author(s) and contributor(s) and not of MDPI and/or the editor(s). MDPI and/or the editor(s) disclaim responsibility for any injury to people or property resulting from any ideas, methods, instructions or products referred to in the content.

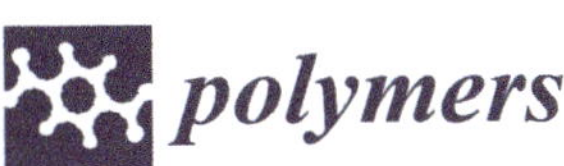 *polymers*

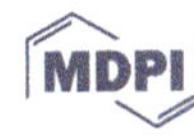

Article

Collagen Membrane Derived from Fish Scales for Application in Bone Tissue Engineering

Liang Chen [1,2,3,4], Guoping Cheng [1,2,3], Shu Meng [1,2,3] and Yi Ding [1,2,3,*]

1   National Clinical Research Center for Oral Diseases, West China Hospital of Stomatology, Sichuan University, Chengdu 610041, China; clworkzone@126.com (L.C.); cgp19940611@foxmail.com (G.C.); dreamingsue@163.com (S.M.)
2   State Key Laboratory of Oral Diseases, Sichuan University, Chengdu 610041, China
3   Department of Periodontology, West China College of Stomatology, Sichuan University, Chengdu 610041, China
4   Department of Periodontology, Peking University School and Hospital of Stomatology, Beijing 100081, China
*   Correspondence: yiding2000@126.com

Abstract: Guided tissue/bone regeneration (GTR/GBR) is currently the main treatment for alveolar bone regeneration. The commonly used barrier membranes in GTR/GBR are collagen membranes from mammals such as porcine or cattle. Fish collagen is being explored as a potential substitute for mammalian collagen due to its low cost, no zoonotic risk, and lack of religious constraints. Fish scale is a multi-layer natural collagen composite with high mechanical strength, but its biomedical application is limited due to the low denaturation temperature of fish collagen. In this study, a fish scale collagen membrane with a high denaturation temperature of 79.5 °C was prepared using an improved method based on preserving the basic shape of fish scales. The fish scale collagen membrane was mainly composed of type I collagen and hydroxyapatite, in which the weight ratios of water, organic matter, and inorganic matter were 20.7%, 56.9%, and 22.4%, respectively. Compared to the Bio-Gide® membrane (BG) commonly used in the GTR/GBR, fish scale collagen membrane showed good cytocompatibility and could promote late osteogenic differentiation of cells. In conclusion, the collagen membrane prepared from fish scales had good thermal stability, cytocompatibility, and osteogenic activity, which showed potential for bone tissue engineering applications.

Keywords: fish scale; collagen; hydroxyapatite; bone marrow mesenchymal stem cells; osteogenic differentiation

Citation: Chen, L.; Cheng, G.; Meng, S.; Ding, Y. Collagen Membrane Derived from Fish Scales for Application in Bone Tissue Engineering. *Polymers* 2022, 14, 2532. https://doi.org/10.3390/polym14132532

Academic Editors: Nunzia Gallo, Marta Madaghiele, Alessandra Quarta and Amilcare Barca

Received: 21 May 2022
Accepted: 10 June 2022
Published: 21 June 2022

Publisher's Note: MDPI stays neutral with regard to jurisdictional claims in published maps and institutional affiliations.

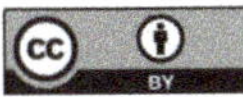

Copyright: © 2022 by the authors. Licensee MDPI, Basel, Switzerland. This article is an open access article distributed under the terms and conditions of the Creative Commons Attribution (CC BY) license (https://creativecommons.org/licenses/by/4.0/).

1. Introduction

Periodontitis is a chronic inflammatory disease that occurs in periodontal tissue and is the main cause of tooth loss in adults. Resorption of alveolar bone is one of the main pathological changes [1]. Traditional periodontal treatment methods, such as scaling and root planning, can only prevent the development of periodontal disease. However, alveolar bone regeneration is difficult to achieve [2]. Guided tissue/bone regeneration (GTR/GBR) is not only the main treatment of alveolar bone regeneration clinically but also the main means of bone augmentation during implant surgery. GTR/GBR is a technique that uses membranes as a barrier to keep gingival connective tissue from contacting the root surface, creating space, and guiding periodontal tissue or bone regeneration [3–5]. Collagen membranes, whose main component is type I collagen and whose most common source is mammals like porcine or cattle, are commonly used as barrier materials in the GTR/GBR.

Collagen is the most important structural protein in most soft and hard tissues of animals and humans, accounting for about 30% of the total proteins in mammals and playing a critical role in maintaining the biological and structural integrity of the extracellular matrix [6]. Collagen regulates cell morphology, adhesion, migration, and differentiation and has low immunogenicity, good biocompatibility, and biodegradability [7,8]. There are currently 29 different types of collagen identified, each with their own amino acid sequences, structures, and functions [9]. Type I collagen has the highest content of all of them, which is found in connective tissue such as skin, tendons, bones, ligaments, and cornea [10], accounting for more than 90% of the collagen in the human body [11]. Type I collagen is being studied for a variety of applications, including health products, cosmetics, hemostatic agents, wound healing, regenerative medicine, and drug delivery [10,12–14]. Skin and tendon tissues derived from mammals such as porcine or cattle are the main sources of type I collagen for biomedical applications [15]. However, mammalian-derived collagen has the following disadvantages: (1) safety: zoonotic diseases such as bovine spongiform encephalopathy and foot-and-mouth disease may be transmitted through mammals [16]; (2) religious restrictions [17]: Islam and Judaism do not use any porcine-derived products, while Hinduism does not use any cattle-derived products; (3) cost: mammalian collagen purification is difficult and expensive [11]. Fish-derived collagen is a potential substitute for mammalian collagen because of the low risk of zoonosis from fish to humans, the lack of religious restrictions, the low cost of fish scales and other aquatic scraps, and the fact that it is safe and easily obtainable [11]. As many as 50–70 percent of by-products were produced in the production and processing of fish products [18], with a large number of fish bones, swim bladders, and scales being discarded as leftovers. A growing number of researchers have focused on fish-derived collagen in recent years [19–21].

The bony fish scales are mainly composed of type I collagen fibers and hydroxyapatite, in which the protein content is 41–84% [22]. Hydroxyapatite enhances type I collagen fibers in fish scales, and the parallel collagen fibers overlap to form a multi-layer structure with a highly ordered three-dimensional structure [23,24]. Fish scales have a similar main composition to human bone and dentin [25], and their highly ordered natural multi-layer structure has good mechanical properties. Each year, about 49,000 tons of fish scale waste are produced during the processing of fish, accounting for 2% of the total weight of the fish [26]. It is necessary to use these fish industry waste to synthesize value-added materials for several different applications, such as energy storage and packaging [27]. If these waste by-products could be used, people could not only reduce pollution but also improve the utilization of fish products and economic benefits [28]. With regard to the research of grass carp (*Ctenopharyngodon idella*) scales, some scholars have tried to apply decellularized grass carp scales to artificial cornea [29,30]. In addition, a study has fabricated bone pins with decellularized grass carp scales and implanted them into the femur fractures of animals. Finally, it demonstrated that decellularized grass carp scales could be a promising implant material for bone repair [23]. Therefore, the purpose of this study is to prepare a decellularized fish scale collagen membrane (FS) from grass carp scales and analyze its structure and composition. Moreover, compared to Bio-Gide® membrane (BG), a common commercial collagen membrane used clinically, we want to explore whether FS has good cytocompatibility and osteogenic activity and to further determine whether decellularized grass carp scales have the potential to be applied in bone tissue engineering.

2. Materials and Methods

All experiments were carried out in accordance with the ethical protocol and guidelines. Ethical approval was obtained from the ethical committees of the West China School of Stomatology, Sichuan University, and the State Key Laboratory of Oral Diseases (ethics code WCHSIRB-D-2020-220).

2.1. Preparation of Decellularized Fish Scale Collagen Membrane (FS)

The preparation method was roughly based on our previous research [30,31] and slightly improved as follows. In brief, about 100 grass carp scales with a diameter of more than 20 mm were selected and cleaned with distilled water to remove ash and impurities from the surface. Under the condition of continuously stirring the solution in the blender, the fish scales were treated with 80 mL of chloroform: ethanol = 1:1 mixed solution for 1 h to remove mucopolysaccharides, proteins, and fats and washed with 80 mL of 5% NaCl solution for 1 h to remove unnecessary proteins on the surface. The scales were then soaked in 100 mL of 10% EDTA solution (Solarbio, Beijing, China) for 4 h and then treated with a 0.5 mol/L acetic acid solution (Kelong, Chengdu, China) for 1 h, which was called decalcified fish scale. Finally, the decalcified fish scales were sprayed with a pepsin solution (Kelong, Chengdu, China) for 1 h to etch the surface. The treated fish scales were soaked in 75% ethanol for sterilization for about 12 h and then stored in aseptic PBS at 4 °C, which was called fish scale collagen membrane (FS). The whole preparation process was carried out at a temperature of 25 °C.

2.2. Structure, Composition, and Denaturation Temperature Analysis of FS

2.2.1. Cell Nucleus Staining of FS

Cell nucleus staining was used to determine whether the material was decellularized or not. Decellularized FS seeded with cells were fixed for 20 min in 4% paraformaldehyde solution (Solarbio, Beijing, China) and then permeabilized for 5 min with 1% TritonX-100 (Solarbio, Beijing, China). After three PBS washes, the decellularized FS were incubated with 4′,6-diamidino-2-phenylindole dihydrochloride (Solarbio, Beijing, China) at room temperature for 20 min to label nuclei. The same procedure was used to treat the decellularized FS sample without being seeded cells. The DAPI stained cells were then observed with a fluorescence microscope (DFC7000T, LEICA, Wetzlar, Germany) at a wavelength of 350 nm.

2.2.2. Morphology and Structure Analysis

After being freeze-dried at −20 °C for 24 h, FS was cut along the surface lines of fish scale with a disposable scalpel and fixed with 2.5% glutaraldehyde (Solarbio, Beijing, China) at room temperature for 20 min and at 4 °C for 2 h. After that, 50%, 70%, 90%, and 100% ethanol solutions were used sequentially for dehydration, with an interval of 10 min each time. After dehydration, the above samples were put into the CO_2 critical point dryer for 1 h and sputter-coated with gold. The longitudinal section and surface morphology were observed and photographed with a scanning electron microscope (Inspect F, FEI, Hillsboro, OR, USA).

2.2.3. Fourier Transform Infrared Spectroscopy (FTIR)

Fourier transform infrared spectroscopy (FTIR) of FS was performed with a Fourier transform infrared spectrometer (INVENIO R, Bruker, Billerica, MA, USA). The spectrometer was equipped with an attenuated total reflection (ATR) accessory with a germanium crystal. The FS were directly placed on the ATR crystal and measured under the following conditions: scan range of 450–4000 cm^{-1}, 16 scans with a spectral resolution of 4 cm^{-1}, and indoor temperature of 25 °C. Hydroxyapatite (Aladdin, Shanghai, China) was served as control.

2.2.4. Thermogravimetric Analysis

Thermogravimetric analysis (TGA) of FS was performed with a thermogravimetric analyzer (TGA/DSC2, Mettler Toledo, Switzerland) under a nitrogen atmosphere. Heating temperature ranged from 30 °C to 1200 °C at a heating rate of 10 °C/min. The data were analyzed and graphed using Origin software.

2.2.5. Differential Scanning Calorimetry (DSC)

The thermal stability of FS was evaluated with DSC. The 10–15 mg sample was sealed in an aluminum crucible and heated from 30 °C to 90 °C at a rate of 5 °C/min under a nitrogen atmosphere. The data were analyzed and graphed using Origin software.

2.3. Culture and Identification of Bone Marrow Mesenchymal Stem Cells (BMSCs)

2.3.1. Culture of BMSCs

Two male SD rats, 3–4 weeks old, SPF grade, weighing 200 g, were purchased from Chengdu Dashuo Experimental Animal Center, and rat BMSCs were isolated and cultured as described previously [30]. In brief, the bilateral tibia and femur were aseptically separated under sterile conditions and bilateral epiphyses were cut off. The medullary cavity was rinsed and bone marrow collected using a 5 mL syringe with α-MEM (Gibco, New York, NY, USA) medium containing 10% fetal bovine serum (Gibco, New York, NY, USA) and 1% penicillin-streptomycin solution (Hyclone, Logan, UT, USA). The cell collection was centrifuged at 1000 r/min for 5 min and was cultured at 37 °C in a humidified atmosphere of 95% air and 5% CO_2. After 24 h, the medium was changed for the first time, and then, it was changed every 2–3 days. The cell proliferation and growth status were observed with the inverted microscope (Olympus, Tokyo, Japan). The third passages of BMSCs were selected for subsequent experiments.

2.3.2. Flow Cytometry Analysis

BMSCs were identified with flow cytometry. Cells were stained with the following antibodies: CD29-APC (BioLegend, San Diego, CA, USA), CD45 PerCP/Cyanine 5.5 (BioLegend, San Diego, CA, USA), CD90-FITC (eBioscience, San Diego, CA, USA). After being incubated for 1 h, cells were washed with PBS 3 times before being analyzed on a BD FACSCanto II cytometer. The experimental data were analyzed with FlowJo 10.0.7 software (Franklin Lakes, NJ, USA).

2.3.3. Osteogenic and Adipogenic Differentiation

To induce osteogenic differentiation, an osteogenic differentiation medium was prepared, which contained α-MEM, 10% fetal bovine serum, 50 μmol/L ascorbic acid (Sigma, Ronkonkoma, NY, USA), 0.1 μmol/L dexamethasone (Solarbio, Beijing, China), 10 mmol/L β-glycerophosphate (Sigma, Ronkonkoma, NY, USA), and 1% penicillin-streptomycin solution. Cells cultured with regular culture medium were used as a control. After 7 days of differentiation, BMSCs were fixed in a 4% paraformaldehyde (Solarbio, Beijing, China) for 30 min and stained with BCIP/NBT ALP color development kit (Beyotime, Shanghai, China). After 21-day differentiation, BMSCs were stained with Alizarin red S staining solution (Solarbio, Beijing, China). After washing with ddH_2O, the cells were observed under an inverted microscope.

Adipogenic differentiation medium consisted of DMEM (Gibco, New York, NY, USA), 10% fetal bovine serum, 0.5 μmol/L 3-isobutyl-1-methylxanthine (Solarbio, Beijing, China), 0.5 μmol/L dexamethasone, 10 μg/mL insulin (Solarbio, Beijing, China), 50 μmol/L indomethacin (Solarbio, Beijing, China), and 1% penicillin-streptomycin solution. BMSCs were cultured in an adipogenic differentiation medium or regular culture medium, and the medium was changed every 2–3 days. After 14 days, the cells were fixed in a 4% paraformaldehyde for 30 min and incubated for 10 min in an Oil Red O (Solarbio, Beijing, China) working solution. After thorough washes with a 75% ethanol solution, the cells were observed under an inverted microscope for the presence of lipid droplets, which were stained red.

2.4. Cytocompatibility of FS and Bio-Gide® Membrane (BG)

2.4.1. Cell Adhesion

FS and BG were trimmed with a punch (12 mm in diameter) and placed onto 24-well culture plates with the striated side of FS facing up and the loose side of BG facing up. BMSCs counting 1×10^5 were seeded on both materials and cultured for 1 h and 6 h at 37 °C in a CO_2 incubator. Cells on the materials were fixed with 2.5% glutaraldehyde (Solarbio, Beijing, China) at room temperature for 20 min and at 4 °C for 2 h. Then ethanol of different mass fractions was dropped onto the materials to dehydrate the cell samples. Finally, SEM was used to observe the morphology of BMSCs.

2.4.2. Cell Proliferation

The effect of cell proliferation was analyzed with the CCK8 assay. The eluate from FS and BG was prepared according to ISO10993-5-2009 [32]. Briefly, the aseptic 25 mm × 25 mm BG was incubated with 31.25 mL α-MEM medium without fetal bovine serum (FBS) for 24 h at 37 °C in a CO_2 incubator, where the extraction rate was 20 mm^2/mL. The eluate extraction was collected and stored for further analysis at 4 °C. The eluate of FS was prepared with the same extraction rate. BMSCs were seeded into a 96-well plate at 1×10^3 cells per well with a 100 μLα-MEM medium containing 10% FBS and cultured in an incubator at 37 °C with 5% CO_2. After a 24 h culture, the medium was replaced with 100 μL FS or BG eluate containing 10% FBS. As blank controls, cells cultured in -MEM medium containing 10% FBS were used. CCK8 was added (10 μL per well), and the plates were incubated at 37 °C for 2 h. The absorbance values at OD 450 nm were measured on the 1st, 3rd, and 5th day using a Multiskan™ FC microplate reader (Thermo Fisher, Waltham, MA, USA).

2.5. Osteogenic Activity of FS and BG

2.5.1. ALP Staining and ALP Activity Assay

FS and BG were trimmed with a punch (12 mm in diameter) and placed onto 24-well culture plates with the smooth side of FS facing up and the dense side of BG facing up. The same size aseptic glass slides were used as the control group. A custom polytetrafluoroethylene ring was used to press the materials around the edges of the plates, causing them to sink to the bottom. Four parallel samples were set up in each group. BMSCs counting 5×10^4 were seeded onto the plates with pre-placed materials and cultured for 24 h at 37 °C in a CO_2 incubator. Then, the medium was replaced with an osteogenic differentiation medium. ALP staining and ALP activity were determined after 7 days using the BCIP/NBT ALP color development kit and the ALP assay kit (Beyotime, Shanghai, China).

2.5.2. Relative Quantitative Assay of Mineralized Deposits

As previously stated, the same number of materials were placed onto 24-well culture plates in the same way. After 21-day osteogenic differentiation, BMSCs were stained with Alizarin red S staining solution, and stained materials were washed with distilled water several times to remove stain residue. The stained samples were then eluted with 10% cetylpyridinium chloride (Aladdin, Shanghai, China). The absorbance values at OD 562 nm were measured using a Multiskan™ FC microplate reader.

2.5.3. ELISA Analysis

ELISA was performed to analyze osteocalcin expression of BMSCs on the different materials. After 21-day osteogenic differentiation, supernatants from cell cultures were collected and detected using the Rat OC/BGP (osteocalcin) ELISA Kit (Elabscience, Wuhan, China). Finally, a Multiskan™ FC microplate reader was used to measure the absorbance values at OD 450 nm.

2.5.4. RT-qPCR Analysis

Osteogenesis-related gene expression quantification was performed with RT-qPCR. FS, BG, and glass slide control were placed onto 24-well culture plates in the same way as previously ($n = 3$). BMSCs counting 5×10^4 were seeded onto the plates and osteogenic differentiation induced for 7 days and 21 days at 37 °C in a CO_2 incubator. Cells were collected after digestion with trypsin (Gibco, New York, NY, USA), and total RNA was extracted using an RNA extraction kit (Bioteke, Beijing, China) at the indicated times. Total RNA samples were reverse transcribed to cDNA using a PrimeScriptTMRT reagent Kit with gDNA Eraser (Takara, Kusatsu, Japan). Real-time quantitative PCR was performed with TB Green® EX TaqTM II (Takara, Kusatsu, Japan) in a QuantStudio 6 instrument (Thermo Scientific, Waltham, MA, USA). The primer sequences are shown in Table 1.

Table 1. Primer sequences.

Gene	Primer Sequence (5′–3′)
OCN	Forward: CGCCAGGGTGAAGAACTA Reverse: TACGCTGTGGAAGCCAA
OPN	Forward: CGGAGACCATGCAGAGA Reverse: CGTAAGCCAAGCTATCACC
RUNX2	Forward: TCGGAAAGGGACGAGAG Reverse: TTCAAACGCATACCTGCAT
ACTB	Forward: CCTCACTGTCCACCTTCCA Reverse: GGGTGTAAAACGCAGCTCA

2.6. Statistical Analysis

SPSS 19.0, GraphPad Prism 8 (San Diego, CA, USA), and Origin 8.5 software (Northampton, MA, USA) were used for data analysis. Statistical analysis was performed by one-way ANOVA. Statistical significance was determined using Bonferroni correction when the variances were homogeneous, and Tamhane's T2 test was used for non-homogeneous variances. A $p < 0.05$ was considered statistically significant (NS, $p > 0.05$, * $p < 0.05$, ** $p < 0.01$, *** $p < 0.001$).

3. Results

3.1. Morphology and Structure of FS

DAPI staining showed that FS was successfully decellularized, and no nuclei were found on the FS (Figure 1B). In contrast, after being seeded the cells, the nucleus appeared on the FS (Figure 1A).

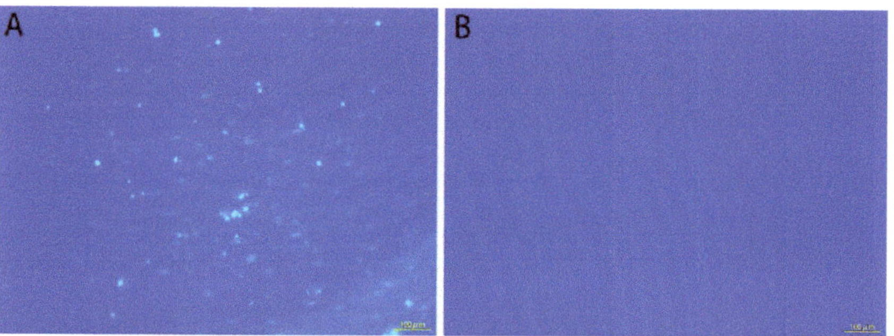

Figure 1. DAPI staining of FS with cells (**A**) and decellularized FS (**B**).

FS is oval and transparent, about 25 mm in diameter with the basic shape of fish scale (Figure 2C). SEM analysis indicates that there were "petal-like" radial ridges and no pores on the surface of FS. The upper surface of FS (Figure 2D) is irregular with curved ridges. On the lower surface (Figure 2F), parallel circular ridges and longitudinal grooves are seen. The lateral surface of FS (Figure 2E) is more uniform with parallel circular ridges forming concentric arcs with the scale focus in the center. FS is a multi-layer structure with type I collagen fibers arranged in parallel and some spherical or cubic crystals embedded between each layer of collagen fibers, as shown in the longitudinal section (Figures 1A and 2A,B).

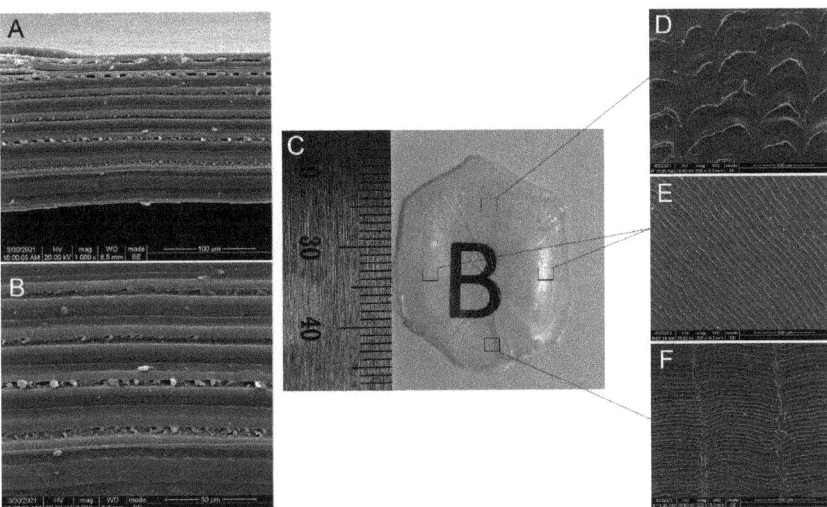

Figure 2. SEM images of surface (**D–F**) and longitudinal section (**A,B**) of FS (**C**).

3.2. Composition and Denaturation Temperature of FS

FTIR analysis (Figure 3A) showed five characteristic bands of type I collagen [33]: amide A (3292 cm^{-1}), amide B (2933 cm^{-1}), amide I (1630 cm^{-1}), amide II (1550 cm^{-1}), and amide III (1236 cm^{-1}). In addition, the weak absorption peak at 3076 cm^{-1} is related to the C-N stretching vibration of amide B, while the 1382 and 1336 cm^{-1} absorption peaks are related to the rocking vibration of -CH$_2$. It was reported that collagen has a complete triple helix secondary structure when the absorption ratio A1235/A1450 cm^{-1} of collagen is about 1.0 [34]. The FS prepared in this study has a ratio of A1235/A1450 cm^{-1} of 1.016, indicating that the collagen in the material has a complete triple helix structure. There are several absorption peaks of FS at 1029–1078 cm^{-1} and 524–623 cm^{-1}, corresponding to the PO$_4$ of apatite crystal. As shown in the figure, the same absorption peaks are present in the absorbance spectra of hydroxyapatite reference. The result suggests that FS is mainly composed of type I collagen and hydroxyapatite.

The thermogravimetric analysis (Figure 3B) revealed that there were three areas of mass loss: 30–178 °C, 178–650 °C, and 650–1200 °C. The first stage of mass loss of 30–178 °C was related to the evaporation of water molecules. The second stage of 178–650 °C was due to the decomposition of organic matter. When the temperature was raised to 1200 °C, the mass no longer changed, and the thermal decomposition of inorganic matter was completed in the third stage of 650–1200 °C. The mass loss curves demonstrated that the mass ratios of water, organic matter, and inorganic matter in FS are 20.7, 56.9, and 22.4%, relatively. Because type I collagen is the organic phase in FS and hydroxyapatite is the mainly inorganic phase, the ratio can be approximately estimated as the mass ratio of water, type I collagen, and hydroxyapatite.

DSC results (Figure 3C) showed a typical endothermic peak at 79.5 °C associated with irreversible denaturalization of collagen protein, indicating that the denaturation temperature of FS was 79.5 °C.

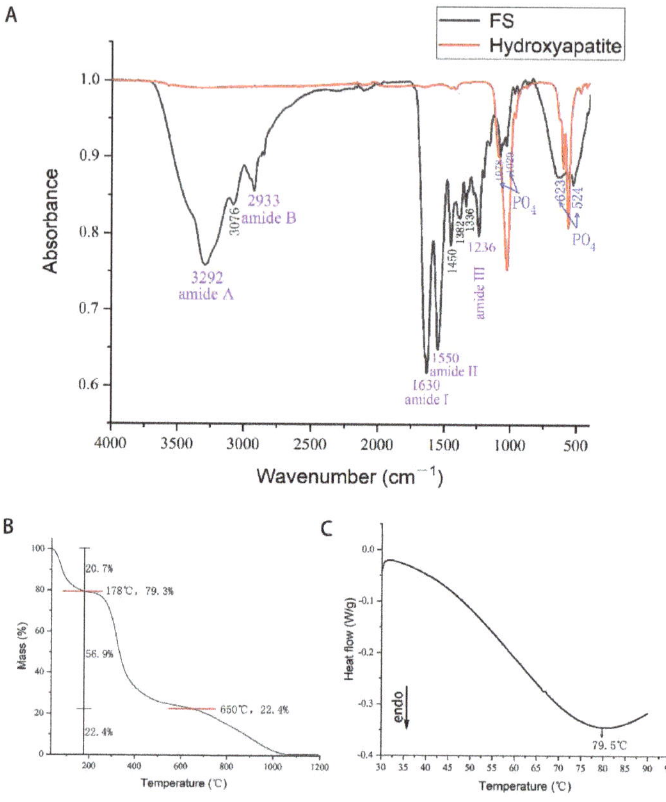

Figure 3. FTIR (**A**), thermogravimetric analysis (**B**), and DSC (**C**).

3.3. Culture and Identification of BMSCs

BMSCs were spindle-shaped and grew in a swirl shape. As shown from the P0-P3 generation cells (Figure 4A), with the increase of passage, the miscellaneous cells gradually decreased, and BMSCs were naturally purified by passage. Flow cytometry analysis suggested that BMSCs of the primary culture were mainly positive for CD90 and CD29 and negative for CD45 (Figure 4B). Cells after 7 days of osteogenic differentiation showed increased ALP staining compared with negative control cells, while cells cultured in the osteogenic medium for 21 days exhibited obvious amorphous calcium deposits by alizarin red staining compared with negative control cells (Figure 4C). The results of Oil Red O staining demonstrated numerous lipid droplets within BMSCs after adipogenic differentiation (Figure 4C). BMSCs expressing specific surface antigens were plastic-adherent and possessed multipotent differentiation potential, which meets the minimal criteria for defining MSCs [35].

3.4. Cytocompatibility of FS and Bio-Gide® Membrane (BG)

Cell adhesion on the materials was observed by SEM (Figure 5). BMSCs on the FS exhibited abundant pseudopods and filopodia at 1 h, and the cells spread fully and extended further pseudopodia at 6 h (Figure 5A). As a contrast, BMSCs were ellipsoidal with no obvious pseudopodia and adhered to the collagen fibers of porous BG, which were the same at 1 h and 6 h (Figure 5B).

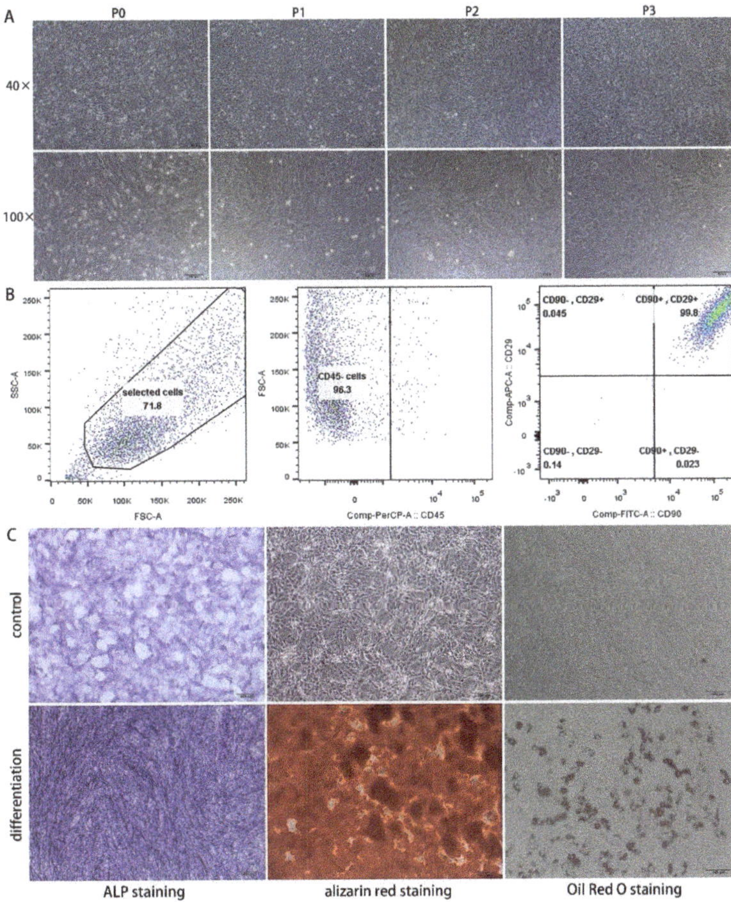

Figure 4. Morphology of BMSCs (**A**), flow cytometry analysis (**B**), and multipotent differentiation (**C**).

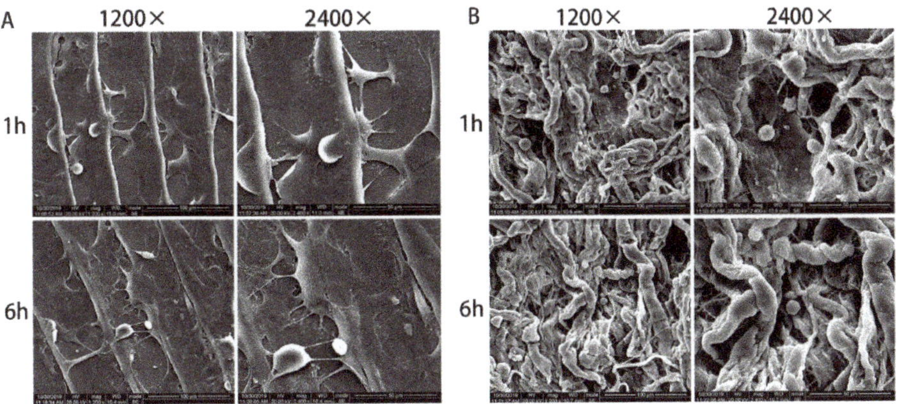

Figure 5. Cell adhesion of BMSCs on the FS (**A**) and BG (**B**).

The results of the CCK8 assay (Figure 6) showed that the cell proliferation in the BG group and FS group was better than that in the control group. The number of cells in the FS group was even higher than that in the BG group on the 5th day, indicating that both FS and BG can promote cell proliferation, and the effect of FS on cell proliferation is stronger.

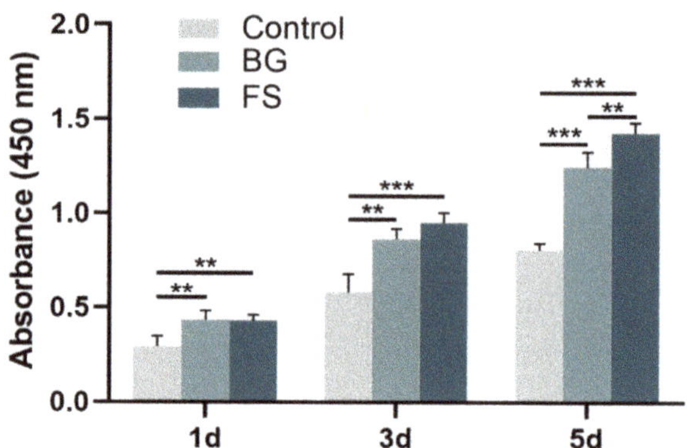

Figure 6. CCK8 assay of control, BG and FS group (** $p < 0.01$, *** $p < 0.001$).

3.5. Osteogenic Activity of FS and BG

ALP staining of osteogenic differentiation at 7 d (Figure 7A) showed that there were obvious dark blue granular in the glass slide control, BG, and FS groups. Because BG was an opaque material, while glass slides and FS were relatively transparent, ALP staining in the BG group was darker under a stereoscopic microscope. ALP activity assay showed that there was no significant difference among the three groups (Figure 7B).

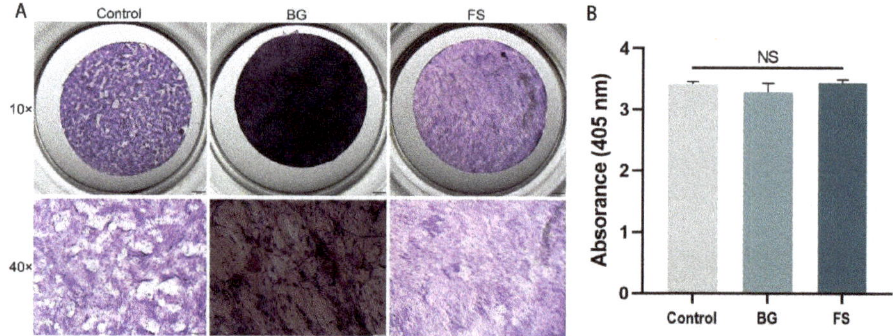

Figure 7. ALP staining (**A**) and ALP activity assay (**B**) of glass slide control, BG and FS group (NS, $p > 0.05$).

After 21-day osteogenic differentiation (Figure 8A), mineralized deposits in the FS group were significantly more than those in the control group ($p < 0.001$) and the BG group ($p < 0.01$), while there was no significant difference between the BG group and the glass slide control group ($p > 0.05$). Similarly, in the results of ELISA (Figure 8B), osteocalcin in the supernatant of cell culture in the FS group was significantly higher than that in the control group ($p < 0.001$) and the BG group ($p < 0.05$), and there was no difference between the latter two groups ($p > 0.05$).

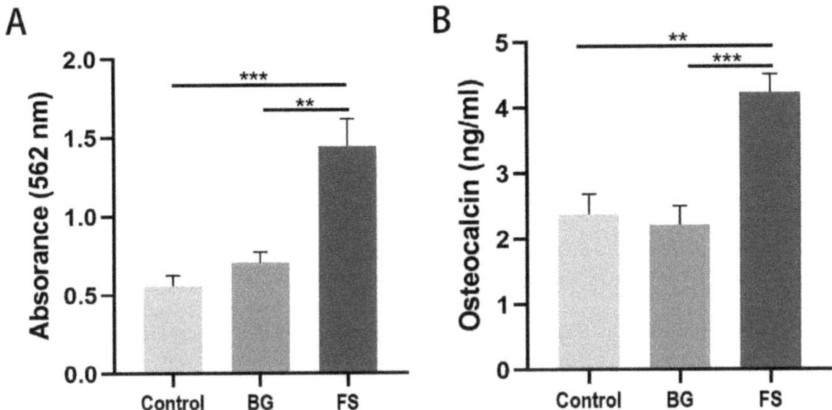

Figure 8. Relative quantitative assay of mineralized deposits (**A**) and ELISA analysis (**B**) of glass slide control, BG and FS group (** $p < 0.01$, *** $p < 0.001$).

At 7 days, there was no significant difference in the expression of osteogenesis-related genes RUNX2, OCN, and OPN among the three groups (Figure 9), which was consistent with the results of the ALP activity assay. After 21-day osteogenic differentiation, the gene expression of RUNX2 ($p < 0.05$), OCN ($p < 0.05$), and OPN ($p < 0.01$) in the FS group was significantly higher than that in the control group, and the expression of OCN ($p < 0.05$) and OPN ($p < 0.01$) in the FS group was significantly higher than that in the BG group. The above results of osteogenic activity suggested that FS did not significantly promote the osteogenic differentiation of BMSCs in the early stage (7 days), but it could promote the late osteogenic differentiation (21 days).

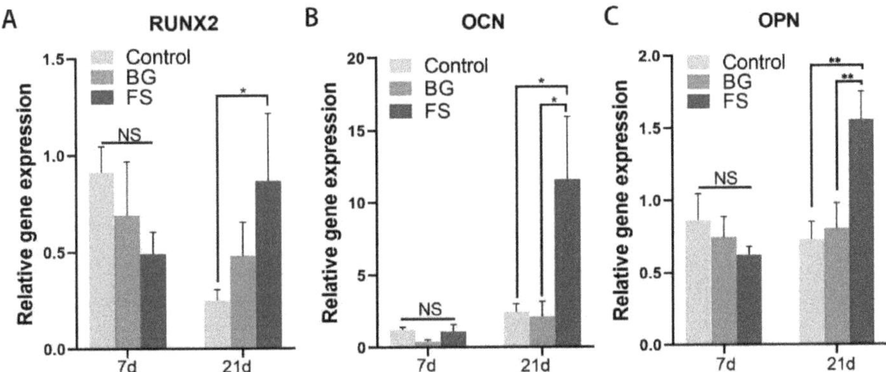

Figure 9. The relative expression of RUNX2 (**A**), OCN (**B**), and OPN (**C**) in the glass slide control, BG and FS group (NS, $p > 0.05$, * $p < 0.05$, ** $p < 0.01$).

4. Discussion

Fish-derived collagen is considered to be a safer substitute for mammalian collagen, but the denaturation temperature of fish-derived collagen is usually lower than that of mammals [11,19], which limits its biomedical application to some extent. The denaturation temperature of collagen in different fish varies due to differences in habitat and body temperature. Collagen extracted from freshwater fish has a higher denaturation temperature than collagen extracted from marine fish [36]. Because freshwater fish collagen contains more imino acids (hydroxyproline and proline) than marine fish collagen, the denaturation temperature of collagen rises with the increase of imino acid content [37]. At present, the most studied freshwater fish is tilapia, which is a tropical freshwater bony fish with a large scale of cultivation, and the denaturation temperature of tilapia collagen is about 37 °C [38], which is equivalent to the human temperature. The grass carp (*Ctenopharyngodon idella*) was selected in this study, which belongs to the freshwater bony fish as tilapia. According to the *China Fisheries Statistical Yearbook 2020*, the annual output of grass carp was the highest among fish, about 5.53 million tons, while that of tilapia was about 1.64 million tons. The denaturation temperature of grass carp collagen was reported to be around 35–39 °C [39,40], similarly high to that of tilapia. In addition, adult grass carp is larger than tilapia generally, and the fish scales of large grass carp can reach more than 25 mm in diameter, while only about 10 mm for tilapia. In terms of utility, larger fish scales can be used to make larger collagen membranes. In this study, the denaturation temperature of FS is 79.5 °C, which is much higher than the human body temperature. It is possible that the high denaturation temperature of FS is due to the fact that the spatial structure of fish scales was preserved during the preparation, and collagen fibrils instead of collagen molecules were obtained. Collagen fibrils are more stable than extracted collagen molecules because intermolecular and intramolecular interactions stabilize the triple helix structure of collagen, and the denaturation temperature of type I collagen in collagen fibrils is usually higher than that in solution [41]. Moreover, hydroxyapatite in FS can improve the structural stability of collagen [42].

To extract collagen from fish scales, it is commonly solubilized in organic acid (usually acetic acid), but the yield of acid solubilized collagen is low, and the use of pepsin can increase the extraction yield of collagen and reduce its antigenicity [43]. In most studies on fish scale collagen, the combined extraction method of acid and pepsin was used [19]. Then, collagen fibers scaffolds for tissue engineering were prepared by a freeze-drying methodology or to be physically or chemically modified [44,45]. However, the natural multilayer and compact structure of fish scales would be destroyed during this collagen extraction process. In addition, decellularization is the key process in the preparation of biomedical materials derived from fish scales, as incomplete decellularization can result in an allergic reaction when the fish scale is implanted [23]. The study's novelty is that the cells and impurities such as ash, keratin, and fat on the surface of fish scales were removed, and FS was successfully prepared by decellularization and decalcification on the basis of preserving the basic shape and spatial structure of fish scales. The natural multilayer structure of fish scales was not damaged, and the collagen fibrils and native mechanical strength have remained. This preparation of decellularization and decalcification is similar to the method of preparing artificial cornea using fish scales [46–48], but the preparation process in this study is simpler and more efficient.

General observation and the result of SEM showed that FS was a multilayer material with the basic shape and structure of fish scale, which is very similar to the fish scales of *Carassius auratus* [25], *Cyprinus carpio* [49], and tilapia [48]. Through the analysis of FTIR spectra, the results showed that the FS prepared from grass carp was mainly composed of type I collagen and hydroxyapatite, which was consistent with the fish scales such as *Pagrus major* [50], *Lates calcarifer* [22], *Carassius auratus* [25], *Cyprinus carpio* [49], *Megalops Atlanticus* [51], and tilapia [52]. After the preparation and treatment of fish scales, the weight ratio of water, organic matter, and inorganic matter is similar to that of decalcified grass carp scale reported before [23], and the mechanical properties of this decalcified fish scale material are significantly higher than that of pure collagen scaffold material [29]. For the mechanical properties, compared to Bio-Gide® membrane, commonly used in the GTR/GBR, which is a kind of non-cross-linked, porcine-derived type I and III collagen membrane with a double-layer structure [53], our previous research [31] found that the thickness of FS is about 0.34 ± 0.05 mm, slightly lower than that of BG 0.44 ± 0.03 mm, but its tensile strength is obviously higher than BG in both dry and wet conditions, and FS degraded more slowly compared with BG.

Collagen derived from fish scales has been shown to have good cytocompatibility in a number of studies [23,54–60]. Similarly in this research, both FS and BG could preserve cellular adherence and well support the growth of BMSCs, indicating their good cytocompatibility. ALP is an important membrane-bound enzyme expressed in the early stage of cell osteogenesis [61,62]. The results of ALP activity assay and osteogenesis-related gene expression at 7 days showed that both FS and BG could not promote early osteogenic differentiation. Relatively, OCN is an essential late marker of osteogenic differentiation [63,64] for the formation of minerals, and the mineralization of the extracellular matrix is the characteristic of late osteogenic differentiation [65]. According to the results of alizarin red staining and ELISA, the mineralized deposits and OCN expression of BMSCs on the FS were higher than those on the BG and the glass slide control. Osteopontin (OPN) is a kind of extracellular matrix glycoprotein, which plays an important role in the process of bone remodeling [66] and is a marker of the intermediate stage of osteoblast differentiation [67]. RUNX2 is a key transcription factor required for osteoblast differentiation [68]. The expression of osteogenesis-related genes in the late stage (21 d) of osteogenic differentiation was significantly higher than that in the BG group and the glass slide control group, indicating that FS could promote late osteogenic differentiation.

In this study, it was found that FS was better than BG in promoting osteogenesis in vitro, and one of the reasons may be the existence of hydroxyapatite (HA). The main inorganic component of human bones and dentin is HA. It has been reported that collagen membrane mixed with HA had better mechanical properties [16], and HA could not only promote the protein adsorption and stimulate the osteogenic differentiation of stem cells [69] but also endow biomaterials with good bioactivity and osteoconductivity [70]. Parmaksiz et al. [71] used HA microparticles and polycaprolactone as binders to assemble bovine intestinal submucosa into multilayer scaffold material. The morphological observation results showed that it had a uniform multilayer pore structure and uniform distribution of HA microparticles. Mechanical tests showed that it had good mechanical stability, and cell experiments showed that it had a good osteoinductive effect on BMSCs even without any external osteogenic inducers. At present, the mechanism of HA promoting osteogenic differentiation is not clear, which may be the action of calcium ions or calcium phosphates from HA [62,72]. Studies have shown that calcium ions are involved in various physiological activities and electrical signal transduction of cell osteogenic differentiation [73], and biomaterials containing calcium phosphate can induce osteogenic differentiation of stem cells through adenosine signaling [74]. On the other hand, the osteogenic activity of FS may also be derived from the collagen of fish scales. Matsumoto et al. [59] found that fish scale collagen can promote the osteogenic differentiation of human MSCs; Studies by Hsu et al. [58] have shown that fish scale collagen can promote chondrogenic cartilage differentiation of human MSCs, and its effect is stronger than that of porcine collagen; Liu et al. reported that hydrolyzed fish scale collagen can directly induce osteogenic differentiation of rat BMSCs [57] and human periodontal ligament cells [75], without the use of any additional inducing reagent, and significantly up-regulate the expression of osteogenic markers (RUNX2, ALP, OPN, and OCN) [57].

It has been reported that the porosity and morphology of materials will affect the effect of bone regeneration in vivo [76]. Generally, the osteogenic effect of perforated barrier membrane is better than that of non-perforated barrier membrane [77]. In addition, macroporous membranes facilitated greater bone regeneration compared with microporous membranes [78]. Due to the differences in morphology and pores between different materials, the materials will be affected by the immune response after being implanted in vivo [3], and it is difficult to compare the effects of different materials on osteogenic differentiation. In the part of the osteogenic differentiation experiment, not only FS and BG were compared but also a glass slide group was set up as a negative control, in which both FS and glass slide had no pores. Considering that there were no obvious pores on the dense side of BG, we put the dense side of BG upward, which can minimize the influence of pores on osteogenic differentiation. The results demonstrated that after removing the effect of pores, BG could not promote osteogenic differentiation of BMSCs (7 d and 21 d), while FS could promote osteogenic differentiation at the late stage (21 d) in vitro. In our previous research [31], FS and BG were implanted into the rat cranial bone defect. The results showed that there was no significant difference in the amount of new bone formation between the FS and BG groups after 4 weeks ($p > 0.05$). At the 8th week after operation, BG was completely degraded, and FS remained partially, and the newly formed bone completely filled in the bone defects in the BG group, which was higher than that in the FS group ($p < 0.05$). The results of osteogenic differentiation in previous animal experiments are inconsistent with this research in vitro, which may be caused by the effect of porosity and speed of degradation. FS has no obvious pores and may not be beneficial to the blood–gas exchange of tissues and cells after implantation in vivo. Moreover, FS degraded more slowly than BG in vivo, which does not match the rate of rat bone regeneration, and the residual FS membrane would occupy the space of newly formed bone. Taken together, the results of our previous animal experiment and this research in vitro suggest that FS may have additional osteoinductive properties compared with BG besides the osteoconductivity. However, because FS has no pores and no appropriate degradation rate for rats, its osteogenic effect in vivo is not as good as that in vitro.

To sum up, BG had good cytocompatibility, but the dense side of BG had no significant effect on promoting osteogenic differentiation of BMSCs on the 7th and 21st day. The cytocompatibility of FS was excellent, and its effect on cell proliferation was superior to that of BG ($p < 0.05$). In addition, FS had no obvious effect on promoting osteogenic differentiation at the early stage (7 d), but it could promote cell osteogenic differentiation at the late stage (21 d), indicating its good cytocompatibility and osteogenic activity, as well as the potential to be used in bone regeneration. In order to achieve good bone regeneration, it is necessary to improve the porosity, pore size and degradation rate of FS in the future so that, when used in vivo, it can not only act as a barrier for epithelium and connective tissue but also benefit blood–gas exchange between tissue and cells on both sides of the membrane.

Author Contributions: Conceptualization, L.C., G.C., S.M. and Y.D.; methodology, L.C.; software, L.C.; validation, L.C., S.M. and Y.D.; formal analysis, L.C.; investigation, L.C. and G.C.; resources, L.C. and G.C.; data curation, L.C.; writing—original draft preparation, L.C.; writing—review and editing, L.C.; visualization, L.C. and Y.D.; supervision, L.C., S.M. and Y.D.; project administration, Y.D.; funding acquisition, Y.D. All authors have read and agreed to the published version of the manuscript.

Funding: This study was supported by the Science Foundation of Sichuan Provincial Department of Science and Technology, China (2020YJ0242).

Institutional Review Board Statement: The animal study protocol was approved by the ethical committees of the West China School of Stomatology, Sichuan University, and the State Key Laboratory of Oral Diseases (ethics code WCHSIRB-D-2020-220).

Informed Consent Statement: Not applicable.

Data Availability Statement: This study did not report any data.

Acknowledgments: We would like to thank the Analytical & Testing Center of Sichuan University for FTIR, TGA, and DSC work, and we are grateful to Yani Xie, Shaolan Wang, and Aiqun Gu for their help with FTIR, TG, and DSC analysis.

Conflicts of Interest: The authors declare no conflict of interest.

References

1. Slots, J. Periodontitis: Facts, fallacies and the future. *Periodontology 2000* **2017**, *75*, 7–23. [CrossRef]
2. De Jong, T.; Bakker, A.D.; Everts, V.; Smit, T.H. The intricate anatomy of the periodontal ligament and its development: Lessons for periodontal regeneration. *J. Periodontal Res.* **2017**, *52*, 965–974. [CrossRef]
3. Chu, C.; Deng, J.; Sun, X.; Qu, Y.; Man, Y. Collagen Membrane and Immune Response in Guided Bone Regeneration: Recent Progress and Perspectives. *Tissue Eng. Part B Rev.* **2017**, *23*, 421–435. [CrossRef]
4. Sallum, E.A.; Ribeiro, F.V.; Ruiz, K.S.; Sallum, A.W. Experimental and clinical studies on regenerative periodontal therapy. *Periodontology 2000* **2019**, *79*, 22–55. [CrossRef] [PubMed]

5. Ramseier, C.A.; Rasperini, G.; Batia, S.; Giannobile, W.V. Advanced reconstructive technologies for periodontal tissue repair. *Periodontology 2000* **2012**, *59*, 185–202. [CrossRef]
6. Ricard-Blum, S. The collagen family. *Cold Spring Harb. Perspect. Biol.* **2011**, *3*, a004978. [CrossRef] [PubMed]
7. Dong, C.; Lv, Y. Application of Collagen Scaffold in Tissue Engineering: Recent Advances and New Perspectives. *Polymers* **2016**, *8*, 42. [CrossRef] [PubMed]
8. Ferreira, A.M.; Gentile, P.; Chiono, V.; Ciardelli, G. Collagen for bone tissue regeneration. *Acta Biomater.* **2012**, *8*, 3191–3200. [CrossRef]
9. Shekhter, A.B.; Fayzullin, A.L.; Vukolova, M.N.; Rudenko, T.G.; Osipycheva, V.D.; Litvitsky, P.F. Medical Applications of Collagen and Collagen-Based Materials. *Curr. Med. Chem.* **2019**, *26*, 506–516. [CrossRef]
10. Chowdhury, S.R.; Mh Busra, M.F.; Lokanathan, Y.; Ng, M.H.; Law, J.X.; Cletus, U.C.; Binti Haji Idrus, R. Collagen Type I: A Versatile Biomaterial. *Adv. Exp. Med. Biol.* **2018**, *1077*, 389–414.
11. Lim, Y.S.; Ok, Y.J.; Hwang, S.Y.; Kwak, J.Y.; Yoon, S. Marine Collagen as A Promising Biomaterial for Biomedical Applications. *Mar. Drugs* **2019**, *17*, 467. [CrossRef] [PubMed]
12. Manon-Jensen, T.; Kjeld, N.G.; Karsdal, M.A. Collagen-mediated hemostasis. *J. Thromb. Haemost.* **2016**, *14*, 438–448. [CrossRef] [PubMed]
13. León-López, A.; Morales-Peñaloza, A.; Martínez-Juárez, V.M.; Vargas-Torres, A.; Zeugolis, D.I.; Aguirre-Álvarez, G. Hydrolyzed Collagen-Sources and Applications. *Molecules* **2019**, *24*, 4031. [CrossRef] [PubMed]
14. Avila Rodriguez, M.I.; Rodriguez Barroso, L.G.; Sanchez, M.L. Collagen: A review on its sources and potential cosmetic applications. *J. Cosmet. Derm.* **2018**, *17*, 20–26. [CrossRef] [PubMed]
15. Sorushanova, A.; Delgado, L.M.; Wu, Z.; Shologu, N.; Kshirsagar, A.; Raghunath, R.; Mullen, A.M.; Bayon, Y.; Pandit, A.; Raghunath, M.; et al. The Collagen Suprafamily: From Biosynthesis to Advanced Biomaterial Development. *Adv. Mater.* **2019**, *31*, e1801651. [CrossRef]
16. Jin, S.; Sun, F.; Zou, Q.; Huang, J.; Zuo, Y.; Li, Y.; Wang, S.; Cheng, L.; Man, Y.; Yang, F. Fish Collagen and Hydroxyapatite Reinforced Poly(lactide-co-glycolide) Fibrous Membrane for Guided Bone Regeneration. *Biomacromolecules* **2019**, *20*, 2058–2067. [CrossRef]
17. Ahmed, R.; Haq, M.; Chun, B.S. Characterization of marine derived collagen extracted from the by-products of bigeye tuna (*Thunnus obesus*). *Int. J. Biol. Macromol.* **2019**, *135*, 668–676. [CrossRef]
18. Morrissey, M.T.; Park, J.W.; Huang, L. Surimi processing waste: Its control and utilization. *Surimi Surimi Seaf.* **2000**, *101*, 127–165.
19. Silva, T.H.; Moreira-Silva, J.; Marques, A.L.; Domingues, A.; Bayon, Y.; Reis, R.L. Marine origin collagens and its potential applications. *Mar. Drugs* **2014**, *12*, 5881–5901. [CrossRef]
20. Ruan, J.; Chen, J.; Zeng, J.; Yang, Z.; Wang, C.; Hong, Z.; Zuo, Z. The protective effects of Nile tilapia (*Oreochromis niloticus*) scale collagen hydrolysate against oxidative stress induced by tributyltin in HepG2 cells. *Environ. Sci. Pollut. Res. Int.* **2019**, *26*, 3612–3620. [CrossRef]
21. Lionetto, F.; Esposito Corcione, C. Recent Applications of Biopolymers Derived from Fish Industry Waste in Food Packaging. *Polymers* **2021**, *13*, 2337. [CrossRef] [PubMed]
22. Sankar, S.; Sekar, S.; Mohan, R.; Rani, S.; Sundaraseelan, J.; Sastry, T.P. Preparation and partial characterization of collagen sheet from fish (*Lates calcarifer*) scales. *Int. J. Biol. Macromol.* **2008**, *42*, 6–9. [CrossRef] [PubMed]
23. Chou, C.H.; Chen, Y.G.; Lin, C.C.; Lin, S.M.; Yang, K.C.; Chang, S.H. Bioabsorbable fish scale for the internal fixation of fracture: A preliminary study. *Tissue Eng. Part A* **2014**, *20*, 2493–2502. [CrossRef] [PubMed]
24. Hsueh, Y.J.; Ma, D.H.; Ma, K.S.; Wang, T.K.; Chou, C.H.; Lin, C.C.; Huang, M.C.; Luo, L.J.; Lai, J.Y.; Chen, H.C. Extracellular Matrix Protein Coating of Processed Fish Scales Improves Human Corneal Endothelial Cell Adhesion and Proliferation. *Transl. Vis. Sci. Technol.* **2019**, *8*, 27. [CrossRef] [PubMed]
25. Fang, Z.; Wang, Y.; Feng, Q.; Kienzle, A.; Müller, W.E. Hierarchical structure and cytocompatibility of fish scales from *Carassius auratus*. *Mater. Sci. Eng. C Mater. Biol. Appl.* **2014**, *43*, 145–152. [CrossRef]
26. Wang, B.; Wang, Y.M.; Chi, C.F.; Luo, H.Y.; Deng, S.G.; Ma, J.Y. Isolation and characterization of collagen and antioxidant collagen peptides from scales of croceine croaker (*Pseudosciaena crocea*). *Mar. Drugs* **2013**, *11*, 4641–4661. [CrossRef]
27. Lionetto, F.; Bagheri, S.; Mele, C. Sustainable Materials from Fish Industry Waste for Electrochemical Energy Systems. *Energies* **2021**, *14*, 7928. [CrossRef]
28. Wang, L.; An, X.; Yang, F.; Xin, Z.; Zhao, L.; Hu, Q. Isolation and characterisation of collagens from the skin, scale and bone of deep-sea redfish (*Sebastes mentella*). *Food Chem.* **2008**, *108*, 616–623. [CrossRef]
29. Feng, H.; Li, X.; Deng, X.; Li, X.; Guo, J.; Ma, K.; Jiang, B. The lamellar structure and biomimetic properties of a fish scale matrix. *RSC Adv.* **2020**, *10*, 875–885. [CrossRef]
30. Cheng, G.; Chen, L.; Feng, H.; Jiang, B.; Ding, Y. Preliminary Study on Fish Scale Collagen Lamellar Matrix as Artificial Cornea. *Membranes* **2021**, *11*, 737. [CrossRef]
31. Cheng, G.; Guo, S.; Wang, N.; Xiao, S.; Jiang, B.; Ding, Y. A novel lamellar structural biomaterial and its effect on bone regeneration. *RSC Adv.* **2020**, *10*, 39072–39079. [CrossRef] [PubMed]
32. ISO. Biological Evaluation of Medical Devices—Part 5: Tests for In Vitro Cytotoxicity. 2009. Available online: https://www.iso.org/standard/36406.html (accessed on 20 May 2022).

33. Akita, M.; Nishikawa, Y.; Shigenobu, Y.; Ambe, D.; Morita, T.; Morioka, K.; Adachi, K. Correlation of proline, hydroxyproline and serine content, denaturation temperature and circular dichroism analysis of type I collagen with the physiological temperature of marine teleosts. *Food Chem.* **2020**, *329*, 126775. [CrossRef] [PubMed]

34. Guzzi Plepis, A.M.D.; Goissis, G.; Das-Gupta, D.K. Dielectric and pyroelectric characterization of anionic and native collagen. *Polym. Eng. Sci.* **1996**, *36*, 2932–2938. [CrossRef]

35. Dominici, M.; Le Blanc, K.; Mueller, I.; Slaper-Cortenbach, I.; Marini, F.; Krause, D.; Deans, R.; Keating, A.; Prockop, D.; Horwitz, E. Minimal criteria for defining multipotent mesenchymal stromal cells. The International Society for Cellular Therapy position statement. *Cytotherapy* **2006**, *8*, 315–317. [CrossRef] [PubMed]

36. Pati, F.; Datta, P.; Adhikari, B.; Dhara, S.; Ghosh, K.; Mohapatra, P.K.D. Collagen scaffolds derived from fresh water fish origin and their biocompatibility. *J. Biomed. Mater. Res. Part A* **2012**, *100*, 1068–1079. [CrossRef]

37. Pati, F.; Adhikari, B.; Dhara, S. Isolation and characterization of fish scale collagen of higher thermal stability. *Bioresour. Technol.* **2010**, *101*, 3737–3742. [CrossRef]

38. Song, Z.; Liu, H.; Chen, L.; Chen, L.; Zhou, C.; Hong, P.; Deng, C. Characterization and comparison of collagen extracted from the skin of the *Nile tilapia* by fermentation and chemical pretreatment. *Food Chem.* **2021**, *340*, 128139. [CrossRef] [PubMed]

39. He, L.; Lan, W.; Wang, Y.; Ahmed, S.; Liu, Y. Extraction and Characterization of Self-Assembled Collagen Isolated from Grass Carp and Crucian Carp. *Foods* **2019**, *8*, 396. [CrossRef]

40. Liu, Y.; Ma, D.; Wang, Y.; Qin, W. A comparative study of the properties and self-aggregation behavior of collagens from the scales and skin of grass carp (*Ctenopharyngodon idella*). *Int. J. Biol. Macromol.* **2018**, *106*, 516–522. [CrossRef]

41. Koshimizu, N.; Bessho, M.; Suzuki, S.; Yuguchi, Y.; Kitamura, S.; Hara, M. Gamma-crosslinked collagen gel without fibrils: Analysis of structure and heat stability. *Biosci. Biotechnol. Biochem.* **2009**, *73*, 1915–1921. [CrossRef]

42. Silva, C.C.; Thomazini, D.; Pinheiro, A.G.; Aranha, N.; Figueiró, S.D.; Góes, J.C.; Sombra, A.S.B. Collagen–hydroxyapatite films: Piezoelectric properties. *Mater. Sci. Eng. B* **2001**, *86*, 210–218. [CrossRef]

43. Ben Slimane, E.; Sadok, S. Collagen from Cartilaginous Fish By-Products for a Potential Application in Bioactive Film Composite. *Mar. Drugs* **2018**, *16*, 211. [CrossRef] [PubMed]

44. Li, Q.; Mu, L.; Zhang, F.; Sun, Y.; Chen, Q.; Xie, C.; Wang, H. A novel fish collagen scaffold as dural substitute. *Mater. Sci. Eng. C Mater. Biol. Appl.* **2017**, *80*, 346–351. [CrossRef] [PubMed]

45. Muthukumar, T.; Aravinthan, A.; Sharmila, J.; Kim, N.S.; Kim, J.H. Collagen/chitosan porous bone tissue engineering composite scaffold incorporated with Ginseng compound, K. *Carbohydr. Polym.* **2016**, *152*, 566–574. [CrossRef] [PubMed]

46. van Essen, T.H.; van Zijl, L.; Possemiers, T.; Mulder, A.A.; Zwart, S.J.; Chou, C.H.; Lin, C.C.; Lai, H.J.; Luyten, G.P.M.; Tassignon, M.J.; et al. Biocompatibility of a fish scale-derived artificial cornea: Cytotoxicity, cellular adhesion and phenotype, and in vivo immunogenicity. *Biomaterials* **2016**, *81*, 36–45. [CrossRef]

47. Lin, C.C.; Ritch, R.; Lin, S.M.; Ni, M.H.; Chang, Y.C.; Lu, Y.L.; Lai, H.J.; Lin, F.H. A new fish scale-derived scaffold for corneal regeneration. *Eur. Cells Mater.* **2010**, *19*, 50–57. [CrossRef]

48. van Essen, T.H.; Lin, C.C.; Hussain, A.K.; Maas, S.; Lai, H.J.; Linnartz, H.; van den Berg, T.J.; Salvatori, D.C.; Luyten, G.P.; Jager, M.J. A fish scale-derived collagen matrix as artificial cornea in rats: Properties and potential. *Investig. Ophthalmol. Vis. Sci.* **2013**, *54*, 3224–3233. [CrossRef]

49. Marino Cugno Garrano, A.; La Rosa, G.; Zhang, D.; Niu, L.N.; Tay, F.R.; Majd, H.; Arola, D. On the mechanical behavior of scales from *Cyprinus carpio*. *J. Mech. Behav. Biomed. Mater.* **2012**, *7*, 17–29. [CrossRef]

50. Ikoma, T.; Kobayashi, H.; Tanaka, J.; Walsh, D.; Mann, S. Microstructure, mechanical, and biomimetic properties of fish scales from *Pagrus major*. *J. Struct. Biol.* **2003**, *142*, 327–333. [CrossRef]

51. Gil-Duran, S.; Arola, D.; Ossa, E.A. Effect of chemical composition and microstructure on the mechanical behavior of fish scales from Megalops Atlanticus. *J. Mech. Behav. Biomed. Mater.* **2016**, *56*, 134–145. [CrossRef]

52. Okuda, M.; Ogawa, N.; Takeguchi, M.; Hashimoto, A.; Tagaya, M.; Chen, S.; Hanagata, N.; Ikoma, T. Minerals and aligned collagen fibrils in tilapia fish scales: Structural analysis using dark-field and energy-filtered transmission electron microscopy and electron tomography. *Microsc. Microanal.* **2011**, *17*, 788–798. [PubMed]

53. Willershausen, I.; Barbeck, M.; Boehm, N.; Sader, R.; Willershausen, B.; Kirkpatrick, C.J.; Ghanaati, S. Non-cross-linked collagen type I/III materials enhance cell proliferation: In vitro and in vivo evidence. *J. Appl. Oral Sci.* **2014**, *22*, 29–37. [CrossRef] [PubMed]

54. Ilyas, K.; Qureshi, S.W.; Afzal, S.; Gul, R.; Yar, M.; Kaleem, M.; Khan, A.S. Microwave-assisted synthesis and evaluation of type 1 collagen-apatite composites for dental tissue regeneration. *J. Biomater. Appl.* **2018**, *33*, 103–115. [CrossRef] [PubMed]

55. El-Rashidy, A.A.; Gad, A.; Abu-Hussein Ael, H.; Habib, S.I.; Badr, N.A.; Hashem, A.A. Chemical and biological evaluation of Egyptian Nile Tilapia (*Oreochromis niloticas*) fish scale collagen. *Int. J. Biol. Macromol.* **2015**, *79*, 618–626. [CrossRef] [PubMed]

56. Jana, P.; Mitra, T.; Selvaraj, T.K.R.; Gnanamani, A.; Kundu, P.P. Preparation of guar gum scaffold film grafted with ethylenediamine and fish scale collagen, cross-linked with ceftazidime for wound healing application. *Carbohydr. Polym.* **2016**, *153*, 573–581. [CrossRef] [PubMed]

57. Liu, C.; Sun, J. Potential application of hydrolyzed fish collagen for inducing the multidirectional differentiation of rat bone marrow mesenchymal stem cells. *Biomacromolecules* **2014**, *15*, 436–443. [CrossRef] [PubMed]

58. Hsu, H.H.; Uemura, T.; Yamaguchi, I.; Ikoma, T.; Tanaka, J. Chondrogenic differentiation of human mesenchymal stem cells on fish scale collagen. *J. Biosci. Bioeng.* **2016**, *122*, 219–225. [CrossRef] [PubMed]

59. Matsumoto, R.; Uemura, T.; Xu, Z.; Yamaguchi, I.; Ikoma, T.; Tanaka, J. Rapid oriented fibril formation of fish scale collagen facilitates early osteoblastic differentiation of human mesenchymal stem cells. *J. Biomed. Mater. Res. A* **2015**, *103*, 2531–2539. [CrossRef]
60. Muthukumar, T.; Prabu, P.; Ghosh, K.; Sastry, T.P. Fish scale collagen sponge incorporated with Macrotyloma uniflorum plant extract as a possible wound/burn dressing material. *Colloids Surf. B Biointerfaces* **2014**, *113*, 207–212. [CrossRef]
61. Nakatsu, Y.; Nakagawa, F.; Higashi, S.; Ohsumi, T.; Shiiba, S.; Watanabe, S.; Takeuchi, H. Effect of acetaminophen on osteoblastic differentiation and migration of MC3T3-E1 cells. *Pharm. Rep.* **2018**, *70*, 29–36. [CrossRef]
62. Chai, Y.C.; Carlier, A.; Bolander, J.; Roberts, S.J.; Geris, L.; Schrooten, J.; Van Oosterwyck, H.; Luyten, F.P. Current views on calcium phosphate osteogenicity and the translation into effective bone regeneration strategies. *Acta Biomater.* **2012**, *8*, 3876–3887. [CrossRef] [PubMed]
63. Karaoz, E.; Aksoy, A.; Ayhan, S.; Sariboyaci, A.E.; Kaymaz, F.; Kasap, M. Characterization of mesenchymal stem cells from rat bone marrow: Ultrastructural properties, differentiation potential and immunophenotypic markers. *Histochem. Cell Biol.* **2009**, *132*, 533–546. [CrossRef] [PubMed]
64. Donzelli, E.; Salvadè, A.; Mimo, P.; Viganò, M.; Morrone, M.; Papagna, R.; Carini, F.; Zaopo, A.; Miloso, M.; Baldoni, M.; et al. Mesenchymal stem cells cultured on a collagen scaffold: In vitro osteogenic differentiation. *Arch. Oral Biol.* **2007**, *52*, 64–73. [CrossRef] [PubMed]
65. Xu, F.T.; Li, H.M.; Yin, Q.S.; Liang, Z.J.; Huang, M.H.; Chi, G.Y.; Huang, L.; Liu, D.L.; Nan, H. Effect of activated autologous platelet-rich plasma on proliferation and osteogenic differentiation of human adipose-derived stem cells in vitro. *Am. J. Transl. Res.* **2015**, *7*, 257–270.
66. Kahles, F.; Findeisen, H.M.; Bruemmer, D. Osteopontin: A novel regulator at the cross roads of inflammation, obesity and diabetes. *Mol. Metab.* **2014**, *3*, 384–393. [CrossRef]
67. Kusuyama, J.; Amir, M.S.; Albertson, B.G.; Bandow, K.; Ohnishi, T.; Nakamura, T.; Noguchi, K.; Shima, K.; Semba, I.; Matsuguchi, T. JNK inactivation suppresses osteogenic differentiation, but robustly induces osteopontin expression in osteoblasts through the induction of inhibitor of DNA binding 4 (Id4). *FASEB J.* **2019**, *33*, 7331–7347. [CrossRef]
68. Toor, R.H.; Malik, S.; Qamar, H.; Batool, F.; Tariq, M.; Nasir, Z.; Tassaduq, R.; Lian, J.B.; Stein, J.L.; Stein, G.S.; et al. Osteogenic potential of hexane and dichloromethane fraction of *Cissus quadrangularis* on murine preosteoblast cell line MC3T3-E1 (subclone 4). *J. Cell Physiol.* **2019**, *234*, 23082–23096. [CrossRef]
69. Zhao, C.; Wang, X.; Gao, L.; Jing, L.; Zhou, Q.; Chang, J. The role of the micro-pattern and nano-topography of hydroxyapatite bioceramics on stimulating osteogenic differentiation of mesenchymal stem cells. *Acta Biomater.* **2018**, *73*, 509–521. [CrossRef]
70. Nazeer, M.A.; Yilgor, E.; Yilgor, I. Intercalated chitosan/hydroxyapatite nanocomposites: Promising materials for bone tissue engineering applications. *Carbohydr. Polym.* **2017**, *175*, 38–46. [CrossRef]
71. Parmaksiz, M.; Elçin, A.E.; Elçin, Y.M. Decellularized bovine small intestinal submucosa-PCL/hydroxyapatite-based multilayer composite scaffold for hard tissue repair. *Mater. Sci. Eng. C Mater. Biol. Appl.* **2019**, *94*, 788–797. [CrossRef]
72. Tavares, M.T.; Oliveira, M.B.; Mano, J.F.; Farinha, J.P.S.; Baleizão, C. Bioactive silica nanoparticles with calcium and phosphate for single dose osteogenic differentiation. *Mater. Sci. Eng. C Mater. Biol. Appl.* **2020**, *107*, 110348. [CrossRef] [PubMed]
73. Petecchia, L.; Sbrana, F.; Utzeri, R.; Vercellino, M.; Usai, C.; Visai, L.; Vassalli, M.; Gavazzo, P. Electro-magnetic field promotes osteogenic differentiation of BM-hMSCs through a selective action on Ca(2+)-related mechanisms. *Sci. Rep.* **2015**, *5*, 13856. [CrossRef] [PubMed]
74. Shih, Y.R.; Hwang, Y.; Phadke, A.; Kang, H.; Hwang, N.S.; Caro, E.J.; Nguyen, S.; Siu, M.; Theodorakis, E.A.; Gianneschi, N.C.; et al. Calcium phosphate-bearing matrices induce osteogenic differentiation of stem cells through adenosine signaling. *Proc. Natl. Acad. Sci. USA* **2014**, *111*, 990–995. [CrossRef] [PubMed]
75. Liu, C.; Sun, J. Hydrolyzed tilapia fish collagen induces osteogenic differentiation of human periodontal ligament cells. *Biomed. Mater.* **2015**, *10*, 065020. [CrossRef]
76. De Santana, R.B.; De Mattos, C.M.; Francischone, C.E.; Van Dyke, T. Superficial topography and porosity of an absorbable barrier membrane impacts soft tissue response in guided bone regeneration. *J. Periodontol.* **2010**, *81*, 926–933. [CrossRef]
77. Lundgren, A.; Lundgren, D.; Taylor, A. Influence of barrier occlusiveness on guided bone augmentation. An experimental study in the rat. *Clin. Oral Implant. Res.* **1998**, *9*, 251–260. [CrossRef]
78. Gutta, R.; Baker, R.A.; Bartolucci, A.A.; Louis, P.J. Barrier membranes used for ridge augmentation: Is there an optimal pore size? *J. Oral Maxillofac. Surg.* **2009**, *67*, 1218–1225. [CrossRef]

MDPI

St. Alban-Anlage 66

4052 Basel

Switzerland

Tel. +41 61 683 77 34

Fax +41 61 302 89 18

www.mdpi.com

Polymers Editorial Office

E-mail: polymers@mdpi.com

www.mdpi.com/journal/polymers

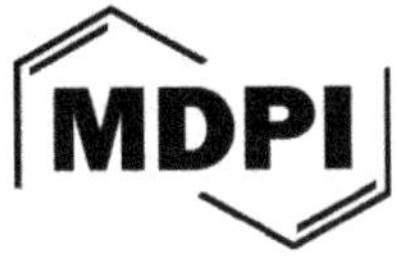

www.ingramcontent.com/pod-product-compliance
Lightning Source LLC
LaVergne TN
LVHW071306170726
843515LV00006BA/1503